CONSUMPTIVE CHIC

CONSUMPTIVE CHIC

A HISTORY OF BEAUTY, FASHION, AND DISEASE

Carolyn A. Day

Bloomsbury Academic
An imprint of Bloomsbury Publishing Plc

B L O O M S B U R Y
LONDON · OXFORD · NEW YORK · NEW DELHI · SYDNEY

Bloomsbury Academic

An imprint of Bloomsbury Publishing Plc

50 Bedford Square	1385 Broadway
London	New York
WC1B 3DP	NY 10018
UK	USA

www.bloomsbury.com

BLOOMSBURY and the Diana logo are trademarks of Bloomsbury Publishing Plc

First published 2017
Reprinted 2017

© Carolyn A. Day, 2017

Carolyn A. Day has asserted her right under the Copyright, Designs and Patents Act, 1988, to be identified as Author of this work.

British Library Cataloguing-in-Publication Data

A catalogue record for this book is available from the British Library.

ISBN: HB: 978-1-3500-0938-7
          PB: 978-1-3500-0937-0
          ePDF: 978-1-3500-0939-4
          ePub: 978-1-3500-0940-0

Library of Congress Cataloging-in-Publication Data

Name: Day, Carolyn
Title: Consumptive chic : a history of beauty, fashion, and disease / Carolyn Day.
Description: London ; New York : Bloomsbury Academic, an imprint of Bloomsbury Publishing Plc, 2017. | Includes bibliographical references.
Identifiers: LCCN 2017006493| ISBN 9781350009370 (paperback) | ISBN 9781350009387 (hardback) | ISBN 9781350009400 (Epub) | ISBN 9781350009394 (Epdf)
Subject: LCSH: Tuberculosis—Social aspects. | Tuberculosis—History.
Classification: LCC RA644.T7 D39 2017 | DDC 362. 19699/5—dc23 LC record available at https://lccn.loc.gov/2017006493

Cover design: Liron Gilenberg
Cover image: "Dropsy Courting Consumption." Coloured etching by T. Rowlandson. (© Wellcome Library, London/Creative Commons)

Typeset by RefineCatch Limited Bungay, Suffolk
Printed and bound in Great Britain

To find out more about our authors and books visit www.bloomsbury.com. Here you will find extracts, author interviews, details of forthcoming events and the option to sign up for our newsletters.

CONTENTS

Contents

LIST OF FIGURES

LIST OF PLATES

List of Plates

ACKNOWLEDGMENTS

This book has been a labor of love that has kept me constantly entertained for more than a decade, and would not have been possible without the assistance of more people than I have room to thank. Most importantly, thank you to my amazing family for believing in me when I chose to change disciplines and follow my heart. I am so very grateful to you, mom and dad, for teaching me to chase my dreams and to persevere in the face of whatever obstacles come my way. Donal, Lorraine, Benjamin, and Emily this book is dedicated to you and is a testament to your love and support. To my beloved niece and nephew, Avalyn and Brennan, thank you for being so excited about Aunt Nee Nee's book and constantly wanting to be a part of the process. Your enthusiasm as I trudged through archives, and thirst for the stories I uncovered, has made the process all the sweeter. It is hard to believe that you are the same age as the project and watching you grow up as the book did has been incredibly special.

The encouragement and assistance I have received from other academics and friends has been invaluable, both to my development as a scholar as well as to *Consumptive Chic*. To my current and former colleagues and wonderful friends, thank you for your constant advice and support as I navigated academic life and the ins and outs of publishing. Special thanks must go to Dr. Mark Smith for your championing of a young scholar and to Dr. Hugh Belsey and Claudia and Robert Maxtone-Graham for their kind assistance with Mary Graham's dress.

I am extremely grateful to Dr. James Secord for encouraging this project when I first stumbled across the idea and words cannot express what the constant support of Dr. George Bernstein has meant to me. Thank you for taking a chance on me, not only as your student but also for being willing to back a dissertation on the strange juxtaposition of fashion and disease. I would also like to thank Dr. James Boyden and Dr. Alisa Plant who championed this book when it was only a dissertation proposal. Your friendship and wisdom have been invaluable and are so appreciated. I have also been the beneficiary of the generosity of so many archivists, but a special thank you must be given to the wonderful staff of the rare books room at the Cambridge University Library who aided me in making the most of my time in the archives. To that same end, thanks to my amazing friend Dr. Renae Domaschnez who made those brief trips possible. Just as I was slated to begin my research, Hurricane Katrina hit New Orleans closing Tulane University and wiping out my funding. Renae rescued me, and my academic career, by offering me a free place to stay on that first trip and on many subsequent visits to Britain. Special thanks must also go to my friend Dr. Steve Mason who has subsequently put me up on numerous research trips making both this and my next book possible.

INTRODUCTION

The tragedy that befell the Cathcart family was repeated in countless households during the eighteenth and nineteenth centuries. A mother, father, son, and two daughters struck down by tuberculosis—but it was the poignant death of the second daughter, Mary, that encompassed the full tubercular repertoire. A beautiful, delicate, kind, intelligent woman beloved by her family, and most especially by her husband, quietly slipped away in 1792 despite every effort to forestall her end. Mary Graham (1757–1792) was the daughter of the ninth Baron Cathcart and the wife of Thomas Graham of Balgowan, whom she married on December 26, 1774. Mrs. Graham evidently captured the attention of Thomas Gainsborough, whose rendering of the recently married eighteen-year-old Hugh Belsey argues "is one of the finest portraits he ever painted."[1] (See Plate 1.)

The couple was devoted to one another and Thomas went to enormous lengths to shore up his wife's health. Although his estate was in Scotland, they spent a great deal of time in the milder climate of England to avoid stressing her delicate constitution. Thomas and Mary also attended a number of heath resorts, undertaking a regimen of sea-bathing at Brighton and visiting Clifton, a popular option for consumptives.[2] When this proved inadequate, they traveled abroad multiple times for Mary's health, visiting a spa in Belgium and going to Portugal in 1780. In 1781, during this trip, Thomas Graham gave the following account of Mary's condition, stating:

> I think it is most probable that we shall not pass next winter at home, though Mrs. Graham continues pretty well, and has borne these fatigues surprisingly. I hope it will not be necessary for her to go abroad again but it may be prudent to put it easily in our power by being in some place in the southernmost part of England, which will likewise be a milder climate than any other in Britain.[3]

They returned to England and rented a home in Leicestershire in an attempt to avoid another sojourn abroad.[4]

Mary's health continued to degenerate and in 1791 the desperate couple made their way to France, in spite of the revolutionary turbulence, hoping the milder climate would prove beneficial. After spending some time in Paris, they settled in Poil just outside of Nice on the advice of Mary's physician Dr. Webster who was traveling with them. Here they remained, until May of 1792, hoping to gain benefit from the sea air.[5] Mary's health continued to decline, and by the summer of 1792, she recognized the inevitability of her death. Choosing to keep her thoughts from her husband, fearing she would cause him even greater distress, she instead spoke to her friend Mrs. Nugent of his "affectionate conduct to me" stating that "a Mr. Graham is not easily found," and expressing concern over "how he suffers" and "how he tries to conceal it from me."[6]

Her physician prescribed a sea voyage and the Grahams set out from Nice on June 19. Nine days before they left, Mary wrote a letter to her husband to be given to him after her death. This note demonstrated her resignation and concern for those she would leave behind. To her beloved Thomas she wrote "Let your comfort be that I could never have lived without you, and am happy to go first."[7] Although she had given up hope of recovery, Thomas's journal provides glimpses of a woman enjoying her time dining on deck, reading *Don Quixote* and even proving a good sailor. He wrote "She was not at all sick & did not mind this gale at all but was rather entertained with the confusion & the awkwardness of those who try'd to get the things put in order."[8] Despite his tender devotion, Thomas was not present when Mary passed away. He had been assured the end was not close by her physician, and on June 26, 1792 went ashore at Hyères to seek lodging, when he returned Mary was gone. Thomas lamented "It is impossible to say how much I regret being absent when this angel breathed her last."[9]

The trials did not end with Mary's death as Thomas ran into trouble trying to get her home from Revolutionary France. On July 14, just outside of Toulouse, the boat was stopped by National Guard and Volunteer soldiers. What followed filled Thomas with abject horror and rage, he wrote that a "riotous mob of half-drunk rascals . . . armed with muskets . . . insisted on seeing the Box that was sealed." Although he had the permission of the town's municipal officer to pass unmolested and despite his attempts to stop them: "With savage violence they broke open everything." They were so brutal the grieving widower found it necessary to have Mary's body examined by Dr. Webster and was deeply relieved to hear "that there was no injury done," however, he wrote "there was a necessity for a new lead coffin."[10]

Thomas Graham never recovered from Mary's death, and could not bear to look upon her countenance—packing up the Gainsborough portrait of her and placing it in storage.[11] He did, however, keep mementos of Mary including his wedding ring, which he wore throughout his fifty-year widowhood and a more tangible reminder of her final days—a dress worn during her last illness. (See Plate 2.) This gown illustrates the wreckage consumption wrought on its emaciated victim, revealing Mary's very slight frame at the end of her illness.[12] It stands as a tangible remnant of a life cut short and as an attempt to memorialize the last days of a lovely young woman sinking under tuberculosis. Rather than just serving as the material evidence of the illness, dress and tuberculous would become connected in a number of active and meaningful ways.

Constructing Tuberculosis

During the late eighteenth and early nineteenth century cultural ideas about beauty intertwined with the disease process of tuberculosis, allowing the ravages of the illness to be presented in an aesthetically pleasing light. How is it possible that a disease characterized by coughing, emaciation, relentless diarrhea, fever, and the expectoration of phlegm and blood became not only a sign of beauty, but also a fashionable disease? The practical application of this rhetoric and the ways in which consumption became both idealized and feminized are the overarching concerns of this inquiry.

Depictions of tuberculosis diverged from those proffered for other diseases like smallpox, cholera, and typhoid; these differences were due in part to the way the illness manifested itself in the body and its social distribution. Although it altered its sufferer physically, it was not disfiguring in the same way that smallpox or cholera was. Instead, as a disease characterized by wasting and pallor, consumption seemed to enhance its victim by amplifying those qualities already established as attractive. Tuberculosis was further distanced from other illnesses in its chronic nature and constant presence. Unlike sudden, acute maladies that manifested in sweeping epidemics, tuberculosis was always present, in all classes at all times. However, beginning at the end of the eighteenth century, mortality from tuberculosis was on the rise, at its peak causing 25 percent of all deaths in Europe, and then after 1850 it gradually declined.[13] This epidemic curve corresponds with the relatively gentle representation of the illness, which shifts by the mid-century.

Between 1780 and 1850 there was a growing correspondence between tuberculosis and rapidly changing concepts of beauty and fashion. The symptoms were not only compatible with popular ideals of beauty, but the dominant presentation of tuberculosis was that of a disease characterized by attractive aesthetics. This was made possible, in part, by a congruence of factors including disease mortality, advances in the approach to illness, and the influence of the key social movements of the era. The cultural expectations that developed for tuberculosis, as a result of these broader changes, were articulated in medical treatises, literature, poetry, and the works that sought to define fashion and the female role. All of these provided examples that connected the hallmarks of beauty with the symptoms of tuberculosis, and as such, reveal a shared consciousness that the disease was aesthetically pleasing.

The Social Context

Illness is not only a subjective experience but also one defined by its cultural location, both geographically and historically. The intricate relationship between society and illness provides a way in which the value-laden concepts of health and disease can function both within and outside the framework of established medical knowledge and biological evidence. Echoing Susan Sontag, Claudine Herzlich and Janine Pierret argue "that in all societies there is a correspondence between the biological and social order."[14] It is through this interaction that "the language of the sick thus takes shape within the language expressing the relations between the individual and society."[15] A large part of this process is determined by changing definitions of the body and its corresponding relationship to health and disease. Susan Sontag's investigation into the role of metaphor in the disease experience—particularly her contrast between the positive Romantic representation of tuberculosis and the stigmatization of certain illnesses (including cancer and AIDS)—was an important step in explicating the ways in which illnesses are culturally created.[16] Social and historical theorists like Michel Foucault have argued that illness is an invention of ideology, society, and economics.[17] Illness, therefore, reflects the intricate mix of circumstances that define life and social value, as well as its own significance in a given time. The varying terminology employed in describing tuberculosis over the centuries reflects the power of linguistic representations in crafting metaphorical descriptions of an illness. These terms also mirror the dominant understandings of the disease and illustrate the persistent confusion over the cause, course, and meaning of tuberculosis. Tuberculosis infections have been classified using a number of idiosyncratic designations and these alterations in language demonstrate one way in which a dialogue evolves to reflect new information and attitudes towards an illness.[18]

The term "tuberculosis" did not come into widespread use until the latter half of the nineteenth century; instead, the disease was identified by a number of other names, including phthisis, consumption, and scrofula (which referred to a non-pulmonary form of the disease). Other terms used include: tabes, inflammation of the lungs, bronchitis, asthenia, lupus, graveyard cough, and hectic fever, to name a few. In 1725 Richard Blackmore expressed the difficulty in categorizing the affliction that accompanied this diverse nomenclature, emphasizing the dominance of ancient medicine in the understanding of disease, by addressing the Greek roots of phthisis. The term was already in common use in the sixteenth century and translates into a wasting away, perishing, or decaying of the body and its use was, in part, an indication of the sweats and emaciation that were characteristic symptoms of the malady's final stages.

Though the term "phthisis" remained in common use well into the nineteenth century, it was increasingly supplanted by "consumption," which was in use by 1660 to denote phthisical decline.[19] This term spoke to the fact that the disease seemed to consume its victim from the inside out, leaving a withered husk and gaunt devastation. Although evocative, the term was neither precise nor exclusive, as it was used to identify a plurality of wasting conditions. In 1847 Henry Deshon complained of the indiscriminate use of the label, stating "The term 'Consumption', as generally applied to denote disease of pulmonic origin, is employed in too vague and indiscriminate a manner . . . 'Pulmonary consumption', or 'phthisis pulmonalis', more correctly applies to the general failure of health dependent upon the formation of tubercle."[20] This curious intermingling of terms and their use as essentially interchangeable entities was indicative of the ongoing confusion over identifying and quantifying the illness; however, the role of the tubercle would become increasingly important in discussions of the illness. (See Plate 3.)

The term "tuberculosis" first appeared in print in 1839, when J. L. Schonlein, a professor of medicine in Zurich, proposed the word as a generic sobriquet for all manifestations of the disease. The root word "tubercle" was, by this point, commonly understood to be the fundamental unit of pathology. The word derived from the Latin term *tuberculum*, which translated into "lump."[21] The term reflected the growing influence of pathological anatomy as medical investigators searched for the exact role the tubercle played in the disease's causation, course, and consequences. In 1852 Henry Ancell laid out the appropriate usage for all associated tubercular definitions.

> The term "Tuberculosis" being employed to designate the constitutional origin of all the local manifestations of Consumption and Scrofula, and "Tubercle" to designate a special morbid element, the word "Tubercular" is generally used where the presence of tubercle is intended to be implied, and the word "Tuberculous" where it is not; but owing to the indefinite employment of these terms by preceding writers, it has been found impracticable to adhere rigidly to any rule.[22]

Nonetheless, the term tuberculosis would not supplant consumption or even phthisis until the turn of the twentieth century.[23] Robert Koch's identification of the *Mycobacterium tuberculosis* bacillus in 1882 proved a crucial step in the acceptance of the germ theory of disease and would eventually ease the way for the term tuberculosis.

Scholarly Construction of Tuberculosis

The scholarly engagement with tuberculosis has itself been a reflection of specific social and cultural concerns—in particular, concerns about class, poverty, and the role of the state. Thus, while scholars have long been interested in the study of the "white plague" they have primarily concerned themselves with explaining its mortality decline, or with analysing the ways in which campaigns to mitigate its effects took place in various countries.[24] The return of tuberculosis as a public health threat in the 1980s, with its tendency to co-infect those with the human immunodeficiency virus (HIV), led to a resurgence of interest and in the 1990s there were a number of works published on tuberculosis in American society.[25]

The threat has not diminished and tuberculosis has once again become an enormous global public health problem. In 2007 there were approximately 1.7 million deaths from tuberculosis and 9.27 million new cases, even more shockingly one-third of the human population is thought to be infected with the *Mycobacterium tuberculosis*.[26] (See Plate 4.) Global efforts at tuberculosis (TB) eradication have been complicated by the growing incidences of MDR-TB (multi-drug resistant TB), the advent of XDR-TB (extensively-drug resistant TB),[27] and by the reliance on decades-old drug therapies.[28] This combination of factors "threatens to return TB treatment to the pre-antibiotic era, when 50% of patients with TB died of the disease."[29] Current therapies for MDR-TB include a combination of between eight to ten different medications and the course of the therapy ranges on average from 18–24 months. Despite these aggressive tactics the treatment regime fails in nearly 30 percent of those cases of XDR-TB.[30]

The continuing concern over tuberculosis is reflected in a number of new scientific works on the subject as well as new histories of the illness.[31] There remains, however, a dearth of works on tuberculosis that concentrate exclusively on Britain, and those that do, like Linda Bryder's *Below the Magic Mountain: A Social History of Tuberculosis in Twentieth-Century Britain* (1988), focus on the late nineteeth or twentieth centuries. In

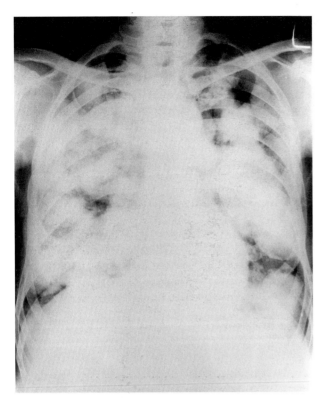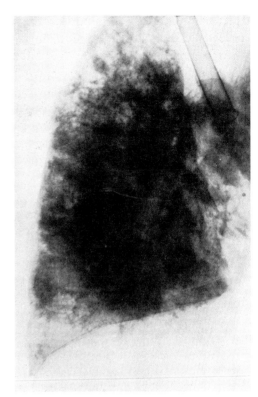

Figure I.1 Left: X-ray of chest showing tuberculosis. Right: Photograph of the lungs of a patient after death from tuberculosis. Francis Henry Williams, *Roentgen Rays in Medicine and Surgery as an aid in diagnosis and as a therapeutic agent* (New York, London: Macmillan, 1903). Wellcome Library, London. Copyrighted work available under Creative Commons Attribution only licence CC BY 4.0 http://creativecommons.org/licenses/by/4.0/

general, works on tuberculosis in the nineteenth century have either looked at the concepts surrounding the illness at the beginning of the century, focusing exclusively on the working classes, or are devoted to assessing the illness in the latter half of the century. These works often acknowledge the existence of the Romantic myth in literature, but this subject was not adequately explored until Clark Lawlor's *Consumption and Literature: the Making of the Romantic Disease* (2006). Lawlor's work addresses the disparity between biological reality and literary interpretation and remains the only work that delves deeply into the "aesthetics" of consumption. However, his focus is primarily literary and fails to adequately delve into the popular applications of that rhetoric or on its correspondence with contemporary beauty ideals. Even the newest works on the subject, for instance, Katherine Byrne's *Tuberculosis and the Victorian Literary Imagination* (2011) and Helen Bynum's *Spitting Blood: A History of Tuberculosis* (2012), only briefly mention the aesthetics of the illness.

There was a definite relationship between female roles, fashion, and beauty that both illustrated and aided the construction of a changing social view of tuberculosis. The nature of consumption's reciprocal impact during the late eighteenth and first half of the nineteenth centuries on upper- and middle-class women, both as individuals and as part of the social body, is the focus of this inquiry. There was a persistent and influential idea during the period that consumption, in its middle- and upper-class incarnations, was a disease that was not only identified by the existence of beauty in women, but one that also conferred beauty upon its sufferer. Thus, tuberculosis was rationalized as a positive affliction for women, one to be emulated in beauty ideals and fashions. Yet there was also a contradiction, since fashions and the way of life of fashionable society were thought to "excite" the disease in upper- and middle-class women who possessed a predisposition to consumption and whose inherent feminine character rendered them more susceptible to the activation of that predisposition. The positive associations with consumption and its "look," permitted the widespread flouting of admonitions against the clothing and fashionable practices believed to cause the disease. Tuberculosis, despite evidence to the contrary, was portrayed as an easy or beautiful way to die. How did these poignant representations of consumption reconcile with its horrific reality? Moreover, why was the illness interpreted aesthetically not only as a sign of strong emotions such as passion and love, or as a mark of genius and spirituality, but also as a marker for physical beauty?

CHAPTER 1
THE APPROACH TO ILLNESS

Tuberculosis Mortality

During the nineteenth century, consumption supplanted the great epidemics (such as plague or smallpox) in the public's imagination. The growing presence of the disease was apparent in England, beginning in the mid-seventeenth century, and its widespread nature was quickly recognized. In the 1674 edition of *Morbus Anglicus: or the Anatomy of Consumptions*, Gideon Harvey expounded upon those most affected. "It's a great chance we find, to arrive at one's grave in the English Climate, without a smack of a Consumption, Death's direct door to most hard Students, Divines, Physicians, Philosophers, deep Lovers, Zelots in Religion, &c."[1] Harvey's title was a nod to the prevalence of the disease in England, translating as it does into "Disease of the English,"[2] and this emerging "social scourge" was accompanied by new imagery.

In general, infectious diseases adhere to an epidemic pattern. Initially, they increase very quickly; then, having attained a certain level, slowly fade in intensity and incidence. Despite the fact that the development and course of tuberculosis is less "flashy" than other contagious illnesses, it still follows a typical epidemic cycle of infection, though the progress is often extraordinarily slow, taking decades rather than weeks or months. In Europe, the epidemic curve for tuberculosis began in the latter part of the seventeenth century and peaked in the middle part of the nineteenth. By the close of the nineteenth century, it was still claiming one-seventh of the world's population and even in 1940 tuberculosis was responsible for a greater loss of life than any other single contagious illness.[3] In Great Britain, for the two hundred years preceding 1840, tuberculosis was a major endemic disease afflicting nearly as many individuals as all other diseases combined.[4] Whatever the actual numbers, there was certainly an eighteenth-century perception of a rise in mortality for consumption. It was widely acknowledged that the illness was pervasive and deadly. For instance, William Black, who wrote several works concerned with medical statistics, stated in 1788: "from one fifth to one sixth of all the mortality in London, is from consumption; which is nearly double to that even of small pox," and that "phthisis, phthisis, phthisis, towering with gigantic bulk" dominated the London funeral catalogues.[5]

Its impact was heightened by the seemingly indiscriminate way in which it claimed its victims, afflicting the denizens of mansions as well as tenements. The disease was rampant in urban centers, but not limited to the city, and showed no respect for gender, status, age, or occupation. In 1818, John Mansford argued consumption was on the rise:

It is as a growing disease that consumption assumes its most important feature. It has with justice been termed the giant malady of the country; and with fearful, and giant-like strides does it gain upon us ... It appears probable ... that the number of deaths from consumption in Great Britain have increased one-third within the last century; and that they have now reached the enormous amount of fifty-five thousand annually.[6]

In spite of the conviction that there was an increase in tuberculosis deaths, determining the specific incidences of consumption remains difficult due to the lack of accurate mortality data, a circumstance complicated by the

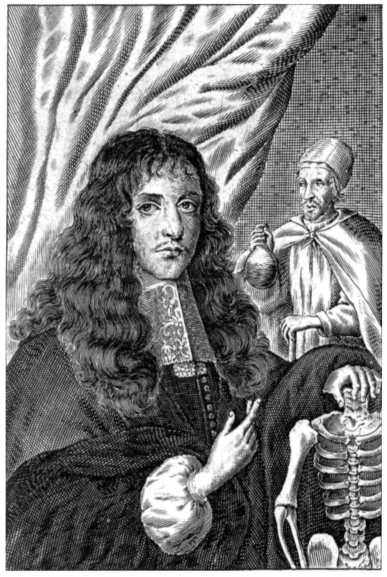

Figure 1.1 Gideon Harvey by A. Hertochs, n.d. Wellcome Library, London. Copyrighted work available under Creative Commons Attribution only licence CC BY 4.0 http://creativecommons.org/licenses/by/4.0/

uncertainty of contemporary diagnosis. Consumption's slow, creeping nature meant that it often remained unnoticed until the latter stages, and its nomenclature further complicates the assessment of mortality. The terms phthisis and pulmonary consumption were used, almost indiscriminately, to indicate a number of unrelated maladies.[7] The designation of consumption was particularly problematic, as it was often applied to any illness accompanied by weight loss.

In spite of these difficulties, it is clear that the nineteenth century can reliably be termed the "age of consumption," whether one cites the disease's actual or imagined impact. It can also be styled the age of medical statistics.[8] Until the nineteenth century, there were no regular or accurate records of quantitative mortality kept in England. That is not to say that there had not been attempts, both by institutions such as hospitals as well as by some cities, to keep records of births and deaths. In 1836 a parliamentary mandate formalized these efforts and led to the creation of a nationwide system of registration of births, deaths, and marriages. The following year, the statistician and physician, William Farr, gave up his medical practice and became temporarily employed by the General Registrar Office to assist in arranging and classifying this information and in 1839 his position became permanent.[9] With Farr's publication of *The First Annual Report of the Registrar General of Births, Deaths, and Marriages*, officials in England began to systematically tracking mortality rates for a variety of diseases, including tuberculosis.

These new statistics bore witness to the nationwide destruction of human life caused by consumption—a situation that did not escape the notice of those chronicling the disease. One such investigator, Henry Gilbert, wrote: "According to the Report of the Registrar-General, pulmonary consumption destroyed more human lives during the six months referred to [July 1 to December 31, 1837], than did cholera, influenza, small-pox, measles, ague, typhus-fever, hydrophobia, apoplexy, hernia, colic, diseases of the liver, stone, rheumatism, ulcers, fistula, and mortification!"[10] Gilbert quickly put these statistics to use, arguing "There is no disease so universal, and none so mortal, as consumption of the lungs. According to the best data, it has been calculated, by medical men, that it causes one-fourth part of all the deaths occurring from disease in Great Britain and Ireland."[11] By 1850 the *Annual Reports* were publicly highlighting the substantial tuberculosis death rates found in large cities.[12] Sizable mortality helped raise public awareness and focused the medical community's attention on the disease throughout the last half of the nineteenth century. In 1882, Robert Koch wrote of consumption's impact, "If the number of victims which a disease claims is the measure of its significance, then all diseases, particularly the most dreaded infectious diseases, such as bubonic plague, Asiatic cholera, etc., must rank far behind tuberculosis. Statistics teach that one-seventh of all human beings die of tuberculosis, and that, if one considers only the productive middle-age groups, tuberculosis carries away one-third and often more of these."[13]

Anatomico-Pathological Approach to Disease

Beyond a growing awareness of the magnitude of the disease, early nineteenth-century attitudes toward tuberculosis reflected the dominance of the anatomico-pathological approach to illness. The eighteenth century witnessed the development of a localized concept of disease, one explored and understood in terms of morbid anatomy. During the 1760s the Italian anatomist, G. B. Morgagni linked sickness to anatomical findings in his work *De sedibus et causis morborum*, helping to establish the idea that medical investigators should correlate symptoms and lesions through autopsy. He was instrumental in altering the theoretical ideology of illness by elevating pathology and the role played by precise, localized lesions. In this new anatomical perspective, the lens of medical investigation was focused on the parts rather than the whole.[14] Increasingly, the symptoms manifested by the living victims of illness were correlated after death with the structural alterations seen post-mortem.[15] The ground-breaking French pathological anatomist Xavier Bichat helped define this outlook and charged physicians to dissect and discover.[16] Underpinning the new approach was the idea that an illness had specific pathological manifestations and investigation of these particulars would provide answers to the cause of diseases. This alteration in the intellectual approach led to a new way of categorizing the process of disease; however, for consumption, the growth in the depth and quality of anatomical information raised more questions than it answered.

In tuberculosis, the anatomico-pathological approach was limited to diagnostics and the identification of the pathological indicators, but failed to elucidate the causes of these morbid presentations. Slowly medical investigators developed new methodologies and tools to scrutinize the disease process not just in the dead, but also in the living body. To this end, the discovery of percussion and development of the stethoscope helped advance the knowledge of tuberculosis and aid in its diagnosis.[17] When Theophile Hyacinthe Laennec created the stethoscope in 1816, he produced an item that would become the primary instrument of the new anatomical approach to medicine. (See Plate 5.) By opening the living body to "dissection" through sound, the stethoscope provided a new vehicle for investigating a diseased individual; pathology could now be performed on the living as well as the dead.[18] The stethoscope and accompanying methodology significantly altered the approach to respiratory ailments, and Laennec applied his new weapon to pulmonary consumption. *A Treatise on the Diseases of the Chest and on Mediate Auscultation* (published in French in 1819 and translated into English by 1821) clearly described the clinical route taken by tuberculosis.[19] In the work, Laennec not only

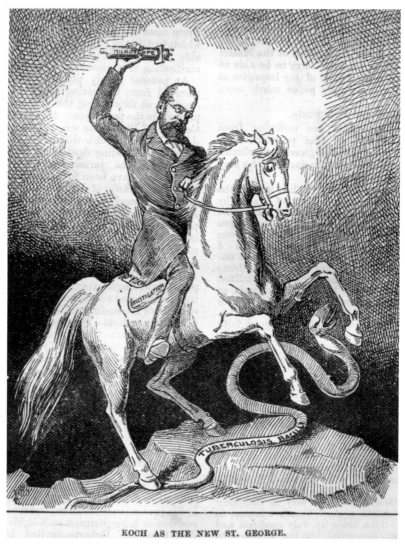

KOCH AS THE NEW ST. GEORGE.

Figure 1.2 Robert Koch as the new Saint George after isolating the tuberculosis bacillus. Editorial #: 3362301 Photo by Hulton Archive/Getty Images.

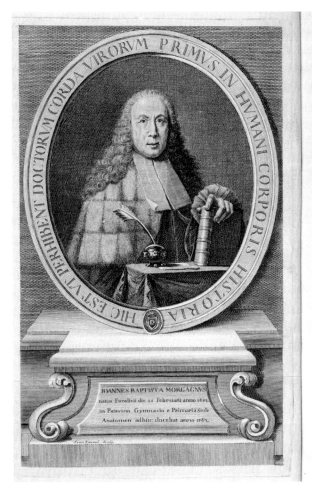
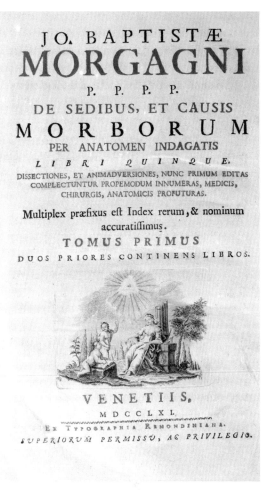

Figure 1.3 Giovanni Battista Morgagni. Title page and frontispiece Giovanni Battista Morgagni, *De sedibus, et causis morborum* (Venice: Remondiniani, 1761). Wellcome Library, London. Copyrighted work available under Creative Commons Attribution only licence CC BY 4.0 http://creativecommons.org/licenses/by/4.0/

established guidelines for diagnosing consumption, but also argued that the tubercle was the signifier of one single malady, whether it was located in the lungs or elsewhere in the body, like the liver or the gut. Laennec proposed a unitary theory of consumption, which became the accepted viewpoint until the discovery of the tubercle bacillus in 1882.[20] In 1843, John Hastings paid homage to Laennec's contributions, stating:

> Although various and varied in their character were the works on Pulmonary Consumption before Laennec's time, his vast discoveries, by means of auscultation, have spread over it a new light, and created another era in its history ... But extraordinary as it may appear, our means of cure seem to have diminished, in proportion as our knowledge of determining the character of Consumption has increased; for at no period of its history has it been so fatal as since the discovery of the stethoscope.[21]

Credence was granted to Laennec's theories by his contemporary Gaspard Laurent Bayle whose work *Recherches sur la phthisie pulmonaire* (1810) also argued that tuberculosis was a precise and specific condition rather than some pervasive generalized wasting disorder that occurred as a result of some earlier malady. Additionally, he asserted that tubercles developed first before any outward symptoms appeared. Bayle insisted that the most visible and recognizable symptoms of tuberculosis indicated the degree of the disease's advance, and that an absence of visible or characteristic symptoms in no way indicated an absence of the disease.[22] Bayle's *Recherches* provided an analysis of the most frequent pathological manifestations and systematically tracked the organic changes produced during the course of the disease process, performing over nine hundred autopsies and combining the results with his own observations. This comparison of pathological and clinical findings led him to conclude that a small tubercle was the origin of the other lesions in consumption. He declared that the further complications observed in phthisis patients, including those seen in the intestine, larynx, and lymph nodes, were the product of consumption and not a separate illness.[23]

Sir Robert Carswell's text on *Pathological Anatomy* (1838) synthesized and evaluated the numerous descriptions of the tubercle by medical investigators like Laennec, Bayle, and Gabriel Andral and assessed the seeming variability of its nature.[24] Carswell was prominent among the British medical men who flocked to France to learn the new anatomico-pathological concepts. There he observed dissections and became familiar with new medical techniques (such as mediate auscultation) while spending time with Pierre Charles Alexandre Louis and Laennec.[25] Carswell is perhaps best known for his stunning illustrations of dissections of the anatomical samples he surveyed in France; additionally he remains important for his work in helping to translate pathological anatomy into a distinct medical discipline in England.[26] Robert Carswell also demonstrated the continued difficulty of accurately determining the cause and course of tuberculosis. He performed dissections and prepared colored drawings of his observations, which demonstrated localized concepts of disease; however, his accompanying case notes presented a more holistic approach.[27] *Pathological Anatomy* raised several questions that continued to plague the medical community about tubercles. (See Plate 6.) What was the origin of these lesions? What were they, and were they related to the disease process of phthisis? One popular theory presented tubercles as small damaged glands whose enlarged state was the result of the injury done by disease. Others saw tubercles as new entities seeded by the disease and growing in a tumor-like fashion. Speculation continued on everything from the size and consistency of tubercles to their origin and location. Investigations into the nature of the tubercle also raised questions over the exact relationship between the tubercles found in the lungs and those in other parts of the body. In 1849, Robert Hull argued "Pulmonary consumption is a systematic malady. A lung may suffer alone, or in common with the viscera of the abdomen."[28] The question remained: was there a relationship between these extra-pulmonary tubercles present in scrofula, for example, and those in pulmonary phthisis?[29] Despite the influence of Bayle and the work of those like Hull, the majority of physicians seem to have viewed these varying pathological symptoms as the result of other, unrelated illnesses.

In an attempt to establish some order over this perplexing wealth of information, medical investigators deliberately categorized different conditions by the type of ulcer, tubercle, or cavity that was present.[30] Cases in which tubercles manifested outside of the lungs had a different designation than consumption and, until the late nineteenth century, they were believed to be distinct but related diseases with their own etiologies and treatments. When Carswell argued that the study of consumption should fall under the aegis of pathological anatomy, he acknowledged the limits of available knowledge and addressed the role played by factors such as the elements and the economy, as well as the acquired or hereditary nature of the illness. But what was this nature? A theory that covered the holes left by the anatomico-pathological approach was necessary, and heredity received the nod for a number of illnesses, including tuberculosis.

There was a widespread acknowledgment of the prevalence and destructive nature of pulmonary consumption, but determining its cause, diagnosis, and treatment proved elusive. In 1808, James Sanders lamented this pervasive ignorance, writing:

One could scarcely perceive from their writings, that authors had ever attempted to relate the symptoms in the order of their occurrence and consistently with the changes which succeed in the constitution; and this probably is the chief cause, that they do not agree with regard to its nature, though of bodies deprived of life by consumption an infinite number has been examined with great patience and anatomical discrimination.[31]

Nearly half a century later the confusion remained, and in 1855 Henry M'Cormac wrote, "For generations phthisis has been the opprobrium of medicine. No disease perhaps has been more patiently investigated, yet none has more frequently baffled inquiry, or has been more extensively abandoned to empiricism and despair."[32]

CHAPTER 2
THE CURIOUS CASE OF CONSUMPTION: A FAMILY AFFAIR

Contagious?

Pathological anatomy advanced the understanding of how tuberculosis manifested in the body; however, it did little to account for variable susceptibility or the source of the tubercles. The theories put forward were diverse and on the European continent, particularly in the south, consumption was generally regarded as a contagious disease, one spread through the air or through contact with either infected persons or materials.[1] Elsewhere—in England for instance—tuberculosis was viewed as the result of a breakdown in an individual's constitution, a flaw that was frequently inherited, passed from parents to offspring like physical characteristics such as facial features and hair color.[2] Contagion theory failed to provide an explanation for all of the observed incidences of consumption and many theorists simultaneously supported the concept of tuberculosis as both a contagious and an heredity illness. Physicians, like Gideon Harvey, emphasized the link between consumption and personal defects, while at the same time embracing the centrality of contagion, stating consumption,

> With all its malignity and catching nature . . . may be connumerated with the worst of Epidemicks, since next to the Plague, Pox, and Leprosie, it yields to none in point of Contagion . . . Moreover nothing we find taints sound Lungs sooner than inspiring the breath of putrid, ulcer'd, consumptive Lungs; many having fallin into Consumptions only by smelling the breath or spittle of Consumptives, others by drinking after them; and what is more, by wearing the Cloathing of Consumptives, though two years after they were left off.[3]

Despite his strong inclination toward contagion, Harvey also wrote that the disease often passes "from Consumptive Parents to their Children," and as such, it is "Hereditary, insomuch that whole families, sourcing from tabefyed progenitors, have made their Exits through Consumptions."[4]

By the end of the seventeenth century there were growing doubts about the validity of contagion theory. In northern Europe, physicians used the evidence that the disease was often relentless and widespread in some families as proof that consumption was the result of a hereditary constitutional defect.[5] By the eighteenth century, there was a definitive split in the belief over the contagiousness of tuberculosis between southern and northern Europe, with a refusal by many in northern Europe to acknowledge the possibility consumption was contagious.[6] In Britain, by the nineteenth century, there was a strong denunciation of the contagion theory as lacking empirical evidence. *A Treatise on Tuberculosis* (1852) stated:

> The doctrine of contagion has, however, at all times been based on very vague and insufficient evidence; such as isolated cases of the disease in individuals who had previously been in constant attendance upon the sick; or in husbands or wives, where both had slept in the same bed until the fatal termination of the disease in the one first affected . . . Against the few facts which tend to support the doctrine of contagion, there are tens of thousands against it.[7]

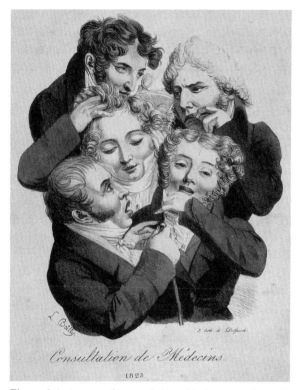

Figure 2.1 A group of young, fashionable doctors. Lithograph by F-S. Delpech after L. Boilly, 1823. Wellcome Library, London. Copyrighted work available under Creative Commons Attribution only licence CC BY 4.0 http://creativecommons. org/licenses/by/4.0/

The disavowal of contagion necessitated the development of other explanative schemes, and the concept of heredity was incorporated into the theoretical repertoire of causation. By the early nineteenth century, many investigators were persuaded that conditions like tuberculosis, gout, and insanity were the end-product of a multifaceted etiology stemming from the action of some murky grouping of environmental factors and influences. Yet fierce debates continued over the various explanations for tuberculosis, ranging from contagion to heredity and from the constitution to the environment. The general consensus was that the blame rested with some inborn susceptibility.[8]

The Constitution

While the anatomico-pathological approach was gaining popularity, a constitutional predilection toward infirmity became the predominant explanation for a variety of chronic illnesses, tuberculosis among them. In 1806 John Reid plainly stated the constitutional case.

> There is however … an acknowledged variety in constitutional tendency to genuine phthisis, from whatever source it may originate. The destroying angel, while requiring general retribution for certain deviations from nature, marks particular individuals for primary sacrifice. Although no one ought

fearlessly to expose himself to the causes of consumption, every one has not an equal cause for fear . . . Natural organization, age, sex and professional or other occupations and habits, may, perhaps, be made to include every peculiarity of disposition to pulmonary consumption, whether native or adventitious; or, in the language of systematics, will comprehend the praedisposing and exciting causes of this formidable and destructive malady.[9]

The "constitutional construction" proposed the body was an ordered structure whose fundamental characteristics were inherited as a whole, resulting in either a strong constitution that was resistant to disease or a weak one that left an individual vulnerable to illness.[10] By placing the constitution at the heart of the explanatory process, physicians crafted a physiological hypothesis of causation that led to the belief that little could be done to correct any inborn constitutional imbalance.

Gradually, certain afflictions came to be intricately tied to hereditary concepts. Horace Walpole (1717–1797) reminisced about the effects of a weakened constitution on his family and his own trials as a child, stating: "[I] was extremely weak and delicate, as you see me still, though with no constitutional complaint till I had the gout after forty, and as my two sisters were consumptive,[11] and died of consumptions, the supposed necessary care of me (and I have overheard persons saying, 'That child cannot possibly live') so engrossed the attention of my mother, that compassion and tenderness soon became extreme fondness."[12] Medical practitioners believed an inherited malady was embedded in the constitution of an individual and could manifest in a variety of ways, as in the Walpole family as both consumption and gout. (See Plate 7.) In his *Treatise on Pulmonary Consumption,* Sir James Clark identified the importance of the constitution: "Before we can hope to acquire an accurate knowledge of consumption, we must carry our researches beyond the pulmonary disease, which is only a secondary affection, the consequence of a pre-existing constitutional disorder, the necessary condition which determines the production of tubercles."[13]

In nearly all of the debates over hereditary disease, the connections between the constitution and heritable disease are plainly evident; but the actual importance of the theoretical web becomes clear when one takes into account how physicians viewed the constitution.[14] Doctors seeking to explain the resistance of certain illnesses—such as tuberculosis, madness, or insanity—to treatment or cure had few options. Reliance solely upon environmental influences and lifestyle, failed to account for the implacability of these illnesses in the face of behavior modification and changes in environmental conditions, which usually produced no permanent improvement. In intertwining chronic illness and the constitution, physicians were able to account for their failure to affect the outcome of diseases like consumption and by maintaining these illnesses were constitutional, physicians were also inclined to view them as hereditary.[15]

Hereditary rationalization carried weight in situations where the disease carried off entire families and when only some individuals were affected, as it was the consumptive constitution that was passed down and not the illness itself. As Thomas Reid argued in 1782, "This disease usually attacks people of a delicate, weak, tender constitution and, as such habits of body are peculiar to certain families; in such cases, it may be with some truth termed an hereditary disease."[16] Consumption was particularly notorious for running through families, like the Brontës, where, tragically, one member after another perished successively of the disease. (See Plate 8.) The two oldest sisters, Maria and Elizabeth, died in 1825 from tuberculosis. They were followed to the grave by Branwell (1848), Emily (1848), and Anne (1849), all of whom perished from consumption. Charlotte passed away in 1855, also believed to be from a tubercular condition complicated by her pregnancy.[17] In January of 1849, Charlotte wrote: "Since September sickness has not quitted the house. It is strange it did not use to be so, but I suspect now all this has been coming on for years. Unused, any of us, to the possession of robust health, we have not noticed the gradual approaches of decay; we did not know its symptoms: the little cough, the small appetite, the tendency to take cold at every variation of atmosphere have been regarded as

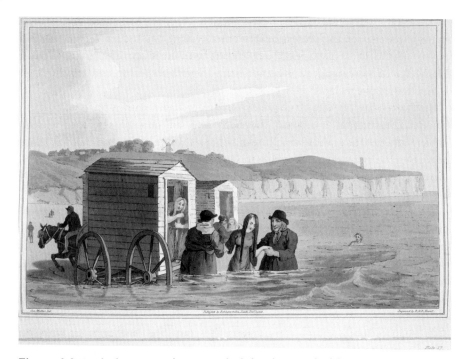

Figure 2.2 Sea-bathing was often prescribed for those with delicate constitutions. "Sea bathing." George Walker, *Costume of Yorkshire* (London: Longman, Hurst, Rees, Orme, and Brown, 1813). New York Public Library Digital Collections [accessed June 14, 2016].

things of course. I see them in another light now."[18] In 1836, Emily Shore remarked on one such family that seemed to be afflicted with a rapidly progressing galloping consumption.

> The bathing women . . . told mamma a few particulars about the family at No. 36. It seems that there is a great mortality among them. As soon as they arrive at the age of twenty they die. The one whose hearse we saw was the fourth of them thus prematurely cut off, and one of them now is expected to have her turn—apparently the pale one, the elder of the two. What they die of we could not make out; probably consumption, though it seems to be a very rapid one.[19]

The frequency of this sort of occurrence, where multiple members of a household suffered from consumption or where entire families perished from the illness, led to the supposition in much of northern Europe that the malady was the consequence of inheriting a flawed constitution.[20] The constitutional construction also provided a convenient explanation for situations where only one member of a family died, as it could be claimed that the victim was the only member to inherit the weak constitution. Nineteenth-century medical practitioners and lay persons alike accepted that consumption was fundamentally an expression of an individual's family legacy and personal circumstances. As J. J. Furnivall wrote in 1835:

> There can now be little doubt, "that the Tubercular Diathesis is in direct proportion to the development of this peculiar constitution," and that the deposition of tubercles is in persons, hereditarily predisposed, much favoured by, and in other, mainly dependent on, a deviation from healthy innervation . . . [which] leads directly to the formation or localization of tuberculous matter.[21]

Heredity and constitutional predisposition, combined with adverse climatic circumstances and living conditions, seemed to provide a convincing substitute for contagion. Physicians argued that if tuberculosis were contagious, everyone in the home would be suffering from the illness. As *On the Nature, Treatment and Prevention of Pulmonary Consumption* stated:

> Consumption is not communicated by any infection, any contagion, any more than a fractured limb is so communicated. It may very well happen however, that persons belonging to the same family, living in the same apartments, exposed to the same deteriorating influences, at once producing the malady and rendering it inveterate when produced, shall in succession be seized with phthisis, so that whole families, as has too often happened, shall be carried off by it. This it is, which has led to the belief not only of the communicability of phthisis from person to person, but also of its transmission in families.[22]

The chief ideological link between notions of the constitution and heritability was not without its contradictions. Although consumption had a penchant for running through families, it did not do so with any predictable consistency. As Thomas Bartlett described in 1855, "As with gout, so with Consumption, it is often found that the disease spares one or two generations, only to appear again in the succeeding ones."[23] To counter this hurdle, the concept of a hereditary predisposition was introduced. This notion provided a theoretical bridge, suggesting that an individual did not inherit the actual disease but instead an inclination or tendency toward the illness, which would only develop under the correct environmental conditions and stimuli.[24]

To account for the role of an innumerable variety of exciting causes in disease, the late eighteenth and early nineteenth centuries saw the rise to prominence of the disease diathesis. In most cases, the term diathesis was used to denote a predisposition to a disease; however, it was also sometimes used to describe an injury to the body which became permanent and was then passed down as the predisposition. As a result, the diathesis could be both the acute injury that created the predisposition, or the predisposition itself.[25] Hereditary sickness emerged as a by-product of the constitutional construction of disease, as a diathesis could either be inherited or acquired during the course of life. In some conditions, such as gout, the diathesis was first thought to be acquired and then passed on. John Murray's *A Treatise on Pulmonary Consumption* addressed the role of parental conformation in the development of hereditary illness, arguing, "As to parentage—the offspring of scrofulous and consumptive, dyspeptic, or gouty parents, will be born into the world with constitutions susceptible of those external agencies which conduct to confirmed Consumption; it is in this way only that Consumption can be said to be hereditary; and thus literally may the 'sins of the fathers be visited on the third and fourth generation.'"[26]

Differences in constitution provided the explanation for the variations observed in mortality rates and in the ways a disease progressed in each individual case. The extensive impact and variable mortality of consumption fueled the search to identify the "tubercular diathesis" and the characteristics that led to a person's innate susceptibility to it.[27] The repeated assaults on a victim's person made by chronic illness had hereditary ramifications, since only recurring actions resulted in a permanent change to the constitutional composition of the body. In 1799 William Grant argued a disease could only become transmissible if widespread alterations occurred in the constitution of the afflicted individual. Similarly, in the early nineteenth century, Horatio Prater argued, "The grand distinction between hereditary and non-hereditary diseases seems to be that the former alter the structure deeply and permanently ... while the latter affect every part superficially."[28] These statements illustrate one of the persistent problems associated with hereditary diathesis—that of defining the exact circumstances under which an illness could result in an overwhelming change in the constitution. The customary response by medical practitioners was an assertion of the importance of the length of the insult. By the nineteenth century, the term "diathesis" had come to refer primarily to chronic

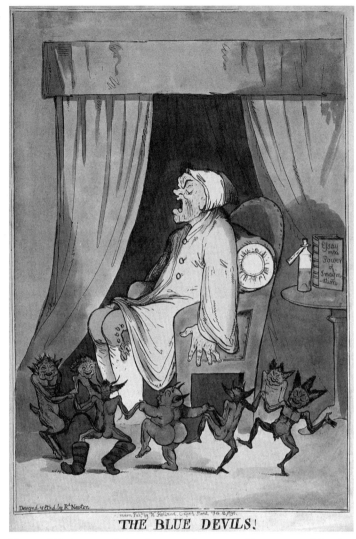

THE BLUE DEVILS!

Figure 2.3 A man suffering from gout (represented by a group of dancing blue devils). Richard Newton (London: W. Holland, 1795). Wellcome Library, London. Copyrighted work available under Creative Commons Attribution only licence CC BY 4.0 http://creativecommons.org/licenses/by/4.0/

rather than acute conditions, particularly those illnesses that either intermittently or progressively exerted an influence on the victim, such as asthma, gout, cancer, epilepsy, insanity, and, of course, consumption.[29]

Beginning in the late eighteenth century and continuing well into the nineteenth, the hereditary explanation of chronic disease became practically universal, touted in medical treatises, nosologies, and textbooks. In 1834, for example, James Clark summed up the feelings on the subject of heritability and tuberculosis, arguing that it was not the disease that was inherited but rather a constitutional predisposition to it. "That pulmonary consumption is an hereditary disease, in other words that the tuberculosis constitution is transmitted from parent to child, is a fact not to be controverted; indeed, I regard it as one of the best established points in the etiology of the disease."[30] Physicians believed that once a chronic disease was firmly established, it was extremely difficult if not impossible to dislodge making hereditary illness synonymous with incurability. The irredeemable nature of these sorts of diseases turned the focus toward prevention rather than cure, and hope in these cases rested on averting the establishment of the diathesis.

Palliate Rather than Cure

As a chronic disease, tuberculosis was located in a framework of predisposition and incurability. Thus, when an 1827 article in *The Lancet* proposed the question "But can consumption be cured?" the answer was inevitable. "Odd bless me, that's a question which a man who had lived in a dissecting room would laugh at . . . for there is no case which, when it has proceeded to a certain extent, can be cured."[31] It was widely believed there was little that could forestall the development of consumption in those possessing the predisposition. The best advice many nineteenth-century medical investigators could proffer was to be born into a family that had no history of the illness. Furthermore, they determined that the origin and pattern of development for phthisis could be a function of the individual's sex, ethnicity, occupation, status, living conditions, or any combination of these factors. In 1808 the *Treatise on Pulmonary Consumption* stated:

> There is nothing absurd in supposing, that the lungs may be often so deficient from their original structure, and such deficiency appears to me to be the only effect of mal-conformation which gives occasion to the disease. Those means which enfeeble the general system, as bad food, excessive venery, vicissitudes of weather, cannot predispose to consumption of the lungs more than to that of any other vices, the predisposition must have been antecedent to their agency.[32]

Complicating the issue of predisposition was the fact that nineteenth-century medical professionals held little hope for a cure once the disease was established, leading to widespread dissatisfaction over the available treatment options. Quack treatments were a constant concern, as unscrupulous individuals purported to have cures for consumption, while desperate victims, like Miss Cashin, were often willing to try anything. This young lady, fearing she might come down with consumption, submitted to a treatment by the quack physician Mr. John St. John Long. He performed a procedure that included rubbing her back with a corrosive, which caused a tremendous sore that then became infected and caused her death in October of 1830. St. John Long was tried and convicted of manslaughter, though escaped imprisonment and instead was fined 250 pounds.[33]

Consumption's extended, and seemingly invisible, period of incubation and vague symptoms often led to routine misdiagnosis until the final stages of the illness. Once the disease was plainly evident, the patient had passed the stage at which medical authorities believed they could affect any alteration. In a letter of condolence to a father who recently lost his daughter to consumption, the author addressed these difficulties.

> I heard nothing of the heavy calamity that you have sustained till the day before I received your letter . . . nor indeed did I apprehend that there was much danger. Your Physicians failed, but I believe in disorders where the lungs are much affected, physical aid will scarcely ever avail.[34]

Purported cures and positive outcomes were generally believed simply to have been cases of curable maladies misdiagnosed, and the effective treatment explained as the result of confusion with another more tractable disease.

The seemingly infinite variety of symptoms led to a plethora of terms for, and types of consumption. The illness could be galloping (a rapidly progressing pulmonary form) or, as William Black described it, "galloping

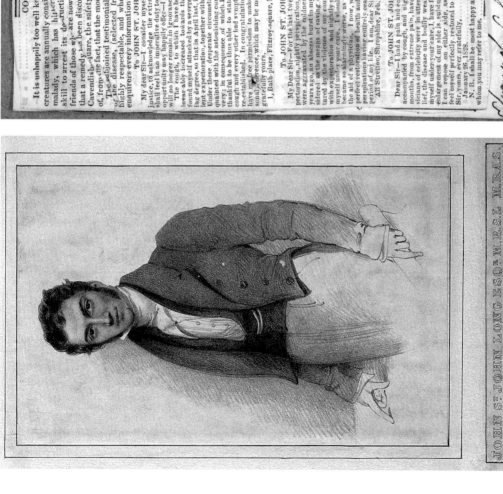

Figure 2.4 Portrait of St. John Long and a Letter from a Consumptive stating "I think it worth your attention" that includes advertisement for the services of St. John Long (1828). John St. John Long. Lithograph. Wellcome Library, London. Copyrighted work available under Creative Commons Attribution only licence CC BY 4.0 http://creativecommons.org/licenses/by/4.0/ & Letter (February 13, 1828) from Jane Somerville to James Somerville Fownes, DD\SVL/3/3/30, Somerset Archives and Local Studies Service (South West Heritage Trust).

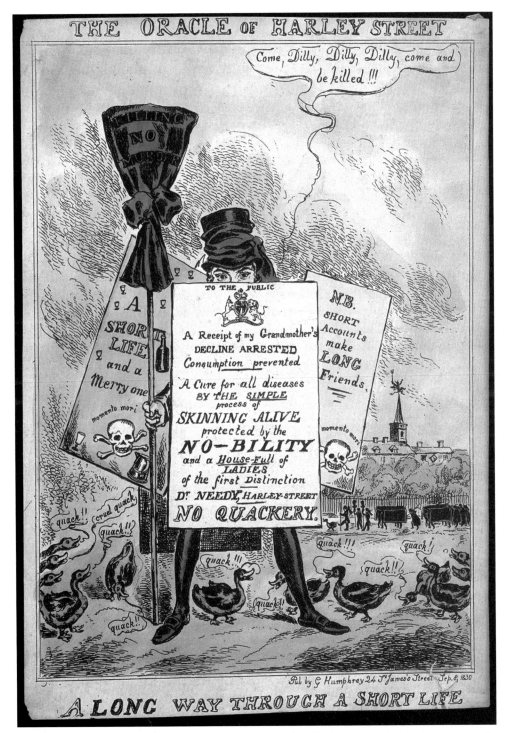

Figure 2.5 St. John Long dressed as a funeral mourner surrounded by ducks and placards advertising the malpractice cases of his in which patients died. "The Oracle of Harley Street." Colored etching by Sharpshooter (?) (London: G. Humphrey, 1830). Wellcome Library, London. Copyrighted work available under Creative Commons Attribution only licence CC BY 4.0 http://creativecommons.org/licences/by/4.0/

the patient to a skeleton in a few months."[35] More typically, however, it developed slowly, with seemingly insignificant or vague symptoms in its early stages. The most common first sign, a chronic cough, was frequently accompanied by pallor. As the illness advanced, the victim developed a loss of appetite and weight. Further indicators included a persistent low-grade fever and night sweats. As the disease progressed, its victims typically presented a combination of symptoms, including a deep cough, wheezing, shortness of breath, a pain in the side, and a low-grade intermittent "hectic fever" which produced a "hectic flush" upon the cheeks. In the advanced stages, the consumption became increasingly visible and the sufferer exhibited signs of emaciation. The eyes became glassy and appeared large as they sank in their orbits, and the cheek bones became prominent. The shoulders elevated and the clavicles projected, forming the characteristic wing-backed appearance. The consumptive was also afflicted with night sweats, loss of strength, debility, and frequent darting pains in the chest or stitch in the side, a rapid pulse, and constipation.

The illness was revealed in the skeletal appearance of its victim, with drawn features and a protruding bone structure. In the latter stages the "hectic fever" intensified, cycling more strongly in the evening hours. The increasingly frail body was wracked by evermore intense fits of coughing, signifying the disintegration of the patient's lungs, a circumstance made even more evident by the appearance of hemoptysis (expectoration of blood and other debris). As the disease advanced, the cough became incessant and was attended with an inclination to vomit; the patient's voice became hoarse, the teeth whitened, and the veins became prominent, the pain in the chest increased, the breathing became more labored and the expectoration of purulent matter also increased until finally ended by the patient's death.

Even when properly diagnosed, the majority of physicians and lay individuals saw it as an affliction with no hope of recovery. In 1840, George Bodington expressed the helplessness and frustration experienced by

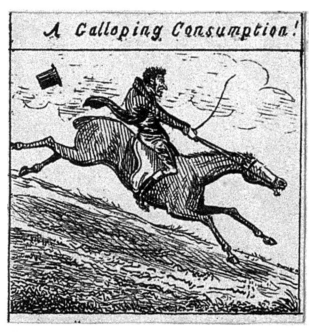

Figure 2.6 Caricature of "A Galloping Consumption." Wellcome Library, London. Copyrighted work available under Creative Commons Attribution only licence CC BY 4.0 http://creativecommons.org/licenses/by/4.0/

doctors when faced with consumption, writing, "Whilst little had yet been done, by way of improvement, in the treatment of the disease: consumptive patients are still lost as heretofore; they are considered hopeless and desperate cases by most practitioners, and the treatment commonly conducted upon such an inefficient plan as scarcely to retard the fatal catastrophe."[36] Accompanying the concern over curability was a widespread dissatisfaction with the available options for treating consumption. Discussions of the current therapies could even be found in *The Magazine of Domestic Economy* (1840) which provides a glimpse of the helplessness the disease engendered in its victims and their families. "Although many nostrums have been from time to time promulgated, and asserted cures for this fatal disease advertised the most respectable of the faculty have long since abandoned all hope from any remedy that medicine can effect."[37] This bleak prognosis reinforced the importance of prevention, but there remained a growing stable of treatments, as no medical practitioner would simply let the disease progress without making any attempt to affect its outcome.

The uncertainty of diagnosis and prognosis narrowed the field of action for the medical practitioner and the victim alike. The consequence was the development of a practical approach to treatment. The management of consumption tended to rest on the experiences with the illness, some dating back to the ancient period, with a corresponding set of traditions and procedures. The most durable prescription was for horseback riding, a therapy popularized by Thomas Sydenham (1624–1689), and one that remained standard long after his death. Sydenham argued that gentle horseback riding was an exercise that provided the correct stimulation for the consumptive, by the dual benefit of exposure to the open air and by strengthening the weakened constitution without overtaxing the system.[38] Riding remained a method for managing tuberculosis well into the nineteenth century.

Sydenham's eighteenth-century successors extended the premise of horseback riding and promoted the beneficial effects of movement by proposing alternative treatments that achieved the advantages of motion. For instance, in 1787 James Carmichael Smyth touted the positive benefits of swinging, arguing it was a mechanism of motion completely "independent of any muscular exertion."[39] For Smyth swinging also furnished an accessible alternative that mimicked the positive results of sailing by providing the benefits of a sea voyage without any of the nasty side effects, like seasickness. (See Plate 9.) Though there was an acknowledged advantage to be gained from sailing, like almost every other aspect surrounding tuberculosis, there was no consensus on the exact nature of that benefit, a circumstance Smyth himself admitted. He conjectured it was the motion achieved during sailing that had "an immediate effect in removing, or at least in suspending the action of coughing," and it was this very motion that swinging duplicated.[40] There was certainly a belief in the effectiveness of sailing in mitigating the effects of consumption. In 1838, a young woman sailing to Spain in hope of restoring her health, wrote, "I continue to be an excellent sailor, and enjoy myself thoroughly on board. My cough is almost gone, and I never wake up feverish and throbbing as I did in England. Really I shall hardly be an invalid when I reach Madeira."[41]

Treatment for consumption was generally limited to recommending a lifestyle and climate conducive to slowing the relentless progress of the illness. One of the most enduring therapies involved removing the patient to a warmer climate. This prescription usually included residency in temperate, sunny surroundings, believed to have the ability to retard the devastation of the lungs that otherwise led to death.[42] King George III reflected the contemporary hope, writing, "in consequence of the Chief Baron's going to Lisbon with his Eldest Daughter whose health requires the change of Climate. The King … desires the Lord Chancellor will acquaint the Lord Chief Baron how ardently He wishes that the Sea Voyage and Mild Air of Lisbon may prove advantageous to the Young Lady."[43] In 1818, John Armstrong addressed the advantages of sailing when combined with removal to a warmer climate. "The best thing that can be done for one in whom pulmonary consumption is suspected, or actually existent in an incipient state, is to send him immediately to a warm climate; and the voyage to the place of his destination should be made rather long, than short, as sailing upon the sea is very useful on many occasions."[44] One such consumptive was Emma Wilson, who chronicled her Italian travels as well as her illness, writing:

Time gets on, but I find no improvement in my health, I daily become weaker, and all my bad symptoms increase rather than diminish. The Celebrated Dr. Stewart is just arrived at Rome … he was the first Inventor of the strengthening System in Consumptive Cases … he thinks me very Ill & hopes to make me soon better under his Strengthening System, but I cannot fill my Journal with an account of how many Pill's [sic] I take.[45]

The benefits of warm, sunny, dry climes remained popular and a move to a more amenable climate continued as an integral part of the therapeutic approach to tuberculosis.

One of the most influential nineteenth-century proponents of climate change was Dr. James Clark. In 1818, Clark accompanied an advanced consumptive to the south of France for treatment, his continental travels inspired his writings and, by 1820, led to a comparative investigation of the medical institutions, climates, and prevalent diseases of France, Switzerland, and Italy. Within a decade, he extended this research to include recommendations on the cure and prevention of chronic complaints and on the role of climate in chronic illness.[46] Clark established a successful practice in Rome, where he treated wealthy English men and women (including the poet John Keats) who sought respite from their illnesses.

Clark's significant and well-received *A Treatise on Pulmonary Consumption* (1835) focused on prevention. He was the first person to not only systematize all of the known information on the disease, but also to make it available to the general public. His work had the added benefit of helping him be appointed as physician to Queen Victoria in 1837.[47] Clark's influence is reflected in George Bodington's *An Essay on the Treatment and Cure of Pulmonary Consumption*: "As regards the causes, origin, and nature of the disease, the work of Sir James Clark, who reaped advantage from the labours of Carswell and other pathologists, is complete and satisfactory."[48] Bodington, however, took issue with Clark's failure to present a comprehensive plan of treatment and argued that he neglected to advance the model of consumption, admonishing the doctor for "leaving the matter, upon the whole, pretty much in the same state he found it."[49]

In 1841, Clark published *The Sanative Influence of Climate*, which offered explicit travel directives for those suffering from consumption and even went so far as to distinguish between the relative advantages of the weather conditions in Nice versus Rome and Madeira versus Pisa.[50] A number of medical investigators used climate as an explanation for the differences observed in the patterns of disease between countries. Comparisons of the behavior of consumption in different geographic locations littered the medical treatises, as did evaluations of its variable impact on certain ethnicities. By way of explanation, "climate" was broadened to include the role played by fluctuations in that climate. This variation came to be considered one of the most significant reasons for the prevalence of consumption in England.

There was also a growing group of drugs and restoratives thought to target certain symptoms of consumption. The focus on therapeutics to allay the effects of tuberculosis, rather than on eradication, was partly the result of the late-stage diagnosis. At this point, symptomatic relief received primacy, as cure was thought impossible.[51] The popularity of certain treatments rested on their ability to ease the patient's ordeal. Many believed that "in a hopeless disease, we are justified in resorting to new expedients when the old ones fail us."[52] It was not uncommon for some of these new treatments to be mentioned alongside tried and true methods. In 1832 a clinical lecture published in *The Lancet* described one physician's attempts to treat the symptoms of tuberculosis:

About nine years ago, a young married lady, who had two children, came under my care with all the symptoms of confirmed consumption, cough, and muco-purulent expectoration. She had occasionally spit a little blood; there were night sweats and colliquative diarroea. I supported her strength with animal food, and some fermented liquor, whenever her pulse could bear it; gentle exercise in the open air, and free admission of air into her rooms. I restrained the diarrhea by catechu, longwood, and sometimes opiates; sometimes applied half-a dozen leeches and blisters, and gave digitalis for a few days, when there was appearance of acute inflammation; sometimes gave bark and soda, sometimes quinine with diluted sulpuric acid, which restrained the sweats.[53]

This account provides just one example of the infinite combination of treatments—both passive and active—employed against consumption. The management of diet, the patient's environment, and the prescription for rest, even having the patient suck chipped ice in an effort to alleviate hemoptysis, were all measures pursued alongside more invasive courses of action, including the application of a variety of therapeutic agents. Asses' milk was a popular component of the consumptive diet, and at one time Thomas Young prescribed a specific daily course of one half pound of suet rendered from mutton as a therapy.[54] Opiates were also commonly employed to assuage the cough and pain customary in the final stages, and though bleeding had waned in popularity, it and the practice of cupping continued, as did the use of leeches.[55] (See Plates 10 and 11.) Other chemicals and therapeutics utilized in treating the various symptoms included calomel, iodine, cod-liver oil,[56] quinine, salicylic acid, digitalis, lead acetate, a variety of emetics, potassium nitrate, antimony sulphate, boracic acid, and creosote, to name a few.[57]

The number of patent medicines steadily grew during the nineteenth century, and an assortment of anti-consumptive agents became available to the public. Additionally, medical practitioners developed a variety of

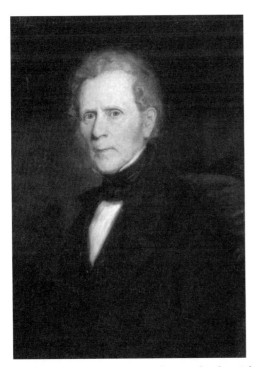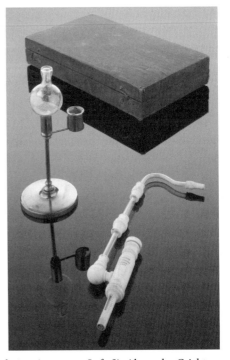

Figure 2.7 Sir Alexander Crichton and Iodine Inhalation Apparatus. Left: Sir Alexander Crichton. Right: French iodine inhalation apparatus for the treatment of tuberculosis, unknown maker c.1830–1870. Science Museum, London, Wellcome Library, London. Copyrighted work available under Creative Commons Attribution only licence CC BY 4.0 http://creativecommons.org/licenses/by/4.0/

inhalation therapies in an effort to tackle the fundamental unit of pathology—the tubercle. These treatments included the inhalation of a variety of balsams, astringents, and resins. In 1823, Sir Alexander Crichton argued for the efficacy of inhaled tar in treating tuberculosis: "The hope which I, in common with a few others, have of late years held out of the curability of consumption, arose entirely from experience, especially for the efficacy of tar vapour and temperature."[58] In the 1830s, the inhalation of iodine vapor became especially popular; later, carbolic acid, creosote, and sulphuretted hydrogen enjoyed acceptance as inhalants.[59] Although treatments were plentiful, there remained a consensus that consumption was "A disease which . . . no remedies in our present state of knowledge can subdue, and which generally leads to a fatal termination."[60]

In the absence of a medical solution, a social one developed, and the attention turned toward prevention which, like everything associated with consumption, was less straightforward than one might have hoped. There was no clear division between the environmental and hereditary causes of tuberculosis; instead, the explanations remained tangled. Generally, an inherited susceptibility was thought to be complicated by an exciting cause, leading to the creation of an acute or persistent illness, which in turn, amplified the likelihood of further illness by magnifying an individual's susceptibility.[61] The hereditary constitution, an individual's physiological fitness, and the quality of the environment, as well as any other strains provided by lifestyle, continued as prominent themes in the working knowledge of the disease.

CHAPTER 3
EXCITING CONSUMPTION: THE CAUSES AND
CULTURE OF AN ILLNESS

In 1855 Thomas Bartlett asserted that "Consumption is a disease which is no respecter of persons; for it seizes alike both upon the high and the low, there being no social position bestowing an exemption from its attacks. There is privilege neither of caste nor sex; and there is no immunity for age, for all . . . are subject to the inroads of this terrible disease."[1] Despite its ubiquity, consumption did not serve as a unifying force, rather it was the subject of numerous discourses and constructed categories of perception and victims were "othered" accordingly. The oppositional representations went beyond a dichotomy between the healthy and diseased body, and included internal differentiations along class and gender lines within the community of sufferers. As Clark Lawlor and Akihito Suzuki argue "consumption becomes a marker of individual sensibility, genius and general personal distinction as the eighteenth century progresses: its heightened representation in literature and art reflects, and to some extent reinforces, its perceived cultural value to the self."[2]

The Personal Environment: Status Symbol

In the nineteenth century, consumption was characterized by two distinct and seemingly unrelated discourses, in which victims from the more prosperous classes were lauded while poorer victims were stigmatized. The management of the malady varied with social status and, in many respects, was treated as a different entity, depending upon the quality and character of its victim. The understanding that tuberculosis was partially linked to social status was crucial in determining the individual's way of life and, as such, his or her environment. Environment became the predominant explanation for tuberculosis in the working classes. This, in turn, fostered a negative perception of the illness in these groups. Instead of victims, members of the lower orders were presented, by social reformers and medical investigators, as the architects of their own demise. In the more prosperous classes, by contrast, consumption was primarily viewed as the consequence of a hereditary defect, one complicated by exciting causes. This more benign presentation of the disease only offered the affluent victim limited control over the circumstances that provoked the illness. Among the lower classes the tubercular diathesis was seen as the result of poor air quality, drunkenness, or material deprivation, all of which were hallmarks of their life circumstances. Given that phthisis was primarily conceptualized as an urban condition, due to its heightened visibility in cities, it logically followed that there was an increased susceptibility to the illness owing to the unhealthy nature of life in the metropolis.[3]

As individuals migrated from rural districts into larger towns and cities searching for work, they encountered living and working conditions that created the perfect environment for sickness to flourish. On this basis, Friedrich Engels argued that living and working situations were responsible for the high incidence of consumption.

That the bad air of London, and especially of the working-people's districts, is in the highest degree favourable to the development of consumption, the hectic appearance of great numbers of persons sufficiently indicates. If one roams the streets a little in the early morning, when the multitudes are on their way to their work, one is amazed at the number of persons who look wholly or half-consumptive.

Even in Manchester, the people have not the same appearance; these pale, lank, narrow-chested, hollow-eyed ghosts, whom one passes at every step, these languid, flabby faces, incapable of the slightest energetic expression, I have seen in such startling numbers only in London, though consumption carries off a horde of victims annually in the factory towns of the North.[4]

Workers faced inadequate housing, insufficient food, and physical toil; circumstances that combined with heavily crowded surroundings in workshops, unhygienic living conditions, and physical and material hardship to provide the perfect setting for the rapid development and proliferation of tuberculosis as well as other devastating illnesses.

Responsibility for outbreaks of a variety of diseases rested with the crowded and horrendous conditions of urban living. Slums were presented as sites of corruption—the antithesis of the open spaces, fresh air, and

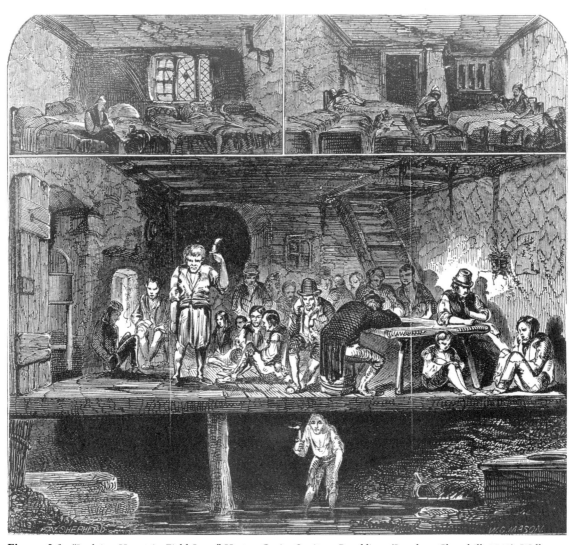

Figure 3.1 "Lodging House in Field Lane," Hector Gavin, *Sanitary Ramblings* (London: Churchill, 1848). Wellcome Library, London. Copyrighted work available under Creative Commons Attribution only licence CC BY 4.0 http://creativecommons.org/licenses/by/4.0/

sunlight peddled by physicians as beneficial in forestalling and treating tuberculosis. *Blackwood's Edinburgh Magazine* addressed the importance of the environment to the health in 1839.

> The Prime essentials to human existence in crowded cities are pure water, pure air, thorough drainage, and thorough ventilation … [and] the facility of taking exercise within a convenient distance. Thus, every city has its public pulmonary organs—its instruments of popular respiration—as essential to the mass of the citizens as is to individuals the air they breathe.[5]

The article highlighted the pertinent physical causes of illness: water, air, sanitation, ventilation, and physical activity, all of which were emphasized time and again in works on tuberculosis.

Consumption could result from any number of internal or external factors including malnutrition, foul air, and emotional misery, all of which were capable of inducing a diathesis.[6] Although these conditions seemed to satisfy investigators seeking to rationalize the abundance of tuberculosis in the working classes, they did little to account for the simultaneous occurrence of lethal consumption among the privileged orders. Thomas Beddoes addressed the impact of the illness in the upper reaches of society.

> It would perhaps be possible to approximate towards an estimate of the number of British families in opulent circumstances, infested by this disease. The members of the two houses of parliament, who have lost either father, mother, brother, sister or child, by consumption, could, I suppose, be ascertained without much difficulty. Now the proportion would probably apply pretty nearly to the gentry at large, their respective habits and constitutions not being materially affected by the difference in wealth.[7]

The roles of injury and inactivity were applied to the upper classes suffering from consumption.[8] Robert Hull admonished the wealthy for what he saw as an emulation of the less fortunate, who were without choice.

> Why should the untethered rich imitate the necessities of the poor? Why should parents, to whom heaven gives the means for flight from undrained houses and lands, reside in the foul atmosphere of crowded cities? In streets, in alleys? Why should a generous nourishment be prohibited to those, whose purses can command it? All agree that scrofula and consumption, a form of scrofula, predominate among the poor. Then they are results of those circumstances, wherein the poor differ from the rich. What are these? Chiefly impure air, scanty food, neglected excretions. Yet the rich incarcerate their consumptives in azotic chambers; keep them low, as if decline were active inflammation; lose sight of the abdominal apparatus and its most potent secretions, as if the lungs, which depend upon the belly within and the atmosphere without, were isolated perfectly from both.[9]

The writings on consumption overwhelmingly presented women of the upper orders as more liable to phthisis than men, largely because of the constraints society placed upon them. Middle- and upper-class women became consumptive by virtue of their inactive lifestyles. As Beddoes remarked, "In opulent families, I impute it in great measure to the indolence of females, that they so much more frequently become the victims of consumption."[10] He even went so far as to raise the power of inactivity to incapacitate above that of air contaminated by small particulate matter.[11] The dissipations that marked the luxurious lifestyle of the wealthier classes were also dubbed significant causes of consumption.[12] In 1832, Charles Turner Thackrah argued "the effects of professional life on the physical state of the upper orders, as produced by their pursuits and habits, are so familiar to a medical practitioner, as to require no direct investigation. They are not, however, the less important. The evils, indeed, of a too artificial state of society are more strongly marked in the upper than in the lower classes."[13] Although poverty and its attendant lifestyle could lead to tuberculosis, the indolent and inactive lifestyle of the wealthy also became one of the most touted causes of consumption, particularly among women.

The devotion to fashion and/or fashionable ways of life, including things such as excessive dancing, or—on the opposite side of the spectrum—the lack of exercise, were all believed to cause tuberculosis. In the early part of the nineteenth century, for instance, as the waltz became popular, many physicians and social commentators

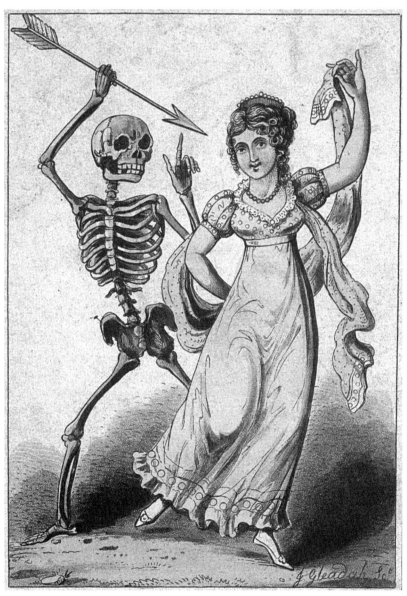

Figure 3.2 Death points an arrow at a female dancer. Aquatint by J. Gleadah, 18–. Wellcome Library, London. Copyrighted work available under Creative Commons Attribution only licence CC BY 4.0 http://creativecommons.org/licenses/by/4.0/

claimed that its movements collaborated fatally with phthisis. In 1814, Hester Lynch Piozzi commented on the choices of one young lady on the occasion of the White's Ball:[14] "Miss Lyddel had the Offer of a Ticket but refused, because she was not half well: Dr. Baillie[15] praised her, and said that 50 Girls more Ill than She—would go at all hazards, and that he expected 40 of them would die in Consequence of such Ardour after Amusement."[16] *The Manual for Invalids* (1829) called dancing a "seductive amusement" that was "very liable to do harm" due to the violence and duration of the exertion. The author remarked, "Indeed, I have frequently known that the foundation of that most fatal malady, pulmonary consumption, has been very clearly traced to the returning home from the ball-room."[17] This association between vigorous exertion and tuberculosis continued well into the nineteenth century. In 1845, *The Medical Gazette* made explicit the connection between dancing and consumption observing "the patient . . . had had repeated attacks of cough, pain in the chest and haemoptysis, the consequence of great exertion in dancing."[18] Thus, the avoidance of illness and individual self-preservation rested increasingly upon the personal environment and individual behavior.

Ephemeral Causes of Consumption

In addition to clearly identifiable causes like environment and lifestyle, there were intangible, ephemeral causes of tuberculosis thought to be equally deadly to those hereditarily predisposed. Consumption seemed to attack the more vulnerable portions of the population with increased vigor, forcing an exploration of other contributing factors presumed to contribute to the illness, such as the mental and emotional. These ephemeral, emotional causes became increasingly central in the explanations of tuberculosis among the upper reaches of society.

The existence of an intimate connection between the mind, the individual, and his or her illness had been recognized since the ancient period, although the relationship had been couched in the terminology of the humors and their interaction with an individual's psyche and soul. Piquant emotions like sadness or excessive joy were thought to trigger illness. By the eighteenth century, a more mechanical approach to the body had replaced humoralism, but the notion that disease was a product of disruption due to either physical, mental, or emotional stresses remained.[19] The unity of function between the spirit and body did not lose its power with the acceptance of an anatomico-pathological approach to medicine. Instead, the focus on solidest thinking, which located disease in tangible bodily structures, particularly the nerves, was applied to the communication between the physical form and the soul. The actions of the solids and fluids replaced the humors, but the passions remained the manner in which the body and the soul met, interacted, and communicated.

Medical investigators sought to elucidate the particulars of the mind–body connection through an examination of the ability of the emotions and mental processes to disrupt health.[20] Laennec was one of the many who tackled the part that an assortment of *causes occasionnelles* played in pulmonary consumption, categorizing the role psychosomatic factors, like the "sad passions," played in tuberculosis and arguing for the destructive nature of deep, abiding, prolonged melancholy emotions.[21] Hereditarians also fell back on the "sorrowful passions" in their explanations of disease; strengthening the idea that tuberculosis was an extension of the victim's nature.[22] Laennec maintained the sad passions accounted for the disease's prevalence in the urban environment. For in the cities people were more involved in a variety of life pursuits, and with each other, and these circumstances provided a greater opportunity for disappointment, sadness, immoderate behavior, bad conduct, and bad morals, all of which could lead to bitter recrimination, regret, and consumption.[23]

Nervous Consumptives

Over the course of the eighteenth century, illness in general, and tuberculosis in particular, were increasingly linked to the functioning of the nervous system.[24] Nerves were conceived of as having an innate sensibility, meaning a "nervous" person could develop consumption and waste away due to the quantity of his or her sensibility and the related psychological dynamics. Emerging models of the nervous system and the role of the "sensible body" were rapidly accepted later in the eighteenth century by a number of renowned physicians and philosophers who pushed for the dominance of the nervous system in the explanations of disease.[25] (See Plate 12.) For example, Albrecht von Haller, the Swiss anatomist, undertook an extensive investigation of the workings of the nerves, arguing that the fibers of the nerves were imbued with an intrinsic property known as "sensibility." For Haller, "sensibility" was the nerves' ability to recognize and react to external stimuli. Tissues that were rich in nerves, including the muscles and skin, also possessed an increased degree of sensibility. Haller classified the "reactive" quality of both the nerves and the muscles, or their ability to respond to outside stimuli, as "irritability." In 1752, Haller published the results of his experiments, which influenced the work of leading Scottish anatomists, like William Cullen, and helped force a key shift in medical theory.[26]

William Cullen's work had a significant impact on the popularity of socio-psychological explanations of disease in England and was part of an extensive movement that pushed for the dominance of the nervous system in the explanations of disease.[27] His work rested upon a patho-physiological approach to the mechanisms and processes of disease—which he believed were controlled by the nervous system. Cullen construed life as the consequence of nervous action, privileging the role of the nervous system in the creation of disease. He promoted the functioning of the nervous system as the source of life, and saw irritability and sensibility as a person's most significant qualities. Cullen argued sensibility was the ability of the nervous system to not only accept sensations but also to convey the body's will, while irritability was a type of "nervous power" located in the muscles. The degree of these qualities differed among individuals. Irritability, in fact, occurred in inverse proportion to an individual's strength. For instance, a weak and debilitated individual would possess an elevated quantity of irritability, while a strong individual would possess less irritability and have a tendency toward torpor. Health was achieved through a balance between the sensibility of the nervous system and the irritability of the muscles. Should the equilibrium break down, creating a deficiency or excess of either of these qualities, disease was sure to ensue.[28] Cullen extended these ideas, arguing that due to the primacy of the nervous system in the proper functioning of the body, all diseases had a nervous component. As a result, a neurosis was more than just a mental disease, it was any illness that resulted from an alteration in the functioning of the nervous system, particularly one that developed as the aftermath of emotion or sensation.[29]

Cullen's one-time student and later detractor John Brown (1735–1788) took the focus on neurophysiology in a different direction. Brown asserted that life rested upon "excitability," and disease transpired when there was either a surfeit or a deficit of this property.[30] For Brown then, illness was the outcome of a disruption in the performance of excitement, and the course of this disturbance determined the type of illness that developed.[31] In his scheme, there were only two basic types of illness. An over excitement of the system produced a "sthenic" disease (like rheumatism, miliary fever, scarlet fever, and measles); while an insufficient quantity of excitement would lead to an "asthenic" disorder (like typhus, cholera, gout, dropsy, and phthisis).[32]

The majority of illnesses were thought to be asthenic in nature, the consequence of debility. Furthermore, an excess of excitement, characteristic of sthenic illness, could be exhausted, ultimately leading to asthenia, or an illness of "indirect debility." The Brunonian system visualized sickness as the product of a general disruption of the patho-physiological processes and asserted that deviation from health was a quantitative and not a qualitative issue.[33] The elevation of the nervous system had implications beyond the biological, as it was

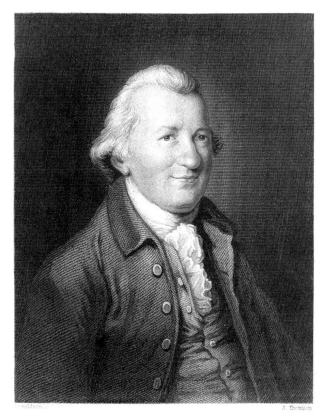

Figure 3.3 John Brown by J. Donaldson after J. Thomson. Wellcome Library, London. Copyrighted work available under Creative Commons Attribution only licence CC BY 4.0 http://creativecommons.org/licenses/by/4.0/

incorporated into the developing "cult of sensibility." Sensibility involved a more refined type of suffering by those in the middle and upper classes and became one of the ways in which the middle class separated itself from the lower orders and constructed its own identity.[34]

Sensibility was heavily embedded in eighteenth-century notions of the body, leading to new strategies of self-presentation and social performance, and sensibility signified the Enlightenment epistemology of the senses as the material origin of consciousness.[35] The nervous system remained the foundation of this psycho-perceptual approach: the nerves transmitted sensations, and the speed of this transaction rested upon the elasticity of the nervous system. The suppleness of the nervous system was thought to be more highly refined among the middle and upper classes, a notion made even more fashionable by popular literature. Sensibility was even employed in the legal context as a defense strategy in some court cases.[36] The adaptability of sensibility and its growing association with consciousness, emotions, knowledge, and refinement led to a continual redefinition of the term as well as its cultural and medical implications.[37] From a medical perspective, cultural issues had biological consequences and there was a growing concern over the effect that this increasingly refined culture had in creating "nervous diseases."

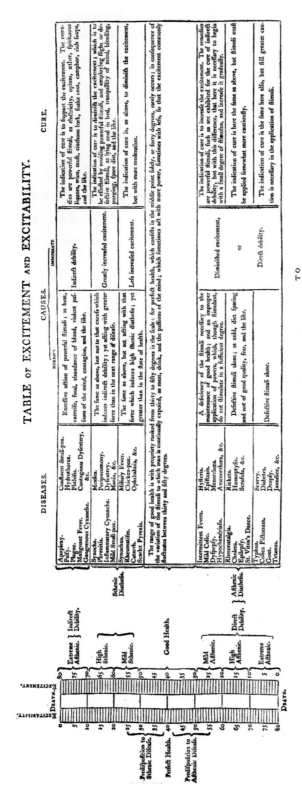

Figure 3.4 Table of Excitability. "Table of excitement and excitability … John Brown. (by) Samuel Lynch," *From The Elements of Medicine of John Brown, M.D.* (London: J. Johnson, 1795). Wellcome Library, London. Copyrighted work available under Creative Commons Attribution only licence CC BY 4.0 http://creativecommons.org/licenses/by/4.0/

Civilizing Consumption

The emergence of "civilized" diseases based on sensibility complemented the pervasive application of the action of the nervous system in explaining the incidence of certain illnesses.[38] At the elite level, the elevation of the nervous system and the corresponding relationship between the mind and body led, according to Lawlor, "to a paradigm shift in which both medicine and literature were dominated by notions of nervous sensibility."[39] Furthermore, Lawlor argues there was a parallel shift in the view of the body away from the notion of mechanistic clock or even the hydraulic machine, and instead toward the image of a string instrument, one that required the maintenance of proper tension in the nerves. Preservation of health could occur if the proper "elasticity" or "tone" in the nerves continued; otherwise, disease ensued.

Physicians expressed a growing concern over the effect that this increasingly refined culture, inhabited by persons of great sensibility, had in creating nervous diseases. The buffeting of the nervous system was creating a scourge of ill health among the upper and middle classes, due to their refined sensibilities and the pre-existing derangement of their nervous systems, which predisposed them to illness.[40] In 1792, William White explicitly elevated the action of the nervous system in tuberculosis, arguing the predisposing causes included "A constitutionally weak system of blood-vessels; a too great irritability of the same" and a "Great sensibility of the nervous system," as a consequence "it chiefly attacks young people; particularly those who are of active dispositions, and shew a capacity above their years."[41]

The idea of a disease of civilization, linked to the nervous system, rose to prominence during the eighteenth century, partly as a consequence of the social dislocation that occurred in conjunction with the explosion of commerce and urbanization.[42] The rapid changes that accompanied progress seemed to be producing parallel pathological alterations. The harmful lifestyles associated with town living included overindulgence of food and alcohol, as well as lack of exercise and insufficient sleep. In addition, there were the pernicious effects of certain fashions, an excessive pursuit of luxury, the business of financial speculation, and the strict etiquette protocols of society in the metropolis. All of these practices created anxiety, depleted energy, and had a deleterious effect on an individual's constitution. The artificiality of urban society was harmful to people on both a mental and physical level and led to the development of these new "civilized" sicknesses. The nervous system explained the observed physiological manifestations of these illnesses. The excesses of civilized society seemingly inhibited the proper communication between the brain and the rest of the body by blocking the action of the nervous fibers, leading to inflammation, pain, chronic feelings of exhaustion and lethargy, symptoms not observed in the sturdy and robust members of the lower orders.[43] Indeed, the idea of a disease of civilization, linked to the nervous system, rose to prominence during the eighteenth century as the British nation gained a reputation across the continent as a hotbed of mental, nervous, and hysterical afflictions. The English came to believe that the price of their prosperity and refinement was sickness and pain, and asserted that the proliferation of "civilized" diseases were a mark of British superiority.[44]

This line of thought was laid out early, in George Cheyne's wildly successful *The English Malady* (1733). The work seemed to paint nervous illness with a new glamor and, by explicitly linking the lifestyles of the elite with conditions provoked by nervous debility, Cheyne implied that fashionability was partly contingent upon the effects of emotional and mental anxiety.[45] His work provided a pathological model of the human body, one dependent on the actions of social factors, especially the "English way of life," upon the nerves. In doing so, he evaded the more repulsive characteristics of disease, helping to make nervous disorders more socially acceptable.[46] For Cheyne, the locus of disease rested in excess. To reach the pinnacle of society, denizens of the upper orders were often forced to surrender their health, physical fitness, and even their figure to the forces of fashion, business, or idle pleasures. Possessing, as they did, acutely reactive nervous systems, they were extremely vulnerable to a number of illnesses and were ensnared in a trap of their own making, in which social

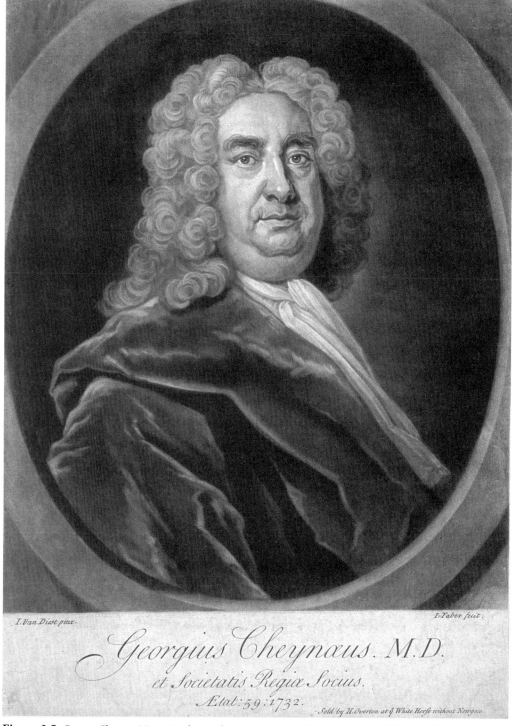

Figure 3.5 George Cheyne. Mezzotint by J. Faber, junior, 1732, after J. van Diest. Wellcome Library, London. Copyrighted work available under Creative Commons Attribution only licence CC BY 4.0 http://creativecommons.org/licenses/by/4.0/

success perpetuated the suffering associated with illness.[47] These "nervous disorders" were the product of civilization and indicated the social and economic accomplishments of the English.[48] In this presentation, nervousness—and, by virtue of association, sickness—were both viewed as symptoms of success.[49]

Cheyne's work on chronic illness was instrumental in the development of the philosophies that governed the perceptions of the interaction between an individual's health and society. His work also helped to explain the oppositional relationship between wealth and health. Urbanization and its corresponding social consequences appeared to be increasing the vulnerability of the population, not just to diseases typically associated with filthy conditions, but also to neuro-pathological illnesses, like tuberculosis. For rich and poor, the city was dangerous to health, a fact widely acknowledged and often lamented. As one mother complained of her daughter,

> I am afraid London does not agree with her, for she never is well there half a year together, this last illness was coming on before she left Town—'tis a grievous suspicion, now I have got such a charming home in Town!—I shall keep her in the Country 'till the end of Octr. & then try Town again—& if I find her ill there again, I fear I must endeavour to Let my dear Downing St. Home, & take a Country Cottage at once, for my Children & Governess—fond as I am of London, there seems a fatality against my living in it.[50]

Similarly, in 1832 Charles Thackrah argued, "Of the causes of disease, anxiety of mind is one of the most frequent and important. Civilization has changed our character of mind as well as of body. We live in a state of unnatural excitement;—unnatural, because it is partial, irregular, and excessive. Our muscles waste for want of action: our nervous system is worn out by excess of action. Vital energy is drawn from the operations for which nature designed it, and devoted to operations which nature never contemplated."[51]

The belief in a mind–body connection helped elevate the status of pulmonary consumption among the upper and middle classes. In the late eighteenth and well into the nineteenth century, the nervous constitution and its associated disorders were being presented in such a way as to make them attractive. Tuberculosis was now perceived as the physical manifestation of a psychological state and a symbol of an elevated aesthetic, physical sensitivity, as well as of a superior spirituality and intelligence. The specific mechanism of action was laid out by George Bodington in 1840 when he argued the first step in developing consumption "consists in nervous irritation, or altered action, or weakened power, in the substance of the lungs, from the presence of tuberculous matter deposited there as a foreign body."[52] In the next phase, the nervous system manifested itself in pathological alterations in the tissues of the body.

> So soon as the nervous power is entirely destroyed in those portions of the lungs where the tuberculous deposits exist, then the destruction of the remaining tissues follows immediately; they die, dissolve down into a half fluid half putrid condition, and are expectorated through the bronchial tubes, leaving cavities in the substance of the lungs . . . Here is then, first, nervous power altered, weakened, or exhausted; then the destruction of the remaining tissues, constituting the main substance of the organ.[53]

J. S. Campbell also wrote of the power of the nervous system and presented a rather attractive description of tuberculosis, writing even "slight causes of excitement, whether mental or corporeal, produce effects on the circulation which are not found in a body naturally robust."[54] He described the physical manifestations of this excitement, stating in a person with a refined nervous system there were "sudden flushes of the countenance from trivial causes of mental emotion, which frequently suffuse the cheek of beauty with a blush originating in a fatal tendency, and hence the sudden but ill sustained fits of transient vigour, very foreign to the nature of the person who exhibits them. It is in constitutions presenting these peculiarities" that one found "a tendency to deposit tubercles."[55] By twining consumption with the refinement of sensibility and presenting it as a product of high society, Campbell romanticized the disease. A person afflicted with such a condition had to be, by implication, fashionable, wealthy, gifted, intelligent, or inspired in some way. In this presentation, nervousness—and, by virtue of association, sickness—were both viewed as symptoms of success. The poor lacked both the material and the psycho-physiological endowment that would make them vulnerable to nervous complaints; as such, a separate dialogue developed to explain the incidence of illnesses such as tuberculosis among them.[56] Diseases, then, were not just the affliction of fashionable people but were themselves becoming fashionable.

The connection between civilization, behavior, disappointment, and illness extended into a belief that a relationship existed between the physical environment, the social status, and the moral character of an individual. Dank, crowded, dark, poorly ventilated housing came to be seen as an environment favorable to fostering tuberculosis in the poor. However, the idea that consumption was a disease of the more refined elements of society informed an alternative narrative about the disease. The various ways in which tuberculosis was perceived, explained, understood, and rationalized provided the justification for opposing discourses of consumption as both a "social scourge" and a Romantic illness.[57] There was a corresponding split in the explanations of tuberculosis by social status. Consumption was, in a number of senses, an archetypical illness of civilization. On the one hand, there was a connection between the disease and the unhealthy living conditions of the urban environment, such as smoke, dust, dirt, and damp. On the other hand, there was a strong tradition that associated the disease with the best and brightest members of society, those intelligent and delicate individuals who seemed so prominent in the ranks of its victims. There was an acceptance by physicians and society alike of an association between the illness and the sophisticated lifestyle pursued by members of the beau monde.[58] The health of the individual now had wider implications as disease became a social problem, and those afflicted were provided a specific place within society—a position assigned not according to their approaching death but instead as a function of their unique quality of life.

CHAPTER 4
MORALITY, MORTALITY, AND ROMANTICIZING DEATH

The Consumptive Performance: Resignation in the Face of Death

Consumption, as an affliction from which neither class, wealth, nor virtue provided any protection, required rationalization in an effort to make the loss of loved ones more bearable. In their attempts to understand something as ambiguous as the social attitudes toward death in the nineteenth century, historians have proposed a variety of interpretations, in part revitalizing the notion of a good death based upon evangelical principles[1] as well as promoting the idea of a culturally beautiful death.[2] Philippe Ariès argued there was an influential cultural archetype in the notion of a "beautiful death," one resulting from the transformation in the approach to illness and death that accompanied the Romantic Movement and presented death as a beautiful experience to be approached with enthusiasm rather than dread.[3] Ironically, Ariès' theory rests primarily upon the approach to death gleaned from the written remnants left by members of the Brontë family while they suffered from the ravages of consumption, again lending weight to the contemporary acceptance of tuberculosis as an easy and even beautiful ending. Patricia Jalland has argued that instead of a "beautiful death" there was a tendency once again toward a "good death," now defined by the principles of evangelicalism.[4] In fact, in the case of tuberculosis there was a reliance upon both, a search for a good and beautiful death—good in the approach to death and beautiful in the outward appearance imparted by the illness itself, as well as in the quality of the soul revealed by the afflicted's handling of their decline and demise. Resignation to the Lord's will, both by the sick individual and his or her loved ones, was an important component of a death from consumption.

Despite the medicalization of disease, tuberculosis remained intertwined with the conception of Divine will, as sin and redemption persisted as prominent features of a consumptive's life and death. The prevailing approach rested upon the Christian ideology of atonement.[5] Boyd Hilton has argued, "The sequence of sin, suffering, contrition, despair, comfort, and grace—shows that pain was regarded as an essential part of God's order, and is bound up with the machinery of judgment and conversion."[6] It is therefore not surprising that sickness, especially chronic illness, came to be characterized by an ideology of atonement, sacrifice, and the redemptive quality of suffering. The Christian sought to bear the burden of sickness well and in doing so, not only responded to the challenges of illnesses with dignity and strength but also gained a measure of control over the experience of sickness, if not over the outcome. This idea of "bearing up" became important, as did the related concept of "dying well."

Minister Philip Doddridge's personal experience with the tragedy of consumption offers a glimpse into the evangelical program for this disease. He provided a heart-rending account of his beloved daughter Betsy's struggle with tuberculosis and death in 1736, just before her fifth birthday. Although Doddridge gave her a funeral sermon entitled *Submission to Divine Providence*, he clearly found this submission a difficult task, and in his diary admonished himself for his adoration of her.[7] The power of this parent's love was evident as was his struggle to accept her fate as God's decision.

> She was taken ill at Newport about the middle of June, and from thence to the day of her death she was my continual thought, and almost uninterrupted care. God only knows with what earnestness and

importunity I prostrated myself before him to beg her life, which I would have been willing almost to have purchased with my own. When reduced to the lowest degree of languishment by a consumption, I could not forbear looking in upon her almost every hour. I saw her with the strongest mixture of anguish and delight; no chemist ever watched his crucible with greater care, when he expected the production of the philosopher's stone, than I watched her in all the various turns of her distemper, which at last grew utterly hopeless, and then no language can express the agony into which it threw me.[8]

Doddridge went on to write of a curious event he attributed to his unwillingness to accept the Lord's will and as punishment for his stubbornness, in this most personal of trials.

In praying most affectionately, perhaps too earnestly for her life, these words came into my mind with great power, "speak no more to me of this matter;" I was unwilling to take them, and went to the chamber to see my dear lamb, when instead of receiving me with her usual tenderness, she looked upon me with a stern air, and said with a very remarkable determination of voice, "I have no more to say to you," and I think from that time, though she lived at least ten days, she seldom looked upon me with pleasure, or cared to suffer me to come near her. But that I might feel all the bitterness of the affliction, Providence so ordered it, that I came in when her sharpest agonies were upon her, and those words, "O dear, O dear, what shall I do?" rung in my ears for succeeding hours and days. But God delivered her; and she, without any violent pang in the article of her dissolution, quietly and sweetly fell asleep, as, I hope, in Jesus, about ten at night, I being then at Midwell. When I came home, my mind was under a dark cloud relating to her eternal state, but God was pleased graciously to remove it, and gave me comfortable hope, after having felt the most heart-rending sorrow.[9]

The importance of submission to the will of God and the Christian idea of death, continued as a significant feature of the approach to the consumptive death through the remainder of the eighteenth and well into the nineteenth century. In 1797, a letter on the death of yet another beloved from consumption shows its continued hold:

The account you give of her death is very affecting, but it is such as must give consolation to every man, who is not so unhappy as to relinquish the hopes of Religion. For my own part, I can honestly say that the more I see of the world the less I think we ought to regret those who are taken out of it, & when I consider the many disappointments & miseries, to which a maturer age is exposed, I cannot but regard the young, who are early called away, as "taken from the evil to come."[10]

The conviction that better things awaited the consumptive in the afterlife, based on the assurance of salvation in the evangelical tradition, lent further weight to the importance of resignation and this acceptance was a central feature in the personal accounts of those consumptives who ascribed to evangelical principles.

Resignation continued as an essential facet of the nineteenth century approaches to the illness and was evident in the writings of the young (Margaret) Emily Shore (1819–1839) about her disease. Even before her diagnosis, she was aware of the possibility that her illness was consumption, and began to prepare for that eventuality.

I get stronger, but my cough gives way very slowly, and my pulse continues high and strong. There is certainly danger of my lungs becoming affected, but we trust that, if it please God, the sea will restore me to health and remove the possibility of consumption. I know, however, that I must prepare myself for the worst, and I am fully aware of papa's and mama's anxiety about me.[11]

Within a month, she once again brought up her concern while being examined by Dr. James Clark. "I had no small reason to apprehend the pulmonary disease had already begun. I prayed earnestly for submission to the Divine will, and that I might be prepared for death; I made up my mind that I was to be the victim of consumption."[12] Clark returned the news that her lungs were not yet affected, but Emily's writing illustrated her conflicted feelings over the limitations placed upon her by illness.

> I feel now quite convinced that I must not exert my mind at all, compared at least with what I should like to do. I cannot read or write without a headache, and writing also gives me a pain in my chest, which I have not, indeed, been free from for some days. It is very painful to me deliberately to lay aside all my studies, and it seems to me that I shall some time hence look back with great regret on the year 1836, the seventeenth year of my life, thus apparently wasted, as far as study is concerned. Yet I ought not to entertain this feeling, for it is God's will.[13]

A year later she lamented, "How appalling is the progress of time, and the approach of eternity!" and acknowledged, "To me, that eternity is perhaps not far distant."[14] She then asked, "let me improve life to the utmost while it is yet mine, and if my span on earth must indeed be short, may it yet be long enough to fit me for an endless existence in the presence of my God."[15] Emily traveled to Spain for her health in 1838, providing a striking account of her visit to the graveyard set up locally for the numerous victims of tuberculosis.[16]

> It was with a melancholy feeling that I gazed round this silent cemetery, where so many early blossoms, nipped by a colder climate, were mouldering away; so many, who had come too late to recover, and either perished here far away from all their kindred, or faded under the eye of anxious friends, who had vainly hoped to see them revive again. I felt, too, as I looked at the crowded tombs, that my own might, not long hence be amongst them. "And here shall I be laid at last," I thought. It is the first time any such idea has crossed my mind in any burial-ground.[17]

The acquiescence to the inevitability of death marked a transition from a way of living to a way of dying, and an acknowledgment of the presence of consumption often led to a process of self-examination as part of the preparation for death. In his diary, the physician Thomas Foster Barham discussed his wife's fears over spiritual preparedness and the effect of consumption upon her personality. In 1836 he detailed her life and death after twenty years of marriage. Although, in the end, his Sarah passed of a fever rather than from tuberculosis, he addressed the effect of that disease upon her during their long relationship. She was particularly concerned "about her religious state: she occasionally complained that she felt her heart cold and dead, and that she wanted something to rouse her spiritual affections: she also at times lamented some little yielding to irritability of temper in domestic vexations."[18] However Barham remarked, "They were indeed little and very transient, a little momentary cloud passing over the sunshine of her habitual serenity and kindness. Such as they were, I have now no doubt that they arose in fact from that state of organic disease which was making a sure though insidious progress."[19] He praised his wife, stating there was "unquestionable evidence that she had given of sincere devotion to him in the steady and conscientious manner in which she had long endeavored to discharge the various duties of her station in life. I pointed out to her that evidence of this kind was more to be trusted than that of excited feelings. In this way, I often restored her tranquility, and happy devotional hours took their turn."[20] As in Sarah Barham's case, notions of preparedness and appropriate behavior, remained laden with moral and religious precepts.

The continued emphasis on the importance of bearing up in a Christian manner while suffering from consumption was even evident in medical accounts of the illness. In 1831 members of the College of Physicians investigated the actions of the diseased body upon the mental state, stating "We were particularly struck with

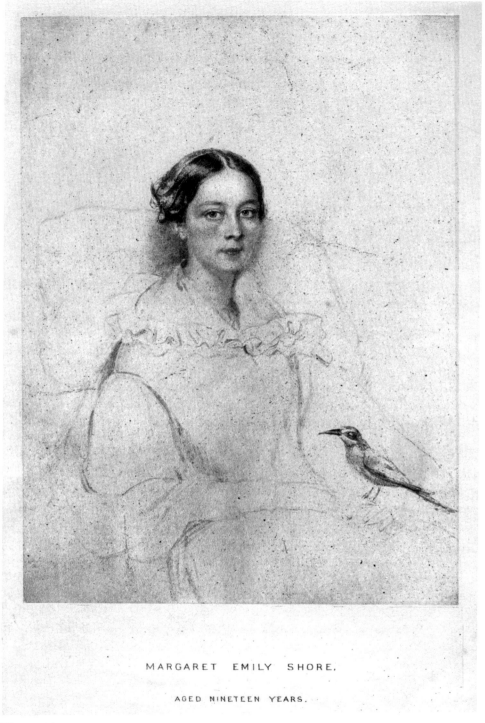

MARGARET EMILY SHORE.

AGED NINETEEN YEARS.

Figure 4.1 Margaret Emily Shore after unknown artist, engraving (c.1838). NPG D11267 ©National Portrait Gallery, London.

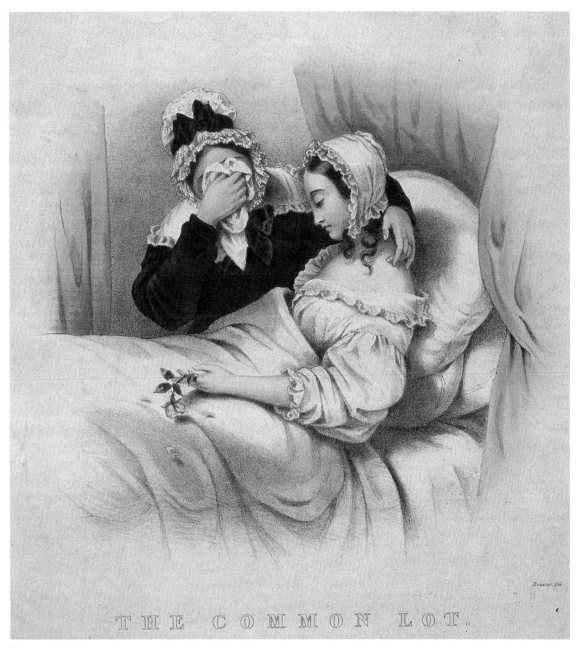

Figure 4.2 "Mourn Not your Daughter Fading." A mother cries in grief while comforting her dying daughter. "The Common Lot," colored lithograph by J. Bouvier. Wellcome Library, London. Copyrighted work available under Creative Commons Attribution only licence CC BY 4.0 http://creativecommons.org/licenses/by/4.0/

the sketch which was given of the cheerfulness of mind often exhibited by the poor victim of pulmonary consumption."[21] It then went on to address the manner in which a victim endured that illness.

> But the Christian bears his sufferings from higher motives, and with a different spirit. It was mentioned by the president as a remarkable fact, that, of the great numbers whom it had been his painful professional duty to attend at the last period of their lives, very few have exhibited an unwillingness to die; except, indeed, from painful apprehensions respecting the condition of those whom they might leave behind. This feeling of resignation, although it might arise in some from mere bodily exhaustion, appeared in others to be the genuine result of Christian principles.[22]

God's will would be re-employed by evangelicals and social reformers to fashion meaning and explain cause, by creating a vision of consumption that linked fate, personality, and inner truth to clarify both illness and death. Consumptives found comfort and meaning for their suffering in the belief that the disease was part of the Lord's will. Additionally, in the homiletic of evangelicalism pain was assigned as central to God's order, so it was a part of the apparatus of evangelical conversion and judgment.[23] Suffering, illness and death were bound up with notions of providence and provided the opportunity to test the victim's faith; as such, submission and resignation were the appropriate response.[24] Yet people still struggled to understand the cause of their condition and why they, in particular, were afflicted. In the search for these explanations, lay understanding of disease causality bumped up against medical etiology, as the quest for meaning was marked by steady exchange between lay and learned opinion.[25] This exchange was particularly important in elevating the influence of Romanticism in the rhetoric surrounding the illness.

Romanticizing Consumption

Many have interpreted Romanticism, at least in part, as a reaction to the Enlightenment's emphasis on rationality, because it elevated "moral passion" above intellectual scrutiny.[26] This elevation of individualism and revival of emotion in literature, the arts, and the broader culture occurred in England roughly between 1780 and 1830.[27] Romantics emphasized creativity, inspiration, and imagination, as well as the relationship between these forces and illness. Many even appeared to root literary intuitiveness in the disease process.[28] Individual exceptionalism could not be had without a cost, and tuberculosis was an acceptable price to pay for extraordinary passion or brilliance. Illness was now an ally, not an enemy, and biological disease in the Romantic presentation became an intricate and treasured part of an individual's personality.[29]

The Illness Intelligence

Sickness in general, and tuberculosis in particular, had a long association with mental exertion, a connection extended in the Romantic period to grant consumption the power of enhancing and freeing the creative sensibilities and imagination.[30] The popularity of sensibility, and the reciprocal actions of the nervous system, implied to contemporaries that the stimulation of the mind had a dampening effect on the energy of the body. For the Romantic, the mind of the languid individual suffering from consumption was enhanced, and mental energy grew as physical torpor increased. When this energy was applied to artistic creativity, health was sacrificed in favor of imagination and ingenuity.[31] The dominant culture of sensibility in the late eighteenth century cemented the notion of the body as the architect of knowledge and victim of its pursuit.

The scholarly, artistic, isolated, and nervous body was both restricted and advantaged by inactivity. Suffering was co-opted by the artistic and scholarly into a self-affirming view of sickness, in which "learned" diseases like melancholia and consumption served as both the symptom and the source of literary achievement.[32] Suffering, illness, and pain did not merely provide the opportunity to fulfill the prescribed evangelical deathbed ritual, but these experiences were also extended to serve as a source of artistic ingenuity, imagination, and intellectual prowess.[33] "The Infirmities of Genius Illustrated" explicitly linked the constitution and literary creativity.

> The "infirmities" of authors, their eccentricities of thought and action, their waywardness, peevishness, irascibility, misanthropy, murky passions, and the thousand indescribable idiosyncrasies, which, in all time, have contradistinguished them from their fellow-men, are proverbial. The anomalies thus so universally conspicuous in the literary character of men of genius . . . are referable to their constitutional (physical) peculiarities and condition: in simple words, that their mental eccentricities result from the derangement of bodily health. That the condition of the mind and the temper of man depends much upon the vicissitudes of health and disease of the corporeal frame.[34]

The Romantic emphasis upon exceptionality and individuality corresponded to a growing stress on the power of passion, love, sentiment, and grief. These notions applied to all aspects of life and death, romanticizing and beautifying the experience of both. Under these conditions death was sentimentalized and suffering, as well as death, were imbued with emotionalism.[35] In the Romantic period, the wasting and emaciation of consumption added a fresh glamor to the artists and poets of the age. Thus, those illnesses thought to result from heightened sensibility were a double-edged sword. They brought the benefit of taste and refinement and elevated their sufferers socially; however, they also doomed their victims to an existence inundated by both mental and physical suffering.[36] Poets were plagued with excessive irritability of their nervous system, which combined with their passionate natures to inundate their bodies with sensations that became pathogenic. The male poet's consumption served not only as an expression of his sensibility, but also as a characteristic of his creative and intellectual distinction, as well as his inability to endure the harshness of the world.[37]

Consumption was the ally of the genius, who was consumed by his excessive emotional and intellectual activity, and exhausted his energy in a single burst that sped him toward death.[38] This was not only a literary convention, but also one that found support in medical treatises, which defined genius as part of the constitutional construction of illness. For instance, in 1774 the *Hibernian Magazine* stated "The finest geniuses; the most delicate minds, have very frequently a correspondent delicacy of bodily constitution."[39] While in 1792, William White listed among the predisposing causes to consumption a "great sensibility of the nervous system" which meant the disease "chiefly attacks young people; particularly those who are of active dispositions, and shew a capacity above their years."[40] Clark Lawlor rightly calls attention to the contributions of Thomas Hayes and Thomas Young to this debate.[41] Thomas Young's *A Practical and Historical Treatise on Consumptive Diseases* (1815), argued, "Indeed there is some reason to conjecture, that the enthusiasm of genius, as well as of passion, and the delicate sensibility, which leads to a successful cultivation of the fine arts, have never been developed in greater perfection, than where the constitution has been decidedly marked by that character . . . which is often evidently observable in the victims of pulmonary consumption."[42] Young was certainly not alone in making these connections, and *A Physician's Advice for the Prevention and Cure of Consumption* furthered these assertions, stating: "It is a common remark too, that those thus unfortunately marked out as the victims of premature disease are, in the majority of cases, remarkable for their high flow of spirits, and for an unusual development of all those moral and intellectual qualities which dignify and adorn human nature."[43]

Consumptive Chic

Tuberculosis and its accompanying symptoms were construed as the physical manifestation of an inner passion and drive. It was the outward sign of genius and fervor that literally lit the individual, providing the pallid cheek with a glow. The consumptive's bright, shining eyes and pink, illuminated cheeks were seen as the outer reflection of the inner soul that was consuming itself, burning hot inside and out.[44] In 1825 the *European Magazine and London Review* dedicated an article to the connection between intellect and illness, asserting:

> It is a striking fact, that genius is often attended by quick decay and premature death … Genius when brought into material union, loves to dwell in the most spiritual form—the pale cheek, the dim eye, and the sickly frame. We seldom find that Promethean fire animating the coarse form of a ploughman. Besides, it heightens the preciousness of the gift when genius is bestowed only for a brief time, irradiating with intellectual light the young and untainted soul, and hurrying the possessor quickly away to an early tomb.[45]

Beyond the pathological alterations accompanying the destruction of the nervous power, there were also physical characteristics corresponding to the presence of a finer and more refined nervous system, ones evident in the consumptive individual. Those persons with a refined nature were thin and possessed a matching fineness and superiority in taste. In contrast, plumpness was associated with a lack of intellect, and the stout and portly were often described as tedious and slow.[46] The notion that mental acuity was fixed in a lack of health continued to dominate the understanding of tuberculosis well into the nineteenth century. For example, in 1851 *The Englishwoman's Magazine and Christian Mother's Miscellany* stated, "Health, perfect and robust bodily health, is, perhaps, rarely found in combination with strong and fully developed intellect."[47]

Romantic symbolism took consumption beyond the simply physical, objective, progression of the disease and gave it an alternative meaning. The consumptive individual became the vehicle through which medical reality intertwined with popular ideology to craft the primary image of the sick individual.[48] Thus, a benevolent view of the disease came to outweigh the far more frightening and disgusting reality of the illness. Clark Lawlor argues "that literary works combined with others (such as visual, religious, and medical) to produce cultural templates for consumption, and that writers provided the way for various groups of people to structure their experience of the disease, whether they be religious, poetic, male or female."[49] The direct relationship between consumption and creative genius was not simply the product of conscious self-fashioning but was part of a wider cultural discourse. The mythology of the consumptive poet was given further impetus by the rise of literary criticism, which, by publicizing the poets themselves, in turn increased the visibility of consumption.[50]

Consumptive Keats

The most famous British example of the Romantic consumptive poet was John Keats (1795–1821), who perished from tuberculosis at the age of twenty-six. He exemplified the Romantic ideology surrounding the disease, and is better remembered for the tragedy of his consumptive death than the progress of his life. In the posthumous treatments of Keats's death, the poet was absolved from responsibility in bringing about his illness. Instead, he was presented as destined to die from tuberculosis, which helped to elevate his death above all the others in the Romantic canon.[51] There was a sense of inevitability to Keats's end, in the way in which his illness was treated both during his life and after his death. His consumption was articulated as a function of his personality, his circumstances, and his talent. Percy Bysshe Shelley, in a letter to Keats on July 27, 1820, made the association between the poet's talent and his illness. "This consumption is a disease particularly fond of people who write such good verses as you have done, and with the assistance of an English winter it can often indulge its selection."[52]

Beyond the connections made by the poets themselves, the link between consumption and intellectual prowess was made explicitly in the mid-1820s in an article which stated "the power of lingering disease to elicit intellect is frequently exhibited strikingly in the development of the mental faculties in victims of consumption, who, when hale and vigorous, were far from being of an intellectual turn."[53] The representations of Keats's life and the attitudes of his contemporaries to his illness and death embody the distorted approach toward the illness characteristic of the Romantic period. They also illustrate the continued difficulties experienced by nineteenth-century medical practitioners in treating a disease they had very little concrete information about, a circumstance that complicated the identification of the illness and its management.

Keats would have been rather knowledgeable about consumption, not only due to the personal tragedy of his family members and later himself, but also as a result of his medical schooling. Keats was a trained apothecary-surgeon and had received instruction at Guy's Hospital (1815–1816) in London while apprenticed to Thomas Hammond. He also studied with Astely Cooper, who was widely held to be the best surgeon in England at the time.[54] The contemporary presentation of Keats as possessing overly delicate sensibilities falters in the face of his enjoyment of, and attendance at, bear-baiting and boxing matches, as well as his forays into brawling which included a win over a butcher's boy at the expense of a black eye.[55]

Keats's story was one repeated in any number of households in England during the course of the nineteenth century, as his family was struck repeatedly by sickness. His uncle and mother both perished from "decline," which could very well have been consumption, and his brother Tom also suffered from the disease.[56] (See Plates 13 and 14.) Keats himself first took ill after a walking trip in the Lake Country and Scotland with Charles Armitage Brown. The strenuous exercise and inadequate food, coupled with a streak of bad weather, probably contributed to the sore throat and cold that Keats contracted, forcing his precipitous return to England via ship.[57] Once home, Keats discovered that Tom was very ill and set about personally caring for him as he lay bedridden throughout the rainy winter of 1818. Despite Keats's best efforts, Tom lost his battle with tuberculosis at the age of nineteen. On December 18, 1818, Keats wrote to his siblings to inform them of Tom's demise. In his letter, he reflected on the final moments of Tom's life and the meaning of his death. "The last days of poor Tom were of the most distressing nature; but his last moments were not so painful, and his very last was without a pang. I will not enter into any parsonic comments on death—yet the common observations of the commonest people on death are as true as their proverbs. I have scarce a doubt of immortality of some nature or other—neither had Tom."[58] Keats further elaborated on the poignancy of lost youth and consumption in his in *Ode to a Nightingale* in 1819: "Youth grows pale, and spectre thin, and dies."[59] The work was most likely an attempt to make sense of the tragedy not only of his brother's illness but also of his own, which by then was already evident.[60]

By 1820, Keats's health was failing and his narrative of his own illness presented the poet as being cognizant of the relationship between his physical and mental states. He consciously constructed a self-image of an individual marked both physically and psychologically by a nervous illness.[61] He acknowledged the role of his temperament in the progression of his malady in a July letter to Fanny Keats. "My constitution has suffered very much for two or three years past, so as to be scarcely able to make head against illness, which the natural activity and impatience of my mind renders more dangerous."[62] For the next several months Keats was plagued by recurring hemoptysis, so he decided to follow the advice of his physician and possibly gain relief from his affliction in the sunny climes of Italy. In September 1820, in the company of his friend Joseph Severn, Keats left for Italy where he sought the counsel of Dr. James Clark, the eminent physician of the English colony in Rome. Clark explicitly referenced Keats's mental exertions in bringing upon his illness and initially believed allaying his mental turmoil would bring a return of health, writing on November 27, 1820: "His mental exertions and application have I think been the sources of his complaints. If I can put his mind at ease I think he will do well."[63]

During the winter, Keats's condition worsened and Severn provided a graphic and disturbing account of Keats's suffering in a letter to Charles Armitage Brown on December 17, 1820.

> I had seen him wake on the morning of his attack, and to all appearance he was going on merrily and had unusually good spirits—when in an instant a Cough seized upon him, and he vomited near two Cup-fuls of blood ... This is the 9th day, and no changes for the better—five times the blood has come up in coughing, in large quantities generally in the morning—and nearly the whole time his saliva has been mixed with it—but this is the lesser evil when compared with his Stomach—not a single thing will digest—the torture he suffers all and every night—and best part of the day—is dreadful in the extreme—the distended stomach keeps him in perpetual hunger or craving—and this is augmented by the little nourishment he takes to keep down the blood—Then his mind is worse than all—despair in every shape—his imagination and memory present every image in horror, so strong that morning and night that I tremble for his Intellect.[64]

Severn's distress is clear and although Clark's letters were more dispassionate, they expressed similar concerns over the patient's mental state, writing on January 3, 1821:

> He is now in a most deplorable state. His stomach is ruined and the state of his mind is the worst possible for one in his condition, and will undoubtedly hurry on an event that I fear is not far distant and even in the best frame of mind would not probably be long protracted. His digestive organs are sadly deranged and his lungs are also diseased. Either of these would be a great evil, but to have both under the state of mind which he unfortunately is in must soon kill him. I fear he has long been governed by his imagination and feelings and now has little power and less inclination to endeavour to keep them under ... It is most distressing to see a mind like his (what might have been) in the deplorable state in which it is ... When I first saw him I thought something might be done, but now fear the prospect is a hopeless one.[65]

Keats finally succumbed on February 23, 1821, and an autopsy revealed the extent of damage to his lungs.

Severn's realistic and gruesome description of Keats's final days does not fit with the eulogistic imagery presented after the poet's death. Most of his contemporaries seemed to agree that disappointment and shattered hopes caused Keats's consumption, but the source of that disillusionment was much debated. Keats's friends, Severn among them, laid the responsibility for his illness on the poet's state of mind. Although the criticism in the *Quarterly Review* was acknowledged, it was Keats's love for Fanny Brawne that was accorded a larger role in creating the mental turmoil that led to his consumption. Both the poet's friends and his critics disputed the role the unfavorable review actually played in Keats's illness and death.[66]

The image of Keats provided by his contemporaries illustrates the power of the Romantic ideology in assessing this illness. Rather than identifying him as an individual who had a great deal of exposure to the disease through his family, he was presented as a delicate person whose sensitivity and weak constitution inevitably succumbed to consumption because he was unable to bear the buffeting of the unrefined wider world.[67] Keats was increasingly represented as having been brought low by an unfavorable critique of his poetry in the *Quarterly Review*, and it was this image of the poet that seemed to be universally accepted even by his detractors. Lord Byron wrote the following to his publisher on hearing of Keats's death:

> You know very well that I did not approve of Keats's poetry ... [but] I do not envy the man who wrote the article; —you Review people have no more right to kill than any other footpads. However, he who

would die of an article in a Review would probably have died of something else equally trivial. The same thing nearly happened to Kirke White, who died afterwards of a consumption.[68]

Byron's allusion to the fate of Henry Kirke White was not the first such pairing with Keats; even before his illness, in 1818 his friend John Hamilton Reynolds had coupled the two in an article.[69] In the work Reynolds lambasted the critics' treatment of Keats, admonishing them to remember their effect upon Kirke White.

The Monthly Reviewers, it will be remembered, endeavoured, some few years back, to crush the rising heart of Kirk[e] White; and indeed they in part generated the melancholy which ultimately destroyed him; but the world saw the cruelty, and, with one voice, hailed the genius which malignity would have repressed, and lifted it to fame. Reviewers are creatures "that stab men in the dark:"—young and enthusiastic spirits are their dearest prey.[70]

The idea that Keats's bout with consumption was precipitated by a brutal attack against his poetry motivated Shelley to style him as Adonais. In the introduction to *Adonais,* Shelley wrote:

The genius of the lamented person to whose memory I have dedicated these unworthy verses, was not less delicate and fragile than it was beautiful; and where cankerworms abound, what wonder, if its young flower was blighted in the bud? The savage criticism on his Endymion, which appeared in the Quarterly Review, produced the most violent effect on his susceptible mind; the agitation thus originated ended in the rupture of a blood-vessel in the lungs; a rapid consumption ensued, and the succeeding acknowledgments from the more candid critics, of the true greatness of his powers, were ineffectual to heal the wound thus wantonly afflicted.[71]

Shelley added to the Romantic mythology surrounding consumptive death with his homage to Keats in *Adonais,* in which he lionized the idea of a youthful demise:

Peace, peace! He is not dead, he doth not sleep—
    He hath awakened from the dream of life—

                . . .

    From the contagion of the world's slow stain
        He is secure, and now can never mourn
    A heart grown cold, a head grown grey in vain;
        Nor, when the spirit's self has ceased to burn,
    With sparkless ashes load an unlamented urn.[72]

Shelley's description of Keats's death speaks to the beauty rather than horror of Keats's end, "Ah even in death he is beautiful, beautiful in death, as one that hath fallen on sleep."[73] This rendition in no way compares with Severn's first-hand account, but it was Shelley's image that triumphed. In his preface to *Adonais,* Shelley waxed lyrical upon Keats's tomb, "in the romantic and lonely cemetery of the Protestants in that city . . . The cemetery is an open space among the ruins covered in winter with violets and daisies. It might make one in love with death, to think that one should be buried in so sweet a place."[74] Shelley would join his friend in that place that made "one in love with death," himself suffering from tuberculosis, though he was spared the consumptive death when he drowned sailing his yacht, the *Ariel,* off the Italian coast.

Keats exemplifies the Romantic ideology surrounding consumptive death in the first part of the nineteenth century; and although the ideology would remain pervasive, the tubercular disease process would increasingly become feminized. Though there would be alterations in the imagery and application of the mythology of consumption, there remained continuity in the notion that the disease provided a serene death. These ideas were still evident in the mid-nineteenth century when Florence Nightingale's *Notes on Nursing* (1859) stated, "Patients who die of consumption very frequently die in a state of seraphic joy and peace; the countenance almost expresses rapture. Patients who die of cholera, peritonitis, &c., on the contrary often die in a state approaching despair. The countenance expresses horror."[75] Representations of consumption, furnished compelling imagery for the individual and the social body that was extended during the nineteenth century to encompass notions of physical beauty and moral inspiration, particularly for tuberculosis in women.

CHAPTER 5
THE ANGEL OF DEATH IN THE HOUSEHOLD

That Sentimental Feeling: Feminizing Consumption

The growing culture of sentimentalism co-opted the Romantic rage for sensibility and applied it to a growing list of defined female attributes. Sentimentalism was not simply a body of literature or an ideal of personal conduct but a set of assumptions that determined, for example, whether or not a man should remove his gloves to shake hands, what kind of bonnet a woman should wear, or how men and women should shed tears for the dead.[1] The seemingly perverse notion of consumptive allure was reinforced in the various literary, social, and medical discourses by sentimentalism. These works confirmed the cultural notion of infirmity as a distinctly feminine quality.[2] Consumption provided one of the main instruments through which femininity was linked to the sort of suffering that was rationalized as both spiritually and morally redemptive. As a result, meaning was given to the illness experience of upper- and middle-class women, a meaning that medicine and social reformers alike had failed to provide. It also supplied yet another way for the women of these classes to distance themselves from the filth, degradation, and related implications that marked the approach to the illness in the lower orders. Evangelical notions of redemptive suffering coupled with Romantic aesthetics to elevate the frail woman laboring under consumption to a position of not only acceptance, but also of emulation—all under the umbrella of sentimentalism.

Sentimentalism defined early Victorian culture in an all-encompassing manner and was situated in a complete refusal, even inability, to recognize reality.[3] Sentimentalism was the Victorian "technique for evading the harsh social realities of expansive industrial capitalism" which dominated every aspect of society from 1830 to 1870.[4] These techniques of evasion and repudiation of the real world set up an ideal condition by which consumption could be elevated into a cultural icon, in the form of the "myth of angelic tubercular femininity" found throughout Victorian literature and society as an ideal of female sensibility.[5] Sentimentalism emerged as an influential force in middle-class culture beginning in the 1830s, and was unsympathetic to the image of Romantic poets and the idea of masculine diseased creativity. These concepts, like the Romantic ideas of suffering for the sake of genius, co-opted the sorts of traits that would increasingly come to be considered exclusively "feminine" during the nineteenth century.

This change was linked to a broader reaction against Romantic ideals, as the early Victorians moved toward earnestness and evangelical Christian religious morality in their social conventions. The Victorian bourgeoisie was deeply religious, and evangelicalism had a seminal role in determining the character of middle-class culture. In the early part of the nineteenth century, an idiosyncratic combination of rationalism and evangelical religious principles was being influenced by Romantic imagery and ideas. The similarities at the core of evangelicalism and Romanticism, as both movements centered on the identity of the individual, made the intermingling possible. Despite the correspondence in approach, there was a move away from the Romantic notion that "moral sentiments" should be cultivated and refined on an individual basis. Instead, the idea that society should have a role in the development and enforcement of moral attitudes became dominant.[6] The ideal that came to delineate the middle-class experience was firmly entrenched in a commitment to the home, and defined the appropriate position and activities of both men and women, roles heavily influenced by religious ideology and practice.[7]

A redefinition of the acceptable roles for women and men occurred during the early portion of the nineteenth century, as did a hardening of the understanding of what was considered suitable for each gender.[8] These increasingly influential notions rested upon a growing philosophy centered on domesticity, one that defined what was both physically and morally suitable to each gender based on the appropriate sphere of action and influence.[9] The nineteenth-century rhetoric of separate spheres embraced the idea that women were inherently affectionate, emotional, and religious, while men were intelligent, vital, and pragmatic. The evangelical revival played a part in elevating the value of domesticity, whereby women occupied the domestic sphere, as virtuous "angels" who provided comfort and moral direction for both their husband and children. The gender-based boundaries tended to highlight the independent healthy male body as a central component of the working world, and as a fundamental attribute of respectable masculinity. On the other hand, respectable femininity was allied to physical frailty, domesticity, and dependence.[10]

Romantic poets were portrayed during the early Victorian period as effeminate, by virtue of their association with heightened sensibility and tuberculosis. This association intensified as the diseases of sensibility increasingly became the purview of women in both medical and social explanations. These notions were well established by 1843, when Lady Morgan spoke on the illness of her brother and alluded to Byron's famous comment on appearing interesting in consumption.[11] Writing to her niece, "Your uncle has made a very perfect

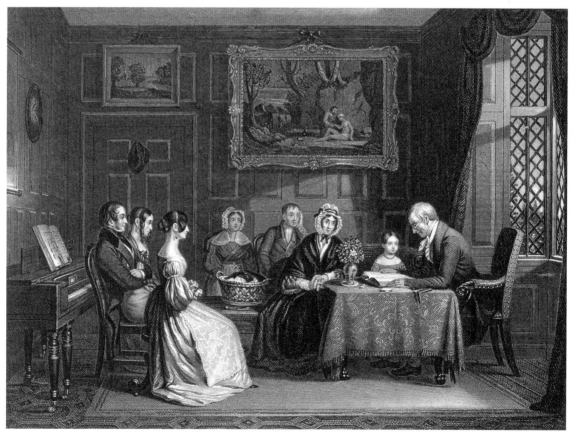

Figure 5.1 A family group in their drawing room at evening prayer. Engraving by William Holl after Edward Prentis (London: Peter Jackson, n.d.). Wellcome Library, London. Copyrighted work available under Creative Commons Attribution only licence CC BY 4.0 http://creativecommons.org/licenses/by/4.0/

recovery from a very alarming illness, but is still rather more 'pale, mild, and interesting' than, in *my* unromanticism, I am desirous to see him!"[12] Literary conventions increasingly intertwined the ideas surrounding female purity with excessive sensibility, a relationship growing in medical, dramatic, and fictitious works. The authors who subscribed to the feminization of sensibility configured consumptive women as reflexive sentimental creatures and passive heroines. During the Victorian period representations of tuberculosis came to revolve around the feminine in both medicine and literature.[13] The feminization of consumption and evidence of its influence can be seen in the less flattering representations of Keats during the 1840s. For instance, an 1848 article discussed an incident in which a woman encountered the poet at a costume ball. The author's response was very different from that of a Romantic era observer.

The scene was less fantastic in those days than it would be now. Not only was it a poetical age … but there was also a poetical foppery prevalent in certain circles, which rendered such a scene more intelligible and less extravagant than it appears to us. This picture of Keats at the feet of the shepherdess seemed very distinctly to represent the sort of lackadaisical, feeble, consumptive poet, who could be 'snuffed out by an article'. Thinking of his early death, his weak lungs, the perpetual recurrence of 'swoonings' and 'faintings' in his poems, and the universally accredited story of the 'Quarterly Review' having hastened his death—we could not help picturing him to ourselves as the sort of man to give way to all fantastical conceits, and to want the very characteristic of greatness—manly sense, and manly strength.[14]

From the sentimentalist point of view, the consumptive male was no longer viewed as a person to be aesthetically pampered; rather, these former heroes were presented as rather effeminate.[15]

Consumption, as a disease heavily influenced by emotion and nervous sensibility, came to have negative connotations when manifesting in men, and was increasingly presented as having a feminizing influence. Tuberculosis remained the product of weakness and excitability, but instead of distinguishing intellectual genius, it symbolized the frailness and fragility associated with women. Extreme sensibility remained the product of an over-stimulated nervous system, but it was increasingly viewed as the result of a lack of control and emotional excess. A connection was therefore created between the sensibility that caused tuberculosis, and those tendencies explicitly viewed as feminine. By virtue of this association, Victorian women not only fell prey more easily to illness but, as a quality of feminine sensibility, sickness became an integral part of female identity.

The discourse of sensibility and suffering guided the feminization of the consumptive death, in which the diseased woman provided the blueprint for the "beautiful death." The link between purity and suffering in the depictions of alluring and attractive females led to an elevation of those who demonstrated consumptive thinness and nervous sensibility, aiding in the process of assigning positive aesthetic representations.[16] These ideas were reinforced by the growing belief that women were the most frequent victims of the malady. As Thomas Hayes had put it as early as 1785, "There is no disease which robs the world of so many useful members of society as Consumptions … for not only men of the greatest talents, but women, of the fairest forms and liveliest sensibility, who might have become shining ornaments to the nations, as well as to domestic happiness, are untimely snatched away, by this cruel distemper."[17]

By mid-century, illness and sensibility were apportioned according to gender, with women having a greater portion of both. As a consequence of the correlation between sensibility and consumption, that illness grew to prominence as both the product of feminine characteristics and as the disease best able to highlight the female character. In 1850, *The World of Fashion* addressed heightened female sensibility and some its consequences:

Consumptive Chic

> No one ever yet accused women of an unfeeling stupidity. The fault, if anything lies in the opposite extreme—an over-refined delicacy. Now, sensibility, whether of joy or misery, arises in proportion to our ingenuity or delicacy of mind. And no one ever yet doubted but that man's mind was of coarser texture than woman's. Afflictions, therefore, fall not so heavily on his, as they do on the more refined disposition of woman. The same delicacy of mind which sheds such lovely luster around every thing in her days of prosperity, and imparts such an exquisite relish to every joy when she does rejoice, casts a deeper shade on her soul in adversity, and gives a keener edge to pain and misery.[18]

The feminization of sensibility, and correspondingly of consumption, fit well with the heavily configured notions of the female role and their assigned place in Victorian society, which were developing as gender boundaries were being re-negotiated during the first half of the nineteenth century.

Consumptive Marriage

The widespread acceptance of the hereditary explanation for consumption meant that the disease was also a part of the nineteenth century discussions of marriage, and freedom from chronic illness was an important criterion for determining an alliance. Advice literature often counseled those entering into matrimony that they had a moral obligation to choose their partners wisely to avoid passing a weak constitution on to their children.[19] For instance, in 1822 *The New Monthly Magazine* stated "Parents who ... transmit their ruined constitutions to their posterity, are like the spider who devours her own young, since with life they communicate to their progeny the seeds of disease, and are the authors of their premature deaths."[20] These warnings seem to have been particularly ignored when the consumptive was female and there were numerous examples in prose and practice that spoke to the exception. For instance, Thomas Foster Barham certainly disregarded these concerns and married a woman with a family history of the disease, writing in 1836:

> My dear Sarah's health had for 2 or 3 years past manifested some signs of decline. She had grown very observably thinner: there was an habitual shortness of breath ... She had also become affected with a considerable mucous expectoration and now and then there had been in this a streak or two of blood ... The remembrance of her mother's early death at about 45 by consumption often dwelt on her mind, and I think her expectation was that she should about the same period of life be taken off by the same disease.[21]

In 1857 "A Sketch of Two Homes" tackled the issue of marriage for the consumptive as a grandfather sought, to no avail, to break the disease cycle by preventing the marriage of his granddaughter who not only had a family history of consumption, but was also already demonstrating a predisposition to the disease. He poignantly recounted his own misery in his appeal to stop the alliance:

> "Young Man ... I pity you! I Pity You ... for once I suffered as you are doing, but—as you have *not* yet done—I prevailed on the woman I loved to marry me. She died of consumption; her daughter also married and died of consumption; Magdalen now is all that is left to me, and though the same terrible disease will kill her, too, she *shall* not marry, and like her mother and grandmother, leave it a fearful inheritance to her children. You have heard me, now ... go."[22]

Despite his angry diatribe, he failed to prevent the marriage, and a year later the husband stated: "It is more than a year ago. I have lived alone with my mistress since; but her *cheek* is hectic and hollowed now, and her step is feeble and slow. Like the rest, she, too is vanishing—a shadow departing from a world of shadows."[23]

The young man in the tale was typical and *Physiology for Young Ladies* suggests that the bulk of the advice against marrying a consumptive was ignored. The author complained:

> Health is but little thought of in matrimonial alliances; though I do remember once to have read, in "A Father's Advice to his Daughters," that they should be careful not to connect themselves with families who have disease … in them. But this is considered quite obsolete now: few think that there is any necessity of attending to this advice.[24]

With the widespread acceptance of heredity as an explanation for consumption, and the centrality of marriage to female identity, how was it possible that a condition like consumption was not only ignored in the choosing of a mate, but also became fashionable to middle-class Victorian women? The answer lies in the influence of contemporary biological definitions of women that led to the development of a culture of sickness.

The Reproductive Body

Evangelical philosophy shaped not only the Christian moralizers who set the requirements for exemplary womanhood, but also the medical men who established an organic foundation for female behavior. According to Carroll Smith-Rosenberg and Charles Rosenberg, "The Victorian woman's ideal social characteristics—nurturance, intuitive morality, domesticity, passivity, and affection—were all assumed to have a deeply rooted biological basis."[25] Femininity was a disputed entity, one that occupied intellectual and religious debates, but in the 1830s the debate became ever more secularized as both male and female roles were gradually transformed into natural biologically defined differences. (See Plate 15.) In the process, they became, according to Lenore Davidoff and Catherine Hall, "the common sense of the English middle class."[26] The decorative role assigned to the woman as the "angel in the house" elevated feminine qualities to the level of the spiritual while placing the masculine firmly in the world.

The role for women created by Christian doctrine was heavily influenced by the idea of atonement, as it connected to disease; therefore, illness became one of the main ways in which femininity intertwined with suffering to provide both moral and spiritual redemption.[27] Women were presented as both "the major source of sin and the primary symbol of purity," having "provoked the Fall and produced the Saviour."[28] Works concerned with sensibility presented the woman suffering from illness as innocent and unsullied, one who's purity made her unable to withstand the onslaught of the vulgar and coarse outside world. This weakness came to be located in the bodily structures, particularly the nerves and this elevation of nervous sensibility resulted in an increased awareness of the aesthetics of illness and death. These gender distinctions became progressively more visible in the portrayal of tuberculosis, with the female experiencing the illness as a result of her inability to withstand the crude world and its disappointments, particularly those in love; while male consumptions were increasingly presented as the product of business failure.[29] Illness, especially consumption, became a part of what it meant to be a Victorian lady. The feminine ideal was also predicated on the institutions of marriage and motherhood, which were socially and medically endorsed as vital to the fulfillment of the prescribed female role.[30]

During the early nineteenth century, consumption was increasingly intertwined with the female reproductive system. In linking consumption to the explicitly and exclusively female experiences of menstruation and pregnancy, medical investigators could account for the greater mortality purportedly observed among women from tuberculosis. This association was made possible by the discourse of sensibility that was supported by contemporary medical theory and supposed women's nervous systems to be more fragile than those of men. As Ornella Moscucci has argued "Reflex theories of nervous organization contained allusions to ideological distinctions between male and female. Gender differences were represented in terms of a different weighting between the controlling and autonomic sectors of the nervous system"[31] The physical appearance of the female provided the necessary evidence: she had a smaller frame and a more delicate muscular system, differences extended to the physiology of the nervous system and thought productive of heightened sensibility.

Robert Bentley Todd's *Descriptive and Physiological Anatomy of the Brain, Spinal Cord, and Ganglions* (1845) laid out the physiological evidence stating "Although Aristotle has remarked that the female brain is absolutely smaller than the male, it is nevertheless not relatively smaller compared with the body; for the female body is, in general, lighter than that of the male. The female brain is for the most part even larger than the male, compared with the size of the body. The different degree of susceptibility and sensibility of the nervous system seems to depend on the relative size of the brain as compared with the body."[32] Physicians and physiologists presented the female system as being more susceptible to the effects of excessive stimulation and prone to irritability, which could more easily result in the exhaustion of her system as a whole and, as such, result in tuberculosis. These notions were reinforced by the growing belief that women were the most frequent victims of the malady. In 1843, John Hastings asserted that "Women are unquestionably more liable to pulmonary consumption than men"[33] while Henry Deshon went so far as to suggest the predisposition to consumption was a direct consequence of "their more delicate and irritable organization rendering them more susceptible of impressions, both mental and physical"[34]

The purpose of female life was defined as the reproduction of the human species, and doctors and social theorists alike viewed women as both the artifact of, and hostage to, their reproductive arrangement. Given that the early nineteenth-century woman was defined in terms of her reproductive potential, the stages of her life were hallmarked by the onset of menstruation, the existence of pregnancy or its potential, and the "change of life" after menopause. Physiologists, like Alexander Walker, argued that the "female character depends on the presence of the ovaries,"[35] and went so far as to claim that in a woman lacking ovaries, all of the female characteristics disappeared, and as menstruation ceased, the breasts vanished and women grew beards. He further asserted that the onset of puberty heralded a "state of excessive susceptibility" in the female and triggered a "superabundance of life, which seeks, as it were to diffuse and communicate itself."[36]

However, this superabundance of life also resulted in an ending of life, as tuberculosis was integrated into this thinking. Medical authors placed the origination of the disease in the disruption caused by puberty, asserting it was at this point that the female was most vulnerable to consumption due to the complexity of her form. For instance, John Reid argued "It is generally known that decided symptoms of phthisis, for the most part, commence about or soon after puberty" because there is "revolution . . . effected throughout the universal frame" one that altered the pulmonary organs and increased "their sympathies with other parts" making the female more susceptible to consumptive illness.[37] It was this increased sympathy between the lungs and the womb that permitted the process of puberty to heighten irritability and cause tuberculosis. Thus, menstruation had significance not just for the development of the reproductive potential in the female but also in the creation of consumption, providing a physical link between the two.

Physiologists argued that the reproductive organs exerted an effect "upon the whole economy of woman."[38] And with puberty the "maiden begins to acquire . . . [an] adaption to purpose" and that "the reproductive organs in woman now no longer subsist in a subordinate condition, but, on the contrary, dominate over the whole animal economy."[39] New talents emerged including "An absolute delirium of imagination—a newly inspired desire of pleasing—emotions of jealousy—not only sexual love, but that of children, and even that of devotion, which then generally bears the impress of connexion with the reproductive organs—and finally, strange and wayward cerebral impressions, caprices of enthusiasm or of antipathy which submit not to her control."[40] By defining women medically, in emotional terms, the chains binding the feminine and a disease caused by sensibility and emotion were further tightened and *The Medico-Chirurgical Review* stated "If a girl is in love, the disturbance of the brain, by the excitement of a passion, may give her a . . . spitting of blood, and . . . consumption."[41]

Although puberty could inflame the passions, the increased vulnerability of women to the disease was, in part, a function of their monthly discharge of blood.[42] And Robert Thomas even listed "immoderate discharge of the menstrual flux" as a predisposing cause of consumption in his *The Modern Practice of Physic*.[43] There was a great deal of speculation over the role played by menstruation in the disease process. Some works argued that the cessation of menstruation served as a causative agent of consumption, while others simply saw it as a symptom. In either case the lack of the relief that menstruation provided was problematic, as amenorrhea (lack of menstruation) was the physical sign of an increased susceptibility to tuberculosis. *The Penny Cyclopaedia of the Society for the Diffusion of Useful Knowledge* acknowledged the difficulty the medical profession had in reading this piece of evidence stating "In females the menstrual discharge almost always ceases when hectic fever is established; and occasionally even before that is the case, which has led to a popular opinion that the disease in such cases arises from the suppression."[44]

This correlation between the menses and hectic fever, provided an avenue of explanation for another symptom that evidenced the presence of the disease, the hemoptysis or spitting of blood that was one of the most notable signs of consumption. Some physicians went so far as to argue that hemoptysis was the evidence of the female body's adaption for amenorrhea and was actually a displaced form of menstruation. In 1835 *An Introduction to Hospital Practice* made the case that hemoptysis "sometimes occurs as a vicarious discharge, when the lungs perform, as far as possible, the function of the uterus. If the menstrual secretion be suppressed, the lungs are overcharged with blood, and an effort is made to evacuate it by these organs."[45] In women who did not demonstrate regularity in menstrual function, consumption and its associated hemoptysis provided a method for the depletion of accumulated blood.[46]

Menstruation however, supplied just one of the ways in which the female reproductive system connected to tuberculosis. A number of medical treatises took as evidence the fact that consumption often seemed to take a hiatus during pregnancy, but hurriedly resumed after delivery, to assert "that the constantly increasing magnitude of the womb, exerts a powerful influence on suspending, and still further in curing, tubercular phthisis."[47] In 1839, Samuel Dickson wrote in his *Fallacies of the Faculty* "Pregnancy has been defined to be a natural process. So is Death!"[48] Although this juxtaposition may seem stark, he goes on to advocate pregnancy as the natural process most capable of securing an escape from the mortality of tuberculosis, stating "The disease most familiarly known to the profession as capable of being suspended, and in some instances cured, by the fever of pregnancy is Consumption. Where all other remedial means have failed, it is the duty of the physician to announce the *possibility* of a cure of this . . . disorder by marriage."[49]

So, while the action of the womb, in readying the body for conception proved problematic for health, the fulfillment of its purpose provided an avenue for regaining that which had been lost. This remission, however, was temporary, and as such required repeated pregnancies to forestall a death from consumption, for although "Phthisis pulmonalis has . . . been found to be considerably retarded in its progress by pregnancy, but when this is over, it hastened to a rapid termination."[50] These notions were supported by physicians, like John Ingleby, who reported cases like that of "A lady, and mother of a very large family, [who] had consumption arrested by eight successive pregnancies. The disease returned in a very marked form after each delivery. As she did not give suck, impregnation speedily recurred, and her temporary comfort was thus ensured."[51] Even more importantly, *Commentaries Principally on Those Diseases of Females Which are Constitutional* argued that the disease actually increased female fertility and aided pregnancy. Stating, most remarkably, "The condition of the uterus, under the influence of tuberculous disease, is one of great proneness to conception, a change which has, in its turn, a reflex action in arresting the progress of the tuberculous affection."[52] Consumption then in its interaction with the female reproductive system aided its own treatment.

If the biological instability of women, brought about by the functioning of the reproductive system, worked in concert with their inherent fragility to create a heightened vulnerability to tuberculosis—it stands to reason that with the loss of reproductive potential there would be a corresponding diminution in the incidence of the illness. After the age of reproductive fruitfulness, those organs of reproduction that were no longer useful were believed to shrivel in the woman leaving, "flaccidity and deformity in its place."[53] She was now a "new kind of being," and with the purpose of female life defined as the reproduction of the human species, there was a physiologically reductionist view that characterized the life of a post-menopausal woman as one of lost purpose and identity.[54] Thus, Alexander Walker stated, "When age finally destroys the energy of the reproductive organs and the faculty of conception, greater power is obtained by the rest of the organization; the mind increases in clearness ... With intellect, the masculine character is assumed."[55] Additionally post-menopausal women, in losing that quality productive of sensibility, were thought to be less susceptible to tuberculosis, evidenced by the widespread belief that consumption was an illness that preferentially attacked the young. *Consumption: What it is, and What it is not* highlighted the tubercular dilemma: "CONSUMPTION!— terrible, insatiable tyrant!—... Why dost thou attack, almost exclusively, the fairest and loveliest of our species? Why select blooming and beautiful youth, instead of haggard and exhausted age? Why strike down those who are bounding blithely from the starting-post of life, rather than the decrepit beings tottering towards its goal?"[56] The answer lay in the interpretation of the evidence, as a heavily feminized disease, tuberculosis struck women at the peak of fecundity, but left unmarked those no longer capable of serving their essential feminine role. Thus, the feminine ideal rested biologically upon both the refined nervous and acutely reactive reproductive systems of women, both of which were intimately intertwined with sensibility.

Sensibility and Feminine Character

Sensibility was presented, in the literature and society, as integral to the feminine ideal on the basis of emotional intensity. It was popularly believed that women were endowed with a superior quantity of this quality and, as such, were defined as creatures of the heart, who acted primarily from their affections, while men were defined as creatures of intellect, motivated primarily by reason.[57] Beyond the emotional association, sensibility also provided an additional connection to disease. Robert Bentley Todd addressed the interdependence: "Thin persons are more susceptible than stout. In diseases which affect the nourishment of the body, the susceptibility increases as the patients grow thinner. The susceptibility and sensibility decreases, on the other hand, with persons recovering from a long illness, gradually as they regain their strength."[58] This correspondence between emaciation and increased sensibility provided yet another link between consumption and the feminine.

Sensibility defined not only personal feelings and emotions but also the physical manifestations of those sentiments. Sentimentalists insisted that women were incapable of hiding their emotions, which made them constitutionally transparent. As a woman progressed through the various stages of chronic illness, sentimentalists maintained the layers of her personality softened, illuminating the woman's true character, which had the added bonus of elevating her spirituality.[59] Women supposedly expressed their emotions in the form of swoons, tears, and, most importantly, in illness.[60] Consumption, then, as a chronic illness provided an avenue that permitted the articulation of a woman's essential being, the truth of her character. A susceptibility to illness, as well as resilience and fortitude under its influence, were important components of the female

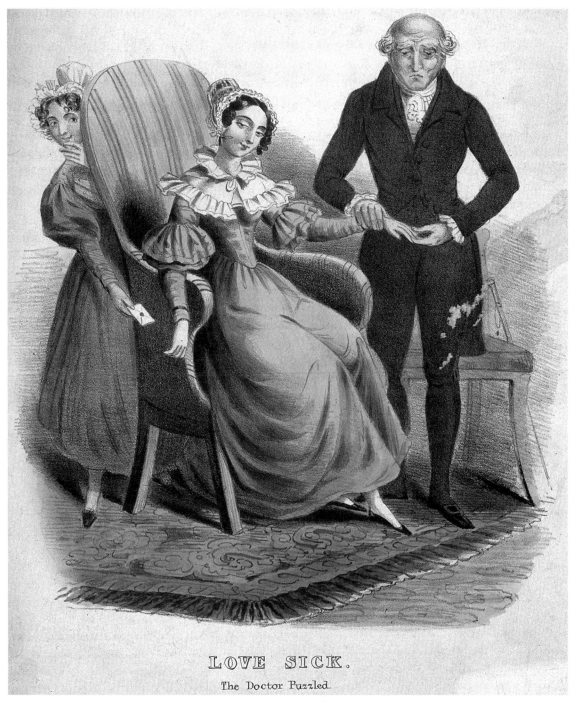

LOVE SICK.
The Doctor Puzzled.

Figure 5.2 A baffled doctor taking the pulse of a love-sick young woman. Lithograph. Wellcome Library, London. Copyrighted work available under Creative Commons Attribution only licence CC BY 4.0 http://creativecommons.org/licenses/by/4.0/

constitution and imparted a certain quality to that illness, defined by character, moral fiber, and spirituality. Additionally, the illness could provide evidence of "emotional authenticity" and was a testament to unadulterated and legitimate suffering. The emaciated body was proof of sincerity of emotion. The body did not lie and so illustrated emotion far more truly than words could ever express.[61] The connection between emotions and consumption was constantly reiterated in medical treatises and literature.[62] For example, James Clark stated,

> Mental depression also holds a very conspicuous place among those circumstances which diminish the powers of the system generally, and it often proves one of the most effectual determining causes of consumption. Disappointment of long-cherished hopes, sleighted affections, loss of dear relations, and reverse of fortune, often exert a powerful influence on persons predisposed to consumption, more particularly in the female sex.[63]

Consumptive illness and death had been a popular literary staple for some time, and the device continued in the Victorian period and was employed in a variety of ways by authors, like the Brontë sisters, who were themselves afflicted with the disease.[64] Clark Lawlor has argued that the use of pallor and delicacy in Victorian literature increasingly came to stand for the occurrence of tuberculosis, though the illness was vigilantly cleansed of its inappropriate and unbecoming symptoms and its young female victim was instead presented as "a sentimental angel."[65] Tuberculosis was also accorded a role as a sign of elevated spirituality and attractiveness, and increasingly the consumptive female became an aesthetic object.[66] The tradition of sensibility that was intertwined with the idea of an individual who was continually hovering on the edge of illness, provided one way in which the regard for the loving, gentle, and sensitive consumptive heroine was elevated beyond the confines of the novel and applied to everyday life. These notions moved past literary devices and were established as medical fact, in an extension of the long-held tradition of mental upheaval as a causative agent of tuberculosis. Richard Payne Cotton tackled the issue in his *The Nature, Symptoms, and treatment of Consumption*.

> Depression of spirits, when long continued and severe, may, even of itself, generate the tuberculous diathesis. How frequently can we date the commencement of phthisis from some reverse of fortune or family affliction, or from something which has deeply affected the mind! We hear of the "broken heart" of affliction; yet this is generally but a metaphor, signifying that sorrow and worldly cares may be destructive of life;—the physician knows too well how easily these may develop a tuberculous state, and how unpromising are the cases thus originated.[67]

There was a widespread acceptance of the cultural discourse of consumption as a product of disappointment in love, one that coincided with the definition of the illness as the product of the female nervous system.

During the first half of the nineteenth century consumption was increasingly interpreted as a function of the sex of the afflicted and meaning was assigned to the disease experience based upon gender. Although the Romantic image of the male poet who fell prey to a consumption as well as his own "irritable sensibility" continued, by the early Victorian period sensibility and, by virtue of its association with that quality, tuberculosis had become explicitly feminine. Observed physiological differences were extended into social expectations and defined femininity, in part, as a function of excess sensibility. These biological notions were then translated into a code of propriety, social sensibility, and physical delicacy, all of which presented women as being precariously balanced on the edge of pathology, and by implication tuberculosis.[68]

CHAPTER 6
TRAGEDY AND TUBERCULOSIS: THE SIDDONS STORY

Already established as an illness of thwarted love, diseased creativity, refinement, and nervous sensibility by the end of the eighteenth century, tuberculosis was increasingly intertwined with ideas of female attractiveness. This association was made possible by the discourse of sensibility that privileged delicacy and was supported by contemporary medical theory that supposed women's nervous systems to be more fragile than those of men. Women were, biologically speaking, starting at a disadvantage. This situation was further complicated by their ever more ornamental and sedentary social roles, which seemed to create the perfect conditions under which consumption might flourish. Thus physicians, authors, and lay individuals alike participated in the identification of tuberculosis with beauty, refinement, and nervous sensibility. Consumptive mythology was powerful, and increasingly an aestheticized metaphor dominated the presentations of the illness.

Consumption was articulated as an illness that was not only beautiful in the physical and spiritual sense, but also as a disease that was associated with love. These notions had relevance in the individual constructions of the disease experience by both the victim of tuberculosis and those witnessing the inexorable progress of the illness. Susan Sontag argued that "many of the literary and erotic attitudes known as 'romantic agony' derive from tuberculosis … Agony became romantic in a stylized account of the disease's preliminary symptoms and the actual agony was simply suppressed."[1] By the latter part of the eighteenth century, individuals were using specific rhetorical imagery to fashion their experiences with consumption. Some elements of this mythology included a reinterpretation of the Christian "good death," which embraced older ideas about consumption as a peaceful exit. In the sentimental incarnation, this gentle death was embellished with notions of beauty and of a young lady victimized by disappointment, particularly in love. In the case of women, descriptions of the causes of consumption and of the death from the illness often included the elevation of both spiritual and physical beauty.

Sarah Kemble Siddons (1755–1831), the most celebrated tragic actress of the eighteenth century, reached the height of her popularity during the latter part of that century.[2] (See Plate 16.) At the same time that she was receiving critical acclaim, she was also facing financial and personal hardship, in part due to Richard Brinsley Sheridan's poor management of the Drury Lane Theatre.[3] Sheridan was constantly in arrears on Mrs. Siddons' salary, and this fiscal instability may have been the motivating force to continue a precedent begun in the summer of 1784. Throughout the late 1780s and 1790s, at the end of the London theater season, Mrs. Siddons set about on a tour of Scotland and the north of England.[4] Whether she actually required the money to supplement the funds Sheridan had failed to pay her or was simply lured by the lucrative profits from these summer tours is unclear. In 1798 however, Mrs. Siddons complained, while absent from her daughter Maria during that daughter's illness, "My grief is that this whim of Maria's [Maria's desire to go to Clifton] separates us for I <u>must</u> wander about to pick up a little money to defray our expenses. I shall be with them about a month and then much away to play at Worcester Glouster [sic] Cheltenham by the Autumn I hope Maria will have had enough of Clifton and that we may be all together at Brighton where I shall play a few nights."[5]

What is clear is that Mrs. Siddons and her brother, John Kemble, had finally reached the end of their patience with Sheridan and at the end of the 1801–1802 season broke ties with the Drury Lane Theatre. Shortly afterwards, beginning in May of 1802, Mrs. Siddons would again leave her family and travel abroad on a performance circuit for more than a year in Ireland. During this excursion, it was Mrs. Siddons elder daughter, Sally, that was too ill to accompany her. Instead, she was attended by the daughter of Tate Wilkinson, the theater manager in York. Martha (Patty) Wilkinson had initially come to the Siddons home as a companion for the eldest Siddons daughter in 1799. She would accompany Mrs. Siddons on her Irish tour of 1802–1803, and indeed would remain her companion until Mrs. Siddons' death.[6] Whatever Mrs. Siddons' motivations, her work accounted for her absences during key points in the illnesses of her two daughters. Mrs. Siddons's busy schedule has permitted unique access to the progress and impact of the illnesses of her daughters, as experienced by her, and chronicled through letters with friends during long absences. Beyond providing a window into the disease process of consumption and its growing association with female ideals, the various theories and treatments of the disease are also apparent. Especially compelling was the part thought to be played by the love triangle involving both girls and the portrait painter Sir Thomas Lawrence. The unhappy consequence was taken by some to be the development, or escalation, of a consumption and the eventual death of the younger daughter.

A Beautiful Predisposition

In 1834 Charles Greville wrote in his memoirs:

> Mrs. Arkwright told me the curious story of Sir Thomas Lawrence's engagements with her two cousins … They were two sisters, one tall and very handsome, the other little, without remarkable beauty, but very clever and agreeable. He fell in love with the first, and they were engaged to be married … after some time the superior intelligence of the clever sister changed the current of his passion, and she supplanted the handsome one in the affection of the artist. They concealed the double treachery, but one day a note which was intended for his new love fell into the hands of the old love, who, never doubting it was for herself, opened it, and discovered the fatal truth. From that time she drooped, sickened, and shortly after died.[7]

As one might expect, the actual course of these romantic entanglements played out a bit differently than in Mrs. Arkwright's accounting. Yet even in contemporary renderings of the affairs between Lawrence and the Siddons daughters, beauty remained a central theme. This focus on attractiveness was especially important to contemporaries as it accounted, in part, for the consumption that caused the "handsome" sister, to droop, sicken, and die. In courting them, Lawrence in fact, first traded in the "clever" and "agreeable" sister, Sarah Martha (1775–1803), affectionately known as Sally, for her younger sister Maria (1779–1798), the one displaying "beauty," before once again swapping his affections as the more attractive Maria lay dying from consumption—hardly a noble portrait of the painter.

Both daughters were thought to resemble their mother in their good looks, although Maria was generally believed to be the more attractive of the two. References to the beauty of Maria began at a young age, as did her mother's concern over the consequences of such loveliness. When Maria was only thirteen, Mrs. Siddons wrote to her friend Mrs. Barrington, "Maria is vastly handsome, I can scarce wish any daughter of mine to be remarkable for beauty, I need not prose to you the reason why."[8] The reason was that beauty was believed to be one of the significant signs of a hereditary predisposition to consumption; moreover, once established, the symptoms were also thought to increase the attractiveness of the sufferer.

Sally, despite Mrs. Arkwright's less than flattering account of her physical charms, was also recognized by her contemporaries as attractive—although, the representations of the elder daughter tended to focus upon her intelligence and character, particularly after her death. For example, the poet Thomas Campbell[9] wrote upon seeing a bust of Sally Siddons that "She was not strictly beautiful, but her countenance was like her mother's, with brilliant eyes, and a remarkable mixture of frankness and sweetness in her physiognomy."[10] Both girls exhibited a certain delicacy of constitution, although Maria, with her greater beauty, was thought to have inherited the full measure of that delicacy.

Paradoxically, Sally was the first to demonstrate a susceptibility to respiratory illness when she was only seventeen. The indications of Sally's tendency to infirmity occur early in her mother's correspondence, as she was "taken *illish*" in October of 1792.[11] Even before this episode, Sally had been placed on a regimen of asses' milk, an accredited remedy for consumption and other respiratory and emaciating ailments.[12] She would suffer several acute attacks of illness before she was struck down by what would eventually be labeled spasmodic asthma. According to her traveling companion, Mrs. Hester Lynch Piozzi, this was a particularly brutal episode as Sally was "seized yesterday with such a paroxysm of asthma, cough, spasm, every thing, as you nor I ever saw her attack'd by."[13] Under the care of Richard Greatheed, Sally improved yet again, and once recovered, there were no concerns expressed that she might suffer any long-term difficulties or have a constitutional predisposition to illness. Sally's medical history seemed to make her the more likely candidate for consumption, as asthma was an accepted antecedent to the disease; however, Sally's "strength" of constitution would be employed to explain her continual triumphs over the bouts of spasmodic asthma that would plague her throughout her short life.[14] In the end, it was the lovely and more delicate Maria who would contract consumption first.

That Lothario Lawrence

It is unclear at what point Thomas Lawrence entered the girls' lives as an object of romantic interest. John Fyvie intimates that Lawrence must have met the girls not long after he established himself in London in 1787, as he quickly made friends with the Siddons family. At this point Maria would have been only eight years old and Sally around twelve.[15] The girls' acquaintance with Lawrence rekindled sometime in 1792 or 1793, when Lawrence then developed a *tendre* for the elder daughter Sally, who was at that time twenty.[16] By end of 1795 or early in 1796, an understanding of romantic intent developed between Lawrence and Sally, (see Plate 17) one that evidently received the support of Mrs. Siddons, although she chose to keep the situation hidden from Mr. Siddons. Lawrence's interest waned, however, and he rapidly transferred his affections to the younger, lovelier sister.

Despite her feelings, Sally seems to have graciously stepped aside in favor of her younger sister, and Lawrence formally proposed to Maria.[17] The suit was refused by Mr. Siddons, both because of Maria's youth, and Lawrence's precarious financial position. Not willing to accept this decision, Maria sustained her relationship with Lawrence for close to two years through clandestine letters and meetings. A liaison made possible by a combination of assistance from Sally Bird and the complicity of Maria's mother, who concealed the relationship to avoid her husband's objections. Maria was permitted to meet with Lawrence with no other chaperone than the unmarried Miss Bird, hardly a likely choice as a companion to ensure respectability.[18] The secret relationship between Lawrence and Maria continued until early in 1798, when Mr. Siddons finally agreed to the match.

What led to this change of heart? In the end, it seems that concern for Maria's wellbeing played a large part in the decision. Maria's health rapidly declined during the winter of 1797–1798. In January of 1798, Mrs. Siddons shared her concerns and fears that she may need to take Maria to Bristol for her health.

Dr. Pearson is decidedly of opinion that the Bristol waters are not proper for Maria at this time; and as any other air will be equally good in the present state of her complaint, and as going thither would be attended with great expense and inconvenience, we have given up that plan . . . The dreaded disorder, he says, has not taken place, but her lungs are in a state of susceptibility for receiving it that required unremitting attention for a great length of time.[19]

The relief over the verdict that Maria's case had yet to progress to consumption was tempered by the looming threat of the disease striking at any time. In May, Mrs. Siddons expressed her continued apprehension over the possibility writing "Maria is still in a state of health which keeps me very anxious for the Consumption has not yet taken place. Yet I am given to understand that her lungs are in that susceptibility of receiving it, that all the vigilance of watchful tenderness may possibly be insufficient to elude its treacherous approach."[20]

The concern over Maria's delicate constitution was an important deciding factor in the Siddonses' agreement to allow their daughter to become engaged to Thomas Lawrence. A suggestion of their anxiety was evident in a letter of January 1798 from Sally to Miss Bird. "Maria determin'd to speak to my Father when she was much worse than she is now; she did, and now he, mov'd by the state in which she was . . . thought it most wise to agree to what was inevitable."[21] Maria's parents were concerned for their daughter's emotional health, and therefore her connected physical state, as well as the possibility of an elopement if they continued to refuse to consent to the match. Once he had given in, Mr. Siddons even tackled the matter of Lawrence's financial problems and made arrangements for his daughter's future by settling the painter's outstanding debts.[22]

Sally was optimistic this new turn of events would have a positive effect on Maria's health despite Pearson's gloomy pronouncements; reflecting the widespread belief that favorable circumstances, including a love affair that ended happily, had the power to forestall the onset of the tuberculosis in an individual constitutionally predisposed to the disease. Hence, she wrote to Mrs. Bird, "Should not this happy event have more effect than all the medicines? At least I cannot but think it will add greatly to their efficacy."[23] For a short time, the decision to allow the engagement seemed to be the correct choice, as Maria's health appeared to improve. On January 28, 1798 Sally remarked to Miss Bird, "I waited to send you news of Maria's return to the Drawing Room, where she has now been for several days, and is recovering her strength and good looks every day. But here she must remain, Dr. Pierson [sic] says, during the cold weather, which means, I suppose, all the Winter."[24]

Sadly, Maria's future was not as easily dealt with as her fiscal security, and her health once again precipitously declined beginning in February of 1798. Compounding her difficulties, within two months of her formal engagement to Lawrence, her fiancée seems to have transferred his affections back to Sally and embarked on a clandestine association with that sister.[25] Sally, however, had not completely forgotten his earlier shabby treatment and inconstancy. The circumstances of their previous relationship still weighed heavily upon her mind. She was also concerned about the effect her renewed relationship might have on Maria, but convinced herself that her sister would not be severely affected because Maria's feelings were not deeply engaged. At the same time, Sally preferred to keep her relationship quiet to prevent the possibility of upsetting her sister and addressed some of these concerns to Lawrence.

I wait but for the time when Maria shall be evidently engaged by some other object to declare to her my intentions, and then there will be no more of this cruel restraint and we may overcome the objections of those whose objections are of importance. You cannot be in earnest when you talk of being soon again in Marlborough Street; *you know it is impossible*. Neither you, nor Maria, nor I could bear it. DO you think that, tho' she does not love you, she would feel no unpleasant sensations to see those attentions paid to another which once were hers? . . . Oh, no! banish this idea. Your absence indeed affects Maria but little—so little that I am convinced she never lov'd—but your presence, you must feel, would place us all in the most distressing situation imaginable.[26]

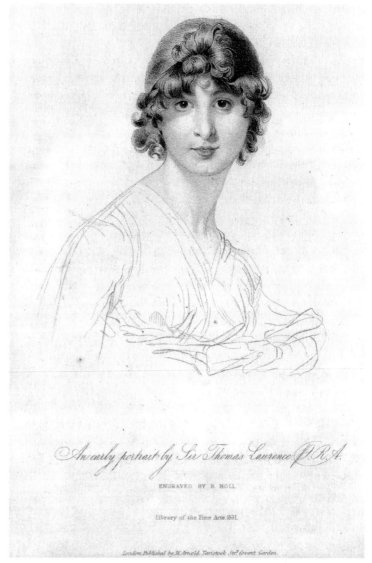

An early portrait by Sir Thomas Lawrence PRA.

ENGRAVED BY R. HOLL

Library of the Fine Arts 1831.

London. Published by M. Arnold, Tavistock Str.t Covent Garden.

Figure 6.1 Portrait of Maria Siddons; after T. Lawrence (Garlick undescribed); illustration to "Library of the Fine Arts" (1831) Stipple. 1933, 1014.543 ©The Trustees of the British Museum.

Sally was obviously emotionally invested, as the mood of the letter turned downright giddy and demonstrated a schoolgirl fascination. She implored Thomas to pass by her parlor window at nine in the morning, as she was "generally writing or reading at that hour."[27] Sally then went on to deal with the sticky situation of his fidelity and unreliability.

> Need I tell you there is *one (if he is but constant)* whose company I would prefer to all the world? . . . I tell you now, before you proceed any further, that *if I love you again* I shall love more than ever, and in that case *disappointment* would be *death*.[28]

This notion that Sally could be disappointed to the point of death was not just an overwrought emotional exclamation, but reflected the well-established belief that disappointments, particularly in love, could lead to the development of consumption and consequently death.

As early as February of 1798, the temperamental Lawrence was once again exhibiting signs of irritability, depression, and restlessness. He finally confessed to Mrs. Siddons his renewed attachment to Sally and his engagement to Maria was officially terminated in March of 1798. The invalid seems to have dealt well with the romantic reversal of fortune and her lover's abandonment.[29] As Sally told Miss Bird,

> Maria bears her disappointment as I would have her, in short, like a person whose heart could never have been deeply engag'd . . . It is now near a fortnight since this complete breaking off, and Maria is in good spirits, talks and thinks of dress, and company, and beauty, as usual. Is this not fortunate? Had she lov'd him, I think this event would almost have broken her heart; I rejoice that she did not.[30]

Sally and Lawrence's association would remain clandestine however, as Mrs. Siddons once again decided to keep yet another relationship a secret from her husband. Despite her apparent acceptance of Sally and Lawrence's renewed relationship at her expense, Maria did however, apportion blame for her illness to the experience and to her erstwhile suitor's behavior. She wrote Miss Bird soon after Sally did, "he himself, if it is possible any feeling can remain in him, will acknowledge how little he deserv'd the sacrifices I was willing to make for him."[31]

Maria's correspondence demonstrated far more concern about her health than her lover's abandonment, and her disease increasingly became the primary focus of her life. On March 14, 1798, she recounted some details of her illness to Miss Bird, writing, "I feel a sad pain in my side."[32] She went on to discuss the difficulty she was having in coping with the reality of her malady. "A relapse is always worse than the original illness, and I yet think I shall not live a long while, it is perhaps merely nervous, but I sometimes feel as if I should not, and I see nothing very shocking in the idea; I can have no great fears, and I may be sav'd from much misery. I fear never creature was less calculated to bear it than I am, and in my short life I have known enough to be sick to death of it."[33] The disease was proving a toll on Maria's emotional, as well as her physical, health. She told Miss Bird, "I look forward with impatience to the time when I shall be myself again, and now I will endeavour to shake off this oppression, and entertain you a little better"[34] Maria's correspondence also provides some insight into the lonely existence often experienced by the consumptive invalid, and a yearning for a return to normalcy.

> I long so much to go out that I envy every poor little beggar running about in the open air. This confinement becomes insupportable to me, it seems to me that on these beautiful sun-shine days all nature is reviv'd, but not me: for it makes me regret the more that I may not enjoy the air, who have so much need of it to cheer me after such an illness . . . I expect to go to a very beautiful place this summer, Clifton, but I look forward to it with no pleasure; for the first time I shall be separated from Sally and my mother both, they go to Scotland, which will be too cold an air for me to venture in. I shall, I believe, be with a Lady at Clifton, where, if I can keep up my spirits, I am more likely to get well than in any other place in England.[35]

As her disease increasingly became the primary focus of her life, Maria's beauty would gain a prominent place in representations of her illness. For instance, a family friend, Mrs. Piozzi, provided an outsider's view of Maria at the time of her engagement's end, writing that "Maria . . . looked (to me) as usual, yet everybody says she is ill, and in fact she was bled that very evening."[36] This failure to recognize Maria's illness was due, in part, to the difficultly of differentiating between the physical appearance of an individual with a hereditary predisposition to consumption and one experiencing an acute attack. The difference in appearance between predisposition and active illness was a matter of degree. In Maria's case, her natural state was considered attractive, and as the disease progressed, the links between the illness and her beauty became more significant and were mentioned more frequently by family and friends.

Mrs. Piozzi's assessment of Maria's illness also demonstrated the difficulty physicians had in gaining acceptance for the anatomico-pathological approach to consumption. In the same letter, she complained about what she termed the "new fangled" approach to the disease and lamented the contemporary therapy. "Shutting a young half-consumptive girl up in *one unchanged air* for 3 or 4 months, would make any of them ill, and ill-humoured too, I should think. But 'tis *the new way* to make them breathe their own infected breath over and over again now, in defiance of old books, old experience, and good old common sense. Ah, my dear friend, there are many *new ways*,—and a dreadful place do they lead to."[37] Her attitude reflected the continued acceptance of older humoral and miasmatic approaches to illness as well as traditional therapeutics, including bleeding and blistering, both of which were used on Maria in the spring of 1798.

As her illness progressed, Maria became increasingly frustrated and focused, in particular, on what she perceived as her failure to bear up appropriately under her affliction. She even expressed concern over the effect that her melancholy was having upon her loved ones. "It appears to me that I should be very like myself if I could but take a walk, and feel the wind blow on me again," she wrote to Miss Bird. "I am indeed doubly unhappy, whenever I cannot keep up my spirits, to see I hurt my Mother and Sally. I am angry with myself though I am conscious of struggling against it."[38] She then berated herself: "Have I not written you a stupid letter? Indeed, it is a great exertion. I hate writing lately, but I shall always be delighted to read your letters when you will send them to me, and perhaps some time I may be rous'd from this low, stupid way, and be able to entertain you better."[39] Maria was concerned about her handling of her illness, particularly what she considered to be her unsuitable feelings in the face of her suffering. In response to her own evaluation, Maria made a concerted effort to modify her behavior, asserting "patience and resignation must be my virtues, and [tho'] they are severely try'd, the reward will, of course, be glorious."[40]

By May of 1798, Mrs. Siddons was very concerned over what she saw as the increasingly slim possibility of Maria's recovery. "The illness of my second daughter has deranged all schemes of pleasure as well as profit," she wrote to Tate Wilkinson. "I thank God she is better; but the nature of her constitution is such, that it will be long ere we can reasonably banish the fear of an approaching consumption."[41] This letter marked Mrs. Siddons's first real acknowledgment that her daughter had a constitutional predisposition to the illness. Mrs. Siddons also provided a glimpse of how heart wrenching it must have been for a mother to watch her beloved child slowly fade before her eyes: "It is dreadful to see an innocent, lovely young creature daily sinking under this distress, you can more easily imagine than I can describe."[42]

The Decline of Maria

With the possibility of a cure slipping away, the family sent Maria to Clifton, which along with the nearby Bristol Hot-wells, was a well-known retreat for consumptives during this period. As a destination for the sick, the town was made more attractive by the social activities available to those seeking not only health but also an alleviation of the boredom often associated with invalidism. Located a mere fourteen miles from Bath and only two miles from Bristol itself, the Hot-wells were situated below the village of Clifton. Rather than detracting from its popularity, the proximity of the Hot-wells to Bath proved advantageous, as the waters at the two spas were believed complementary and serviced separate illnesses. Bath's waters were touted as stimulant in nature and so beneficial to digestive complaints, while the waters of the Hot-wells were supposedly sedative and particularly beneficial in cases of inflammatory disease such as consumption. The status of the Hot-wells was enhanced by the timing of its season, which filled the space between the two popular seasons at Bath and provided an additional warm weather option, beyond the summer season at Tunbridge Wells. The popularity of Clifton was bolstered by the daily summer coach service running between Bristol and Bath that began in 1754, as well as affordable post-chaise journeys to the Hot-wells.[43] *The New Bath Guide* (1799) stated, "The season for drinking the water is from March to September, when the place is much frequented by the nobility and gentry."[44] William Nisbet's, *A General Dictionary of Chemistry* (1805) provided slightly later dates, asserting that "from May to October is the favourite period of the season for the enjoyment of Bristol wells, but the mildness of the climate should always tempt to a longer residence, and on this account it should form the spot for the invalid to spend the winter, if obliged to pass it in Britain."[45] Dr. William Saunders, in his treatise on mineral waters, confirmed Nisbet's dates, maintaining that "the season for the Hot-wells is generally from the middle of May to October, but as the properties of the water are the same during the winter, the summer months are only selected on account of their benefits arising from the concomitant advantages of air and exercise, which may be enjoyed more completely in this season."[46]

By the mid-eighteenth century, the Hot-wells at Clifton was a fashionable resort frequented by the social elite. In 1789, Dr. Andrew Carrick described the place: "The Hot-wells during the summer was one of the best-frequented and most crowded watering-places in the kingdom. Scores of the first nobility were to be found there every season."[47] In 1793, Julius Caesar Ibbeston pronounced the village of Clifton as "one of the most polite of any in the kingdom."[48] He went on to enumerate the advantages of the Hot-wells: "The wells have the necessary attendant of such a place, gaiety. The resort to them is great, and during the summer months, a band

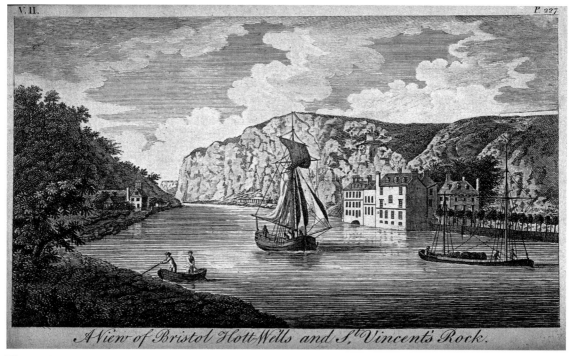

Figure 6.2 Hot-well House and St. Vincent Rocks. Line engraving, early eighteenth century. Wellcome Library, London. Copyrighted work available under Creative Commons Attribution only licence CC BY 4.0 http://creativecommons.org/licenses/by/4.0/

of music attends every morning. Here is a master of ceremonies, who conducts the public balls and breakfasts, which are given twice a week."[49] Dr. William Saunders called the resort "peculiarly calculated for the pleasure and comfort of the invalid."[50] The Hot-wells water was reputed to be effective in cases of pulmonary consumption, either as a cure or as a palliative. Saunders stated that although the idea of a cure was unlikely, the Bristol water "alleviates some of the most harassing symptoms in this formidable disease."[51] Robert Thomas's *The Modern Practice of Physic* (1813) argued that the "benefit . . . should not be attributed wholly to the waters."[52]

> The horse exercise, which is taken daily by such patients, on a fine airy down . . . the salubrity of the air; the healthfulness of the situation, and the frequent attendance on the different amusements which are furnished at these wells, prove beyond all doubt the most powerful of auxiliaries. Places of public resort are food to the mind of convalescents, and serve to keep it in the same active state that exercise does the body, preventing thereby that indulgence in gloomy reflection, to which the want of cheerful scenes and agreeable company is apt to give rise in those who have an indifferent state of health . . . Nay, I am decidedly of the opinion that at least three-fourths of the cure attributed to all mineral waters, ought rather to be placed to the account of a difference in air, exercise, diet, amusement of the mind, and the regulations productive of greater temperance, than to any salutary, or efficacious properties in the waters themselves.[53]

A consumptive in *The Lounger's Common-Place Book* (1799), however, offered a very different view of how to approach the disease and of Clifton.

> I will try every resource which experience, judgment and qualified professors can point out; but once convinced that my disease is a consumption. I will fly from quackery as a pest, and from the apothecary as an unnecessary appendage; and not possessing a sufficient fortune to carry a ship load of friends with me to Lisbon, I would submit with all possible content to the circumstances of my situation, and moderately indulging in whatever food my stomach would take, pass the short remains of life in the bosom of my family. For death in any form, is far preferable to being dismissed to cough a man's heart out in a solitary gravel pit, or to being exhausted by a journey to Clifton, with ghastly undertakers, thrusting their cards of *funerals performed*, into the post-chaise; apothecaries anticipating nitre powders, spermacaeti drafts, silk hat-bands, and long bills; and carpenter's apprentices taking measure of a skeleton as he walks down the street, and *wondering the gentleman remains so long*.[54]

The Siddons family arrived in Clifton in the summer of 1798, according to Sally, due to Maria's "strong desire to come here."[55] Shortly thereafter, Mrs. Siddons embarked upon a tour of the Midlands with Sally, leaving Maria in the care of Mrs. Pennington, who resided in fashionable Dowry Square.[56] Maria seems to have taken full advantage of all that Clifton and the Bristol Hot-wells had to offer, as she immediately began "to drink the Waters, and to ride double."[57] While on tour Mrs. Siddons made numerous inquiries and comments concerning Maria's health. On July 26, she wrote to Mrs. Pennington, "I know she went to a Ball, I hope it did her no harm. This weather has prevented her riding too; tell me about her pulse, her perspirations, her cough, everything!"[58] Her concern over the burden that Maria's social activities were placing on the invalid was clear, as was her anxiety over the possibility of her daughter not being able to accomplish the prescribed horseback riding.[59] Despite her unease, Mrs. Siddons remained hopeful that Clifton and the Bristol waters would prove beneficial to Maria's constitution. The reports on Maria's condition establish the picture of a young woman who, if not on the mend, was at least enjoying the entertainments available in Clifton.[60] Thus Sally wrote Miss Bird on July 17, "Maria sends good accounts of herself, and has been allowed to go to two balls, tho' not to dance."[61] The belief that this activity was an exciting cause of consumption may have contributed to the decision that the frail girl would not be permitted to dance.

By the end of July 1798, Mrs. Siddons seems to have accepted the seriousness of her daughter's illness, and her fears increased as Maria began to fade. She expressed her gratitude to her friend Mrs. Pennington for the solicitous care of her daughter, writing "The dear creature . . . says that she cou'd not have been so happy in any other situation absent from us as with you . . . How sadly unfavorable is the weather, but let me hope it is settled with you, and that she is able to take her rides!"[62] Mrs. Siddons' letter also reflected the commonly held notion that the changes produced by the progress of consumption were attractive upon the face of its victim, as she wrote "of watching each change of her lovely, varying, interesting countenance."[63]

By August, Mrs. Siddons's letters to Mrs. Pennington revealed her resignation to, and acceptance of, Maria's fate. "Mine is the habitation of sickness and sorrow. My dear and kind friend, be assur'd I rely implicitly on your truth to me and tenderness to my Sweet Maria. I do not flatter myself that she will be long continued to me. The Will of God be done; but I hope, I hope she will not suffer much!"[64] She also addressed her fears for her elder daughter's future, writing on the state of Sally's constitution. She was clearly concerned that delicate health would affect Sally's marriage prospects, despite Lawrence's renewed affections.

How vainly did I flatter myself that this other dear creature had acquired the strength of constitution to throw off this cruel disorder! Instead of that, it returns with increasing velocity and violence. What a sad prospect is this for her in marriage? For I am now convinc'd it is constitutional, and will pursue her thro' life! Will a husbands [sic] tenderness keep pace with and compensate for the loss of a mother's, her unremitting cares and soothings? Will he not grow sick of these repeated attacks, and think it vastly inconvenient to have his domestic comforts, his pleasures, or his business interfered with by the necessary and habitual attentions which they will call for from himself and from his servants? Dr. Johnson says the man must be almost a prodigy of virtue who is not soon tir'd of an ailing wife . . . To say the truth, a sick wife must be a great misfortune.[65]

Like her mother, Maria was increasingly anxious not only about her own illness but also about Sally's future. Maria was plagued by anxiety and depression, which increased as her body weakened, as did her apprehension over Sally and Lawrence's love affair. Whether out of concern for Sally's happiness or her own jealousy, she became convinced that the union must be prevented and no amount of pleading or cajoling on the part of Mrs. Pennington allayed her concerns. Mrs. Pennington quickly relayed the invalid's deteriorating mental and physical state to her mother, who responded by sending Sally to Clifton. After her arrival, Sally related Maria's condition to Miss Bird:

I found my poor dear Maria, much worse than when I left her; she was rejoic'd to see me, and my presence has so reviv'd her, she seems so happy to have me with her that I thank Heaven we so immediately determin'd upon my setting off for the Wells. Yet my dear friend, this is but momentary comfort, for it is but too evident we have but little hopes, alas! None, I fear, for the future. The Gentlemen who attend upon her assure us there is no immediate danger, and tell us of persons who have been much worse and yet have recover'd; but I am certain they have no hopes of Maria's recovery, and I am prepared for the worst.[66]

To complicate the situation, Lawrence returned to center stage. Concerned that Sally might be denied to him, he rushed to Clifton to plead his case. In a letter to Mrs. Pennington that warned of his approach, Mrs. Siddons touches upon Lawrence's possible guilt over his harmful effect on both her daughters and was

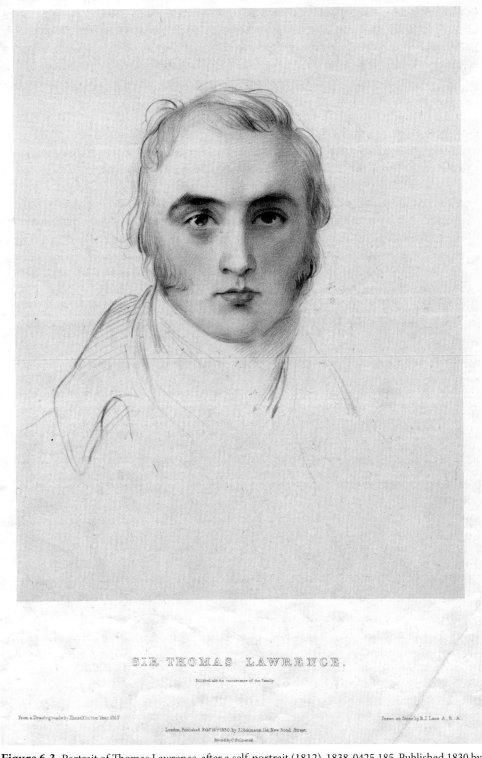

SIR THOMAS LAWRENCE.

Figure 6.3 Portrait of Thomas Lawrence, after a self-portrait (1812). 1838, 0425.185. Published 1830 by J. Dickinson. © The Trustees of the British Museum.

especially troubled over how Lawrence's presence and behavior might distress Maria.[67] She wrote, "the effect on my *poor Maria*! Oh God! His mind is tortured, I suppose, with the idea of hastening her end. I REALLY, my dear friend, do not think so, and if one knew where he was, to endeavour to take this poison from it, he *might* be persuaded to be quiet. Dr. Pearson premis'd from the *very beginning* all that has or is likely to happen to her. But the agonies of this *poor wretch*, if he thinks otherwise, must be INSUPPORTABLE."[68]

In going to Clifton, Lawrence was intent on ensuring his relationship with Sally continued. In a letter to Mrs. Pennington pleading his case, Lawrence acknowledged the charges against him with respect to Maria's consumption. "My name is Lawrence, and you then, I believe, know that I stand in the most afflicting situation possible! A man charg'd (I trust untruly in their lasting effect) with having inflicted pangs on one lovely Creature which, in their bitterest extent, he himself now suffers from her sister!"[69] However, he excused his actions and placed the blame for Maria's ill health upon the invalid and her constitution.

> Miss Maria's situation is, I know, a very dangerous one. *If it is* REALLY *render'd more so by feelings I may have excited, the least mention of me would be hazardous in the extreme.* If it is not, and her complainings on this head are but the weakness of sick fancy, perhaps of Hope, wishing to attribute her illness to any other than the true fix'd CONSTITUTION and alarming cause, still it will be giving an additional distress to her Sister, and afford another opportunity for wounding me with a real, THO' NOT INTENTIONAL, Injustice.[70]

Mrs. Pennington, agreed to meet with the artist but refused to allow him access to either sister, despite his threats of suicide and of running away to Switzerland should he be denied by Sally.[71] Mrs. Pennington apparently relented enough, however, to promise Lawrence updates on the invalid's condition.[72]

While dealing with Lawrence's thoughtless behavior and Maria's worsening illness, the Siddons family was once again reminded of the fragility of their eldest daughter. In September of 1798, Sally was struck down by yet another respiratory attack.

> To the great increase of my cares and anxiety, she has been, for the last week, totally confined to her chamber, and her sweet faculties, for the greater part of that time, locked up by the power of that dangerous medicine, which alone relieves her from the effects of the dreadful constitutional complaint, for which there Appears to be no efficient remedy.[73]

Upon hearing of the seriousness of Sally's attack, which required such high doses of laudanum that she was rendered unconscious for lengthy amounts of time,[74] Lawrence wrote to Mrs. Pennington reassuring her of his devotion.

> Never have I lov'd her more, never with so pure an ardour, as in the last moment of sickness I was witness of (the period she must remember), when, in spite of the intreaties [sic] of her dear Mother and Maria, I stole into her room, and found her unconscious of the step of friend or relation; her faculties ic'd over by that cursed poison, and those sweet eyes unable to interpret the glance that, at that instant, not apathy itself could have mistaken. No, my dear Mrs. P., if her days of sickness trebled those of health, still she should be mine, and dearer than ever to my heart, from the sacrifice of this distrustful and selfish delicacy to confidence and love; from this generous pledge of her esteem and trust in the *heart* of the man she loves.[75]

Although Mrs. Pennington was able to put Lawrence's mind at rest with respect to Sally, Maria's situation was increasingly desperate.[76]

By September, it was obvious that it was but a matter of time before Maria's illness proved fatal. Mrs. Siddons, finally free of her theater commitments, arrived in Clifton on September 24 and moved her daughter across Dowry Square, via sedan chair, to her own lodgings. According to Mrs. Clement Parsons, Mrs. Siddons's fame combined with the tragedy of the unfolding situation to provide the perfect fodder for the gossip columns of the society papers, and journalists jumped on the story as the word spread.[77] Lawrence condemned these journalistic vultures who circled around the dying girl's house in search of a story, writing to Mrs. Pennington, "those unfeeling Blockheads, the Newspaper Writers, have been torturing us with the death at full length. Would to God there was a penalty that might teach them humanity!"[78]

Had these journalists only been privy to the drama unfolding in Maria's sickroom, their prurient interest would have been satisfied. Maria's final moments were not only filled with the ravages of disease, but she remained determined to end the connection between Sally and Lawrence. Mrs. Pennington's correspondence confirmed Lawrence's worst fears: "in her dying accents—her last solemn Injunction was given & repeated some Hours afterwards in the presence of Mrs. Siddons."[79] These deathbed pronouncements were solely concerned with Sally's future, or more correctly with preventing Sally's marriage to Mr. Lawrence. According to Mrs. Pennington, Maria entreated, "Promise me, my Sally, never to be the wife of Mr. L—I <u>cannot BEAR</u> to <u>think</u> of <u>your</u> <u>being so</u>." Sally tried her best to avoid making such a promise, and attempted to distract her sister from her purpose saying, "dear Maria, think of nothing that agitates you at this time." Maria denied that the subject upset her, "but that it was necessary to her repose to pursue the subject." When Sally said "Oh! it is impossible," by which she meant that she was unable to "answer for herself," Maria took the exclamation to mean that it was the marriage that was impossible and responded, "I am content, my dear Sister, I am satisfied."[80] Maria had placed her sister in an untenable position, claiming that she was only acting out of concern for Sally's welfare. Yet Sally was now in an insupportable situation, one made more so by the exchange with Mrs. Siddons that followed.

When Mrs. Siddons returned to Maria's side, the girl, according to Mrs. Pennington, "desired to have Prayers read & followed her angelic mother, who read them, and who appear'd like a blessed spirit ministering about her, with the utmost clearness, accuracy, & fervor."[81] Maria's mind did not long remain on her devotions, however, as she turned once again to the subject of Lawrence. She implored her mother to ensure that he had done as promised and destroyed her letters.

> "<u>That man</u> told you, Mother, he <u>had</u> destroy'd my Letters. <u>I</u> have no opinion of his honor, and I entreat you to demand them" . . . She then said, "Sally <u>had promised her NEVER</u> to think of an union with Mr. L" & appeal'd to her Weeping Sister to confirm it—who, quite overcome, reply'd—"I did <u>not</u> promise, dear, dying Angel—but I <u>WILL</u> & <u>Do</u>, if you require it."—"Thank you, Sally; my dear Mother—Mrs. Pennington—bear witness. Sally, give me your hand—you promise never to be his wife—Mother, Mrs. Pennington—lay your hands on hers" (we did so).—"You understand? bear witness." We bow'd, & were speechless. —"Sally- sacred, sacred be this promise "—<u>stretching</u> out her <u>hand</u>, & pointing her forefinger—"<u>REMEMBER ME</u>, & God bless you!"[82]

And so it was done. As Sally could not honorably deny her sister's final request, she asked Mrs. Pennington to make it clear to Lawrence that she intended to abide by her promise. "And what after <u>this</u> my <u>Friend</u>, can <u>you</u> say to <u>SALLY</u> Siddons? <u>SHE</u> has entreated <u>me</u> to give you this detail—to say that the impression <u>IS</u> sacred, <u>IS</u> indelible—that it <u>cancels</u> all <u>former</u> bonds and Engagements—that she entreats you to submit, and not to prophane the present awful season by a murmur."[83] Maria finally succumbed to consumption on October 7, 1798 and was buried on October 10 at the old Parish church (St. Andrews) in Clifton.[84]

A Beautiful Ending?

Mrs. Pennington's recounting of Maria's illness and death to friends, family, and erstwhile suitors broadly conformed to the general expectations of consumption in the sentimental tradition. Even a month before the end, she was applying sentimental rhetoric to Maria's illness, describing her decline in the following manner: "The Lamp emits each day a rather more feeble ray. Yet all is lovely and interesting!"[85] Mrs. Pennington's detailed descriptions of Maria's final hours revealed the difficulties faced by those seeking to accommodate the dominant representations of consumption, which tended to rest on stylized description, with the brutal progress of the disease. In a clear departure from the notion of a gentle death, she wrote of Maria that "her pains were almost incessant," however, in the same sentence she also stated that "her intellects seemed to gain strength & clearness."[86] Thus, despite occasionally delving into the terrible realities of a death from consumption, Mrs. Pennington mostly stuck to the sentimental script. In a letter written the day after Maria's death, Mrs. Pennington described a deathbed scene worthy of the best novel, as well as one in keeping with the tradition surrounding tuberculosis. "If ever Creature was operated on by the <u>immediate</u> Power & Spirit of God," she wrote, "it was Maria Siddons, in the last 48 hours of her life."[87]

Maria's disease and death were also accorded a full measure of beautification, although the reality was quite different. Up until the very end, Maria's beauty had been unquestioned and her countenance had only been referred to as interesting or lovely. However, in her final days, even Mrs. Pennington could not deny the devastation consumption had wrought upon the young girl, writing, "Not one trace of even *prettiness* remaining—all ghastly expression, and sad discolouration!!"[88] Despite this unflattering description, it was not the havoc produced by the disease that prevailed in Mrs. Pennington's accounts of the final moments of Maria's life. Instead, she wrote of the power of the disease to elevate the girl's beauty beyond even what she had possessed in life. She told Lawrence, "Yet this dear, faded creature, in her latter hours, resumed a Grace & Beauty that, in true Interest, surpass'd her most blooming days."[89] Indeed, she even went so far as to state that a few hours before her death Maria possessed a countenance "that the Painter or the Sculptor with all their art could never reach!"[90]

Mrs. Pennington softened the truth of Maria's death from tuberculosis by claiming it enhanced both her spiritual and physical attractiveness. This perceived power of consumption to beautify its victim, was common in the sentimentalized mythology of the disease and was one that Mrs. Pennington mined again and again in her letters to Lawrence.[91] She wrote that Maria's "<u>last</u> attitude! . . . was Beauty & Grace itself!!—Such a Serenity! Such a divine composure! She took leave of us all with tenderness unbounded."[92] Despite her apparent serenity, there was an acerbic moment, as the subject of Lawrence once again cropped up. Maria laid her death at his door declaring, "Oh! my dear Mother, there will be no Peace but in breaking all tyes with <u>that man</u>. He has . . . been my death."[93] Mrs. Pennington seemed to be in accord with this statement, believing that Lawrence bore some responsibility for the girl's demise, and implored the painter to master his "Passions" and "let not Maria Siddons have died in vain."[94] This link between a disappointment in love and consumption was a commonly cited cause of the illness and certainly part of the literary traditions involving the disease.[95]

Mrs. Pennington went a step further by comparing Maria's death to those of a wealth of sentimental consumptive heroines. Writing, "we have read the death-bed scenes of Clarissa & Eloisa, drawn as they are by the Hands of Genius & embellish'd with all that skilful & powerful fancy . . . believe me they are faint Sketches compared with those last Hours [of] Maria Siddons, where Nature supplied touches that Art cou'd never reach."[96] Clarissa and Eloisa were references to characters in Samuel Richardson's novel of the same name, first published in 1748, and Jean-Jacques Rousseau's Eloise.[97] The choice of Clarissa as comparison for Maria was particularly pertinent, as the heroine's death from consumption embraced all the various traditions associated with that disease. Her death in the novel was an intricate composition that reflected the gendered debates

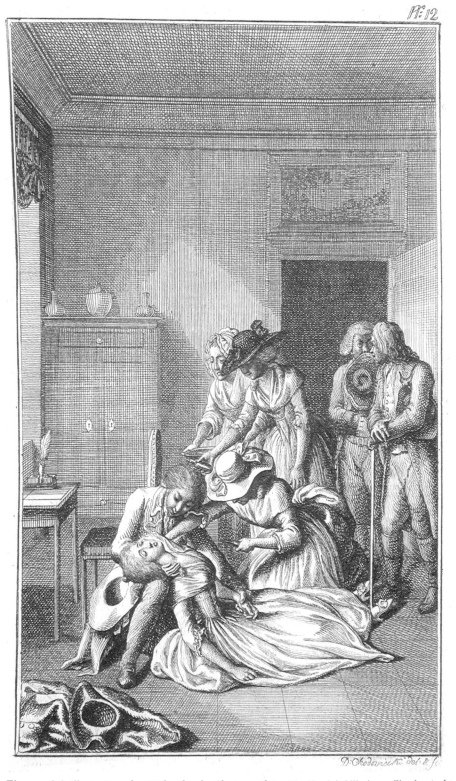

Figure 6.4 Illustration for Richardson's *Clarissa*, Plate 12. Daniel Nikolaus Chodowiecki (Germany, 1785). LACMA Image Library.

surrounding consumption during the period. Although difficult to diagnose and lacking a clear articulation of the actual ailment, Clarissa was brought low by a variety of factors that point to the disease, including providing a role for grief as a cause of the affliction and the utilization of the term decline, which was a common metaphor for tuberculosis.[98] Certainly, Margaret Ann Doody contends that consumption was the cause.[99] While Clark Lawlor has argued that Clarissa's consumptive death became an archetype in Britain, one that "combines a good death and the typically female death of pining for a lost love object in a form of Neo-Platonic ascension from secular to religious love."[100] Clarissa's death, he states, expanded the prescribed consumptive death beyond the older deathbed traditions to encompass not only the Protestant tradition of the "good death," but also elements of sensibility by providing a role for love, melancholy, and the passions. For Lawlor, Clarissa provided the template for any future sentimental representations of the death of a female from consumption, and he asserts that, "by providing an extended process of aestheticised consumptive death, Richardson showed a new way of understanding the relationship between disease and gender."[101] Clarissa's deathbed, styled a "happy exit,"[102] was described in detail in the work. Witnesses remarked, "we could not help taking a view of the lovely corpse, and admiring the charming serenity of her noble aspect. The women declared, they never saw death so lovely before; and that she looked as if in an easy slumber, the colour having not quite left her cheeks and lips."[103]

The accounts of the death of Maria Siddons drew upon a sentimental formula, grounded in a cycle of images and deathbed tableaux, literary and visual, reaching back to Richardson's novel.[104] Maria's death moved all those who witnessed her final moments or heard of them. Hence, her loved ones constructed an illness narrative that spoke to the dominant representations of consumption, and there seemed to be a conscious decision on the part of family and friends to insert Maria into the sentimental traditions so prevalent in accounts of the disease, and in doing so to provide meaning beyond the rather sad end of a young girl. Mrs. Pennington's reading of Maria's illness would dominate all of the other posthumous accounts.

Although Mrs. Siddons was present for her daughter's death, her impressions during the course of Maria's illness came primarily from Mrs. Pennington's and Sally's readings of the situation. Like her friend, Mrs. Siddons also wrapped a blanket of sentimentality around her deceased daughter, writing to Mrs. Barrington twelve days after Maria's death,

> This sad event I have long been prepared for, and bow with humble resignation to the decree of that merciful God who has taken the dear angel I must ever tenderly lament the loss of, from this scene of certain misery to his eternal and unspeakable blessedness . . . Oh that you were here that I might be able to talk to you of a Death-bed. In dignity of mind & pious resignation, forsaking all that the imaginations of Rousseau of Richardson have given as in those of Gloria [Eloise] or Clarissa Winslow [Harlowe] —for this was I believe from the immediate power and inspiration of the <u>Divinity himself.</u>[105]

Mrs. Piozzi, the friend of both Mrs. Pennington and Mrs. Siddons, also provided a reading of Maria's death that not only fully participated in the application of the rhetoric of the consumptive heroine but also consciously admitted to doing so. Mrs. Piozzi even went so far as to write to Mrs. Pennington that the death of Admiral Nelson would "not be half as much regretted as is the lovely object of your late attention."

> Every letter I receive . . . is filled with her praise, and breathes an unfeigned sorrow for her loss. Virtue well tried through many a refining fire, Learning lost to the world she illuminated, and Courage taken from the Island protected by her arms, excites not as much sorrow as Maria Siddons, represented to every imagination as sweet, and gentle, and soothing; as young in short, for in youth lies every charm.[106]

Just ten days after this letter, in which she fully participated in sentimentalizing Maria's death, Mrs. Piozzi admitted to another correspondent that the representations and virtues granted posthumously to Maria Siddons may not have been entirely accurate and instead had been assigned in proportion to her "youthful beauty." Again, Maria's youth and beauty were integral in the readings of her consumptive death and Mrs. Piozzi wrote:

> Have you seen the death of a charming girl in the papers, whose long and severe sufferings interest all her friends, and have half broken her sweet mother's heart! Maria Siddons! More lamented, I do think, than virtue, value, and science all combined would be. But she had youthful beauty; and to that quality our fond imaginations never fail to affix softness of temper and gentle spirit, every charm resident in female minds.[107]

Other parts of Maria's deathbed performance also call into question the sentimentalized aspects of her final days. Arguably her emotional blackmail of Sally into giving up any future with Lawrence was mean-spirited, petty, and vindictive, despite her professed motivation of protecting her sister. Maria's aunt, Mrs. Twiss, conceded that Maria's behavior had been less than noble at the end and labeled her actions as extortion; while Sally believed that Maria had been motivated "as much by resentment for <u>him</u>, [Lawrence] as care and tenderness for <u>her</u>."[108] Despite the inconsistencies of Maria's behavior with sentimental deathbed performances, and the acknowledgments of the conscious application of sentimental virtues to her final days and death, overwhelmingly the posthumous treatments of the young woman match the fanciful representations of a death from consumption in contemporary literature. In the end, Maria Siddons was laid to rest with an epitaph as sentimental as the descriptions of her death proved to be. It was crowned by a verse taken from Edward Young's epic poem *Night Thoughts* (1742). "Early, bright, transient, chaste as morning dew, She sparkled, was exhaled, and went to Heaven."[109]

Mrs. Siddons's grief did not end with Maria's death, as Sally also succumbed to a chronic respiratory illness in March of 1803. Sally and Maria's deaths affected the ways in which Mrs. Siddons viewed her remaining daughter, Cecilia, and she wrote to a friend, "alas! She [Cecilia] too has I fear that fatal tendency in her Constitution which has already cost us so many hours of afflicting Anxiety—She is at present quite well, but so was dear Maria too, at her age."[110] In another letter in the summer of 1803, Mrs. Siddons once again lamented her daughters' deaths and expressed a growing concern for her only remaining daughter.

> Two lovely creatures gone; and another is just arrived from school with all the dazzling, frightful sort of beauty that irradiated the countenance of Maria, and makes me shudder when I look at her. I feel myself, like poor Niobe, grasping to her bosom the last and youngest of her children; and, like her, look every moment for the vengeful arrow of destruction.[111]

Fortunately, despite Cecilia's beauty, this pronouncement proved untrue. Mrs. Siddons' remaining daughter outlived her.

The chasm that existed between the gruesome biological manifestations of consumption and the comparatively positive representations employed as part of the socio-cultural strategies for experiencing that illness are evident in the assessment and representations of the death of Maria Siddons. The dichotomy between the reality of a consumptive death and the sentimentalized presentation of that end were apparent not only during Maria's illness and death, but also in the reactions of her family. Sensibility melded with concepts of beauty and consumption to aid in orchestrating a disease experience and deathbed in which love, disappointment, constitution, and beauty were all explicitly linked in a manner consistent with the ever more powerful rhetoric of consumption.

CHAPTER 7
DYING TO BE BEAUTIFUL: THE CONSUMPTIVE CHIC

During the late eighteenth and early nineteenth centuries, there was a recognition of consumption's connection to aesthetics, and a belief that the disease actually had the ability to create or enhance beauty. Tuberculosis became the site of a battle between professional and popular ideologies of disease—a conflict that played out both in beauty practices and dress. Nineteenth-century notions of respectability and prescribed gender ideologies were of particular importance in shaping these developments. In the upper- and middle-class incarnation, representations of consumption presented the illness as the author of a feminine beauty that was identified with its condemned victims as their lives trickled away. Instead of the afflicted becoming unrecognizable as she deteriorated, the wasting associated with the disease was twinned with ideas of beauty. In other depictions, particularly in the lower classes, consumption was set forth as an illness that disfigured and provided a striking symbol of hard labor. For instance, Thomas Beddoes remarked, "The disorder, however, shews itself in a different form, especially in poor families, where children are fed on water-gruel and potatoes. The countenance is then pale, bloated, and what medical writers term *cachectic*. The upper lip is particularly tumid. The eyes are dull instead of bright. Privation and pain necessarily produce ill temper, and sometimes stupidity."[1]

In the first half of the nineteenth century, the belief that a sensitive nature was a cause of the illness remained; however, both the consumptive look and the notion of sensitivity as a cause moved away from the Romantic male and came to be identified almost exclusively with respectable women. Women possessed an excess of physical sensibility, which translated into a code of propriety and social sensibility, one attributed to nervousness and physical delicacy. These features balanced the nineteenth-century female precariously on the edge of pathology.[2] During this period, there was a tubercular moment during which consumption became the dominant "fashionable disease," and the one most closely connected to beauty and fashion for women. Clark Lawlor asserts that "By the end of the eighteenth century, consumption" was "the glamorous sign of female beauty."[3] Likewise, Roy Porter has acknowledged, that "bright young things, seeking public attention, positively sought to look tubercular, as if delicacy and a tenuous grasp on life made them all the more appealing . . . Through association with fine sensibility and the cult of youth, the tubercular look—indeed tuberculosis— was becoming positively *de rigeur*."[4]

This curious convergence of illness and aesthetics was not just the product of literary minds but was also reinforced in the works of medical men, and those concerned with social instruction. The representations of consumption were remarkably positive, and ignored the unpleasant realities of a disease characterized by wasting, incessant diarrhea, coughing, and the expectoration of blood and phlegm. *The London Medical and Surgical Journal* certainly participated in perpetuating this ideology in 1833 writing,

> Some diseases are borne in silence and concealment, because their phenomena are calculated to excite disgust; to others, the result of vicious courses, the stigma of disgrace is attached; unsightly ravages of the human frame, or the wreck of the mental faculties, inspire us with horror rather than with sympathy; but consumption, neither effacing the lines of personal beauty, nor damaging the intellectual functions, tends to exalt the moral habits, and develop the amiable qualities of the patient.[5]

Consumptive Chic

Increasingly, those women who suffered from consumption were lauded for their delicate (almost otherworldly) beauty that was characterized by pallor, slenderness, and transparency.[6]

From Corpulent to Consumptive Chic

Consumption was not the only disease to influence popular ideas and fashions. Like tuberculosis, dropsy became the focus of the clinical, anatomico-pathological approach to disease, and also had its own set of cultural themes.[7] Dropsy and consumption provide differing illustrations of the ways in which the diseased body was viewed. A renal illness (later termed Bright's disease), dropsy was, like consumption, widespread, fatal in its final phases and produced visible alterations in the patient's body. The characteristic signifier of consumption was a wasting and emaciation that weakened and shriveled the body; dropsy, however, manifested in the severe bloating of its victim.[8] The extreme and opposite nature of the symptoms led these diseases to be utilized as foils for one another in caricatures. Although an obvious exaggeration, caricature, as Peter McNeil asserts, moves beyond social commentary and can also represent "contemporary understandings of idealized aesthetics." Drawing on Hannah Greig, he further states that caricature connects not only to fashion but "also rested upon a metropolitan notion of the beau monde, in which the elites could recognize references to each other."[9] While Dror Wahrman has argued that caricature draws "on recognizable social behavior" and represents "the excess rather than the antithesis of acceptable . . . modes of behavior."[10] As a consequence, caricature, like literature, medical treatises, and fashion periodicals provides another media form through which popular notions of consumption and fashion could be negotiated and represented. Dropsy also provided an early example of an illness being blamed for creating a fashion. In 1793, The Times asserted that the "pigeon-breasted" fashion of the day was an emulation of the disease.

> The Fashion of dressing at present is to appear *prominent*; and the *stays* are made accordingly. This is holding out a wish to be thought in a thriving way, even without the authority of the *Arches Court* of Canterbury—something in the French way—a philosophical desire to be *conspicuously great* with MISCHIEF, without regard to law of reason. The idea was first sent forward by a few *dropsical* Ladies.[11]

Dropsy's role in defining fashion was short-lived however, and increasingly tuberculosis would be the illness most connected with fashion and beauty, its rise to prominence aided by the growing backlash against dropsical corpulence and excess flesh in descriptions of beauty.[12] (See Plates 18 & 19.)

In the second half of the eighteenth century there was a growing fashion for thinness and there arose, according to Roy Porter, "a new cult of the lithe, limber, slim body indicative of delicacy and fineness of sensibility."[13] Litheness would, by the latter part of the eighteenth century, become visible in sartorial choices,[14] and the growing stress on the desirability of a thin body for women in particular, was allied to the emerging culture of sensibility in helping to define refinement. As a result, by the nineteenth century, consumption, beauty, and intelligence were intimately related in the popular imagination. Bodily conformation was connected to intellectual capacity, and corpulence was increasingly deemed unattractive, particularly as it was believed to enfeeble mental energy. "Fat and stupidity" were conceived as "inseparable companions" and used synonymously.[15] These judgments were not limited to medical texts but were also delineated in popular works. For instance, an 1824 article in *The New Monthly Magazine and Literary Journal* presented the new view of the nerves, intelligence, and the sensibility of the individual suffering from corpulence, arguing, "The insensibility and stupidity of corpulent persons go hand in hand with this disease [corpulence]; for the fat covers and buries the nerves."[16] Other works proposed that on an anatomical level, fat itself was "totally insensible";

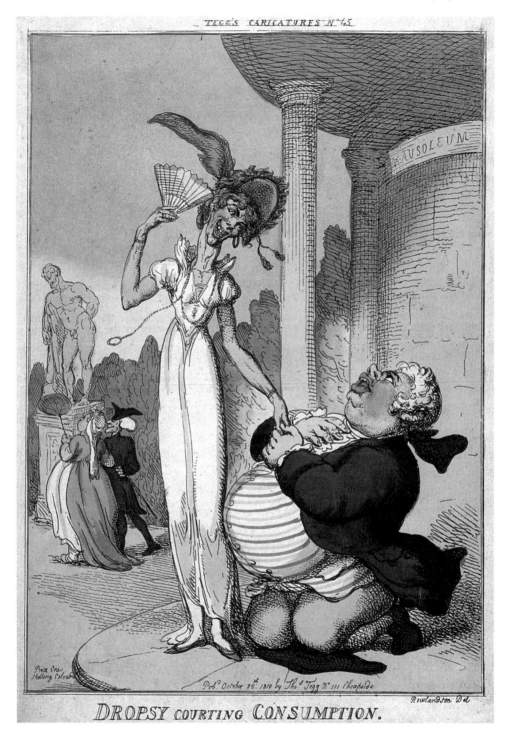

Figure 7.1 "Dropsy Courting Consumption." An obese man wooing a tall lean woman outside a mausoleum; representing dropsy and consumption. Colored etching by T. Rowlandson (London: Thos. Tegg, 1810). Wellcome Library, London. Copyrighted work available under Creative Commons Attribution only licence CC BY 4.0 http://creativecommons.org/licenses/by/4.0/

corpulence then "ought to be as anxiously remedied . . . for it is no less an enemy to health, than to beauty of the figure."[17] The physiologist Alexander Walker took this notion even further stating, "Fat women . . . have not only less sensibility and irritability of the skin, but of the organs of sense generally . . . thinner animals on the contrary have more acute sensibility and among women, more brilliant eyes."[18] In connecting thinness to the feminizing quality of sensibility, these works tightened the connections between femininity and the desirability of a thin body. All of these notions combined with the long tradition of consumption as an easy death, to create a vision of tuberculosis as imparting a slender and delicate appearance that enhanced rather than destroyed the beauty of the female form.[19]

Fashionable Illness

During the eighteenth century there was an extensive examination by physicians like George Cheyne, Thomas Beddoes, and James Makittrick Adair of the relationship between certain illnesses and the quality of sensibility associated with the fashionable elite.[20] Diseases like melancholia, gout, and consumption became associated with the refined members of society and, as Adair suggested, the "great and opulent" were subject to the whims of fashion "in their choice of diseases."[21] Sir William Temple lamented the practice in 1809, likening the popularity for illness and their treatments as being "very much seen or heard of at one season, disappearing in another."[22] As diseases could be fashionable, they also became targets for emulation. Adair certainly carped that "people of no rank and slender means" attempted to transgress social boundaries by "fashionably ruining themselves."[23]

As a fashionable illness, consumption was distinguished by a translucent white complexion. Despite admitting that the disease was "the king of terrors and paleness," *The Lady's Magazine* emphasized beauty as the dominant representation of this illness for its readers in a 1790 essay. According to the author, "in the last stage of a consumption a lady may exhibit the roses and lilies of youth and health, and be admired for her complexion—the day she is to be buried."[24] Consumption's allure lay in the fact that its symptomology operated within the established parameters of attractiveness. Rosy cheeks and lips coupled with pale skin were qualities with an established pedigree in the definitions of beauty. They were also the product of phthisis. The delicate red of the hectic flush, illuminating the consumptive pallor, were symptoms by which the disease could be identified.

The tubercular appeal was also intensified by the growing rhetoric equating women with fragility, a notion then explicitly connected to beauty.[25] In the first half of the eighteenth century, physicians like George Cheyne helped lay the groundwork for the assertion that "refinement meant delicacy"[26] and that beauty relied on the appearance of delicacy.[27] These connections were strengthened in 1757 when Edmund Burke argued that beauty was a socially affirmative quality, one he defined as any attribute that inspired affection. The beautiful was characterized by delicacy; it was tranquil, composed, bright, gentle, and joyful. Burke's assertions complemented those made by physicians and social commentators. In 1774, *The Lady's Magazine* weighed in on this debate, arguing "Many disorders incident to the higher ranks of life, among the ladies especially, of our own nation, are, doubtless, owing to that false delicacy which . . . bestows in return that pallid hue, those irritable nerves, and those general principles of weakness and a diseased constitution, so very prevalent in the sex." The author went on to state "that delicacy is an essential in the composition of female beauty, and that strength and robustness are contrary to the idea of it, nay even fragility is consistent with it. The beauty of women is greatly owing to their delicacy or weakness."[28] While George Keate's *Sketches from Nature* (1790) acknowledged the dominance of Burke's approach, "Robustness and strength do not raise in us the sense of beauty . . . Delicate and almost fragile things are beautiful," he then explicitly linked "delicate-transparent

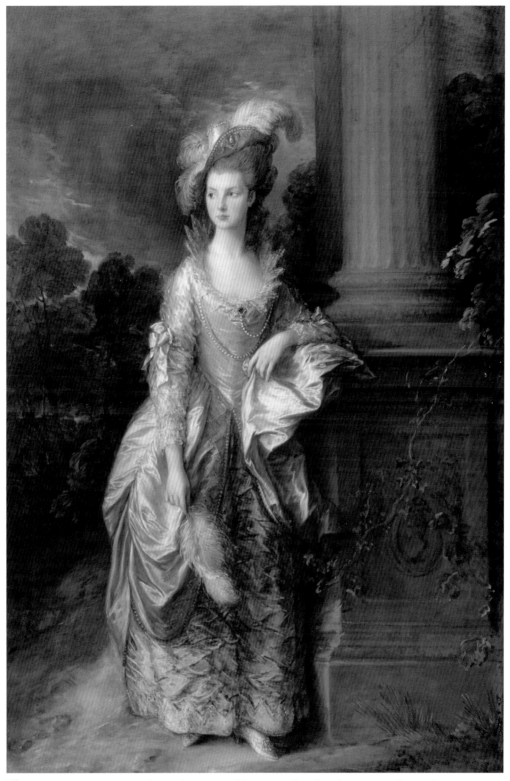

Plate 1 Hon. Mrs. Mary Graham. *The Honourable Mrs Graham* by Thomas Gainsborough. Acc. No. NG 332. Credit Bequest of Robert Graham of Redgorton 1859. © The National Gallery, Scotland.

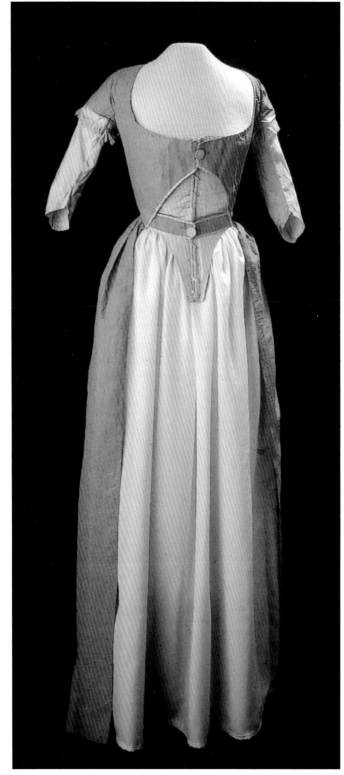

Plate 2 Day Dress worn by Hon. Mrs. Graham, c.1790–1792 (Private Collection). Reproduced with the kind permission of Claudia and Robert Maxton-Graham.

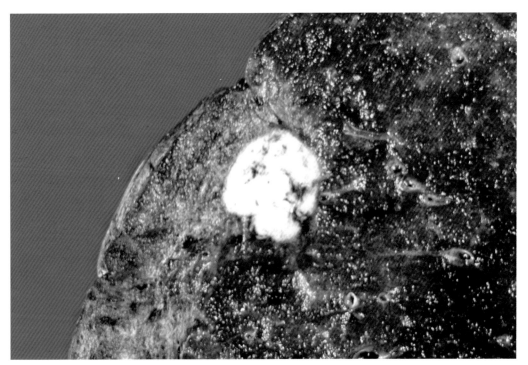

Plate 3 Pulmonary tubercle. Cross-section of lung showing a large, well defined tuberculous lesion. Wellcome Library, London.

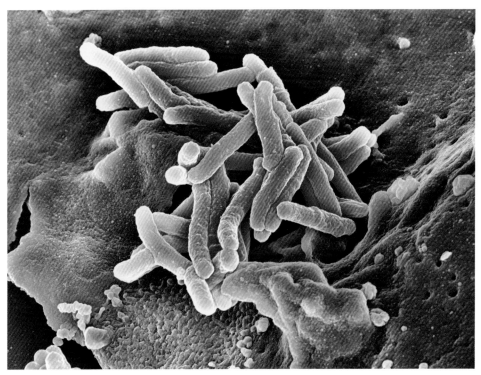

Plate 4 Macrophage engulfing TB bacteria. Colored scanning electron micrograph (SEM) of a macrophage white blood cell engulfing a tuberculosis (*Mycobacterium tuberculosis*) bacterium (orange). Science Photo Library/Getty Images.

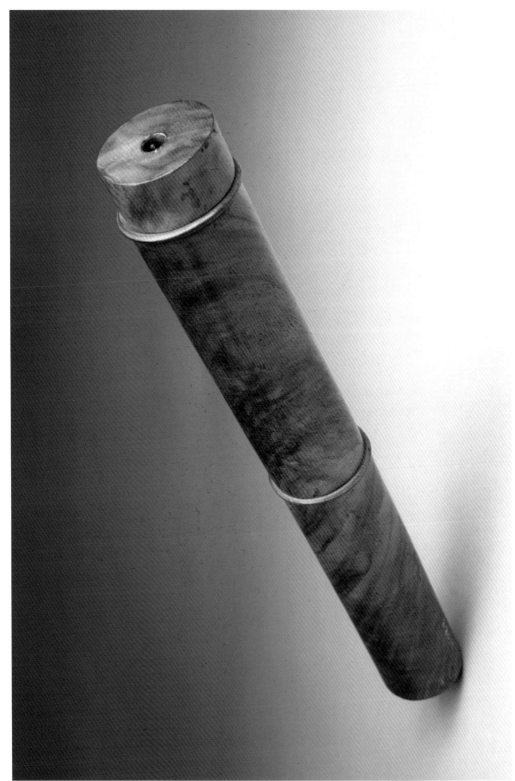

Plate 5 Laennec-type monaural stethoscope. Wellcome Library, London. Copyrighted work available under Creative Commons Attribution only licence CC BY 4.0 http://creativecommons.org/licenses/by/4.0/

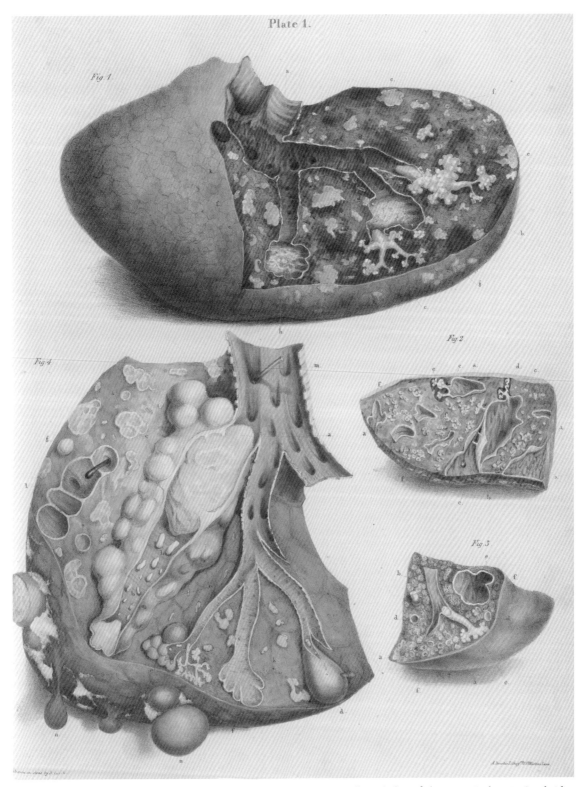

Plate 6 Robert Carswell's illustration of the tuberculous lung. Carswell, *Pathological Anatomy*, Path.a.32, Cambridge University Library.

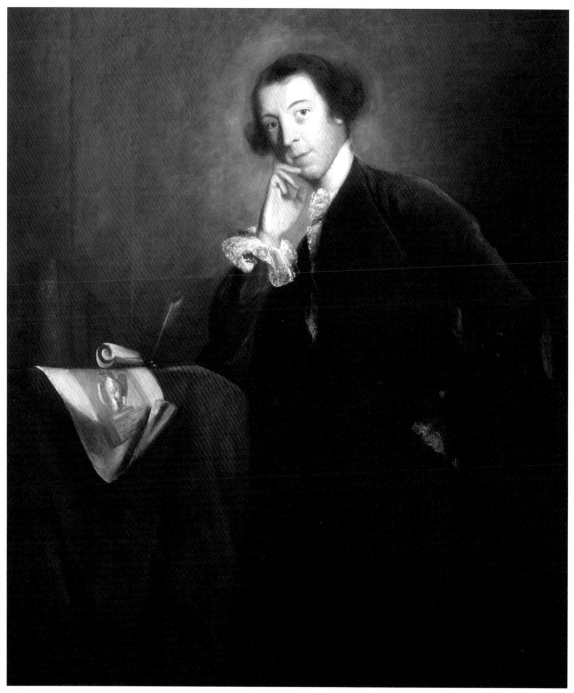

Plate 7 Horace Walpole by Sir Joshua Reynolds, c.1756–1757. NPG 6520. © National Portrait Gallery, London.

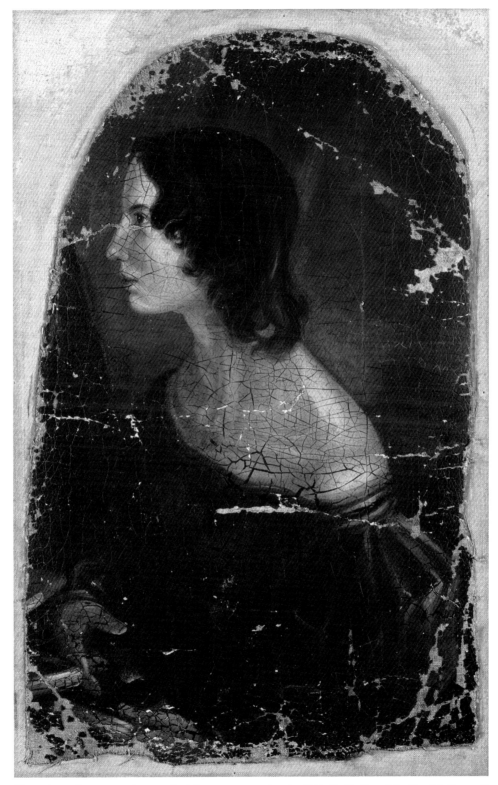

Plate 8 Emily Brontë who perished from consumption in 1848. Emily Brontë by Patrick Branwell Brontë, NPG 1724, © National Portrait Gallery, London. (The sitter is in dispute and may actually be Anne who also perished from consumption in 1849.)

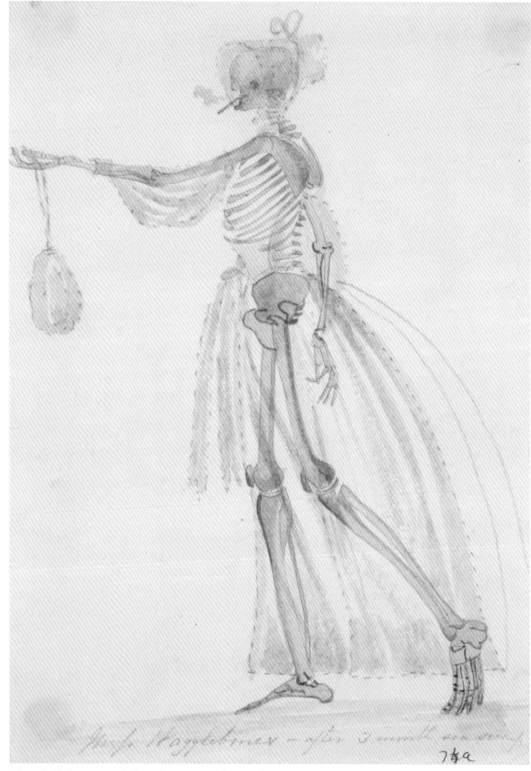

Plate 9 Skeleton in pink dress. "Miss Wagglebones-after 3 month's sea-sickness." © The British Library Board, John Brownrigg Belasis, WD 1478 page 74a. Pencil, watercolor, c13512-96.

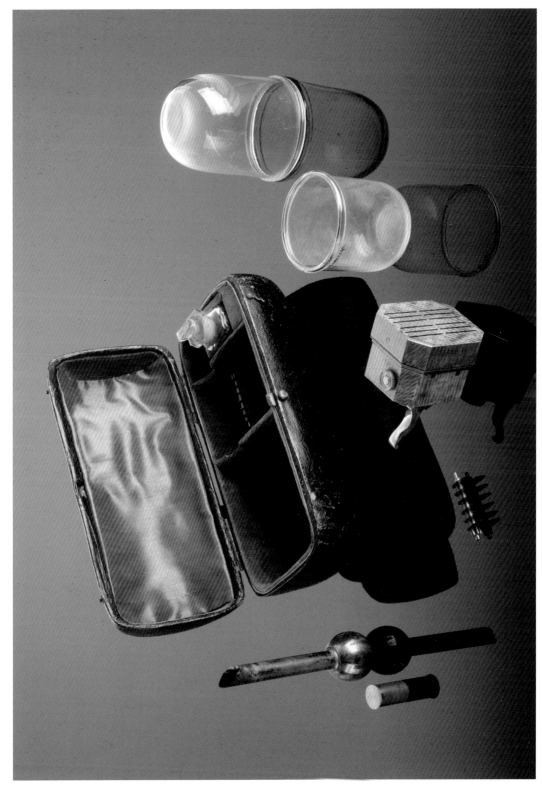

Plate 10 Cupping set with scarifier. Science Museum A606733. Wellcome Library, London. Copyrighted work available under Creative Commons Attribution only licence CC BY 4.0 http://creativecommons.org/licenses/by/4.0/

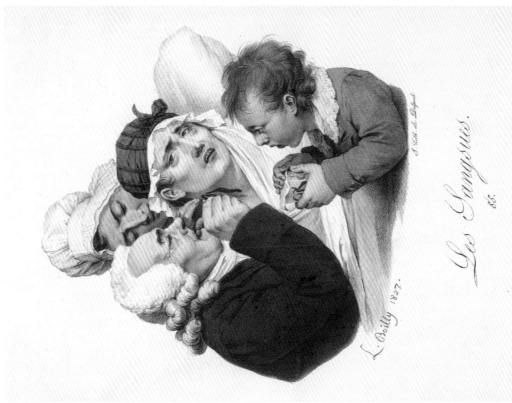

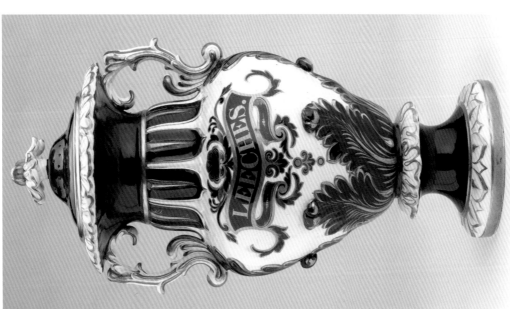

Plate 11 Leeches. Left: Pharmacy leech jar by Alcock at Hill Pottery, Burslem, England, 1831–1859. Science Museum A43107. Right: Louis Boilly after François Séraphin Delpech. A faint-looking woman is supported as the doctor carefully applies the leeches to her neck. (Paris:1827). Wellcome Library, London. Copyrighted work available under Creative Commons Attribution only licence CC BY 4.0 http://creativecommons.org/licenses/by/4.0/

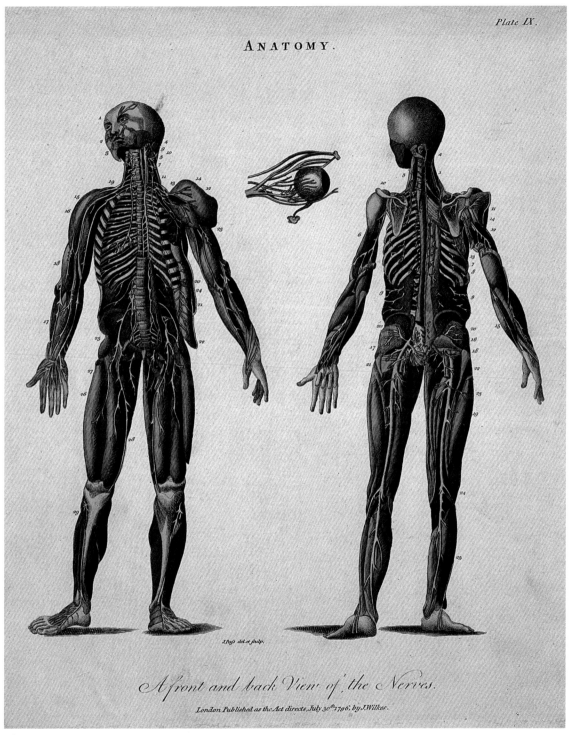

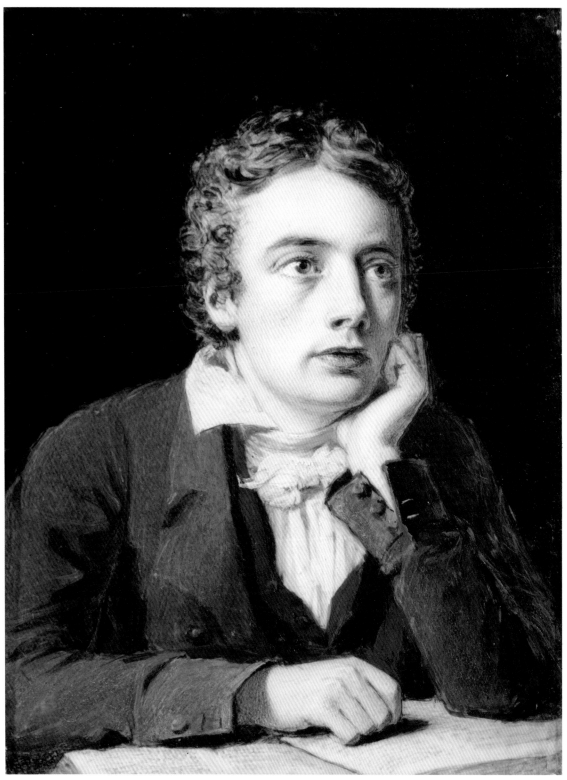

Plate 13 John Keats by Joseph Severn, 1819. © National Portrait Gallery, London.

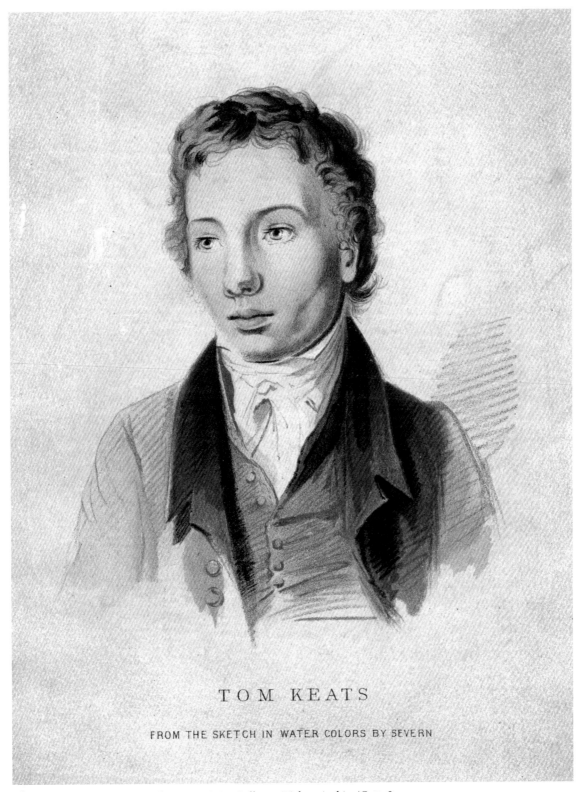

TOM KEATS

FROM THE SKETCH IN WATER COLORS BY SEVERN

Plate 14 Tom Keats, nineteenth century. Print Collector/Hulton Archive/Getty Images.

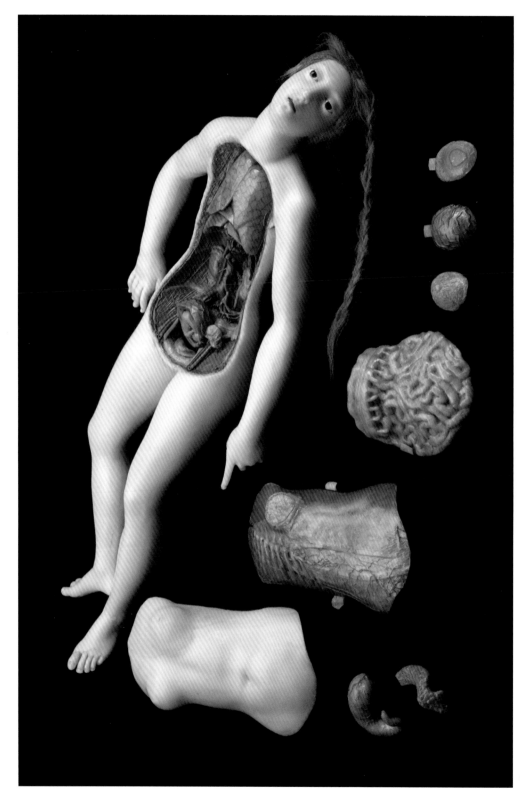

Plate 15 Wax anatomical Venus. Inspired by artistic positions, "Venuses" or female wax anatomical models demonstrated more than simple physical differences between men and women but also demonstrate the gendered perceptions of the period. Maker: Susini, Clemente, made in Florence, Italy (1771–1800). Science Museum A627043. Copyrighted work available under Creative Commons Attribution only licence CC BY 4.0 http://creativecommons.org/licenses/by/4.0/

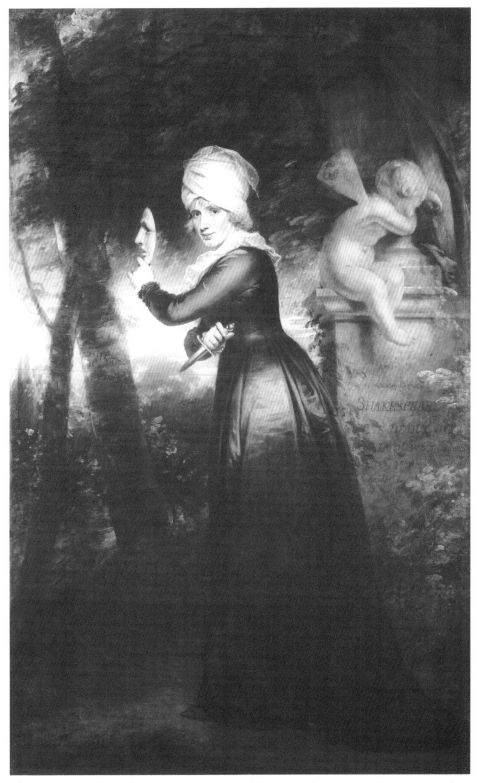

Plate 16 "Mrs Siddons with the Emblems of Tragedy." Sarah Siddons by Sir William Beechey, oil on canvas, 1793. NPG 5159. © National Portrait Gallery, London.

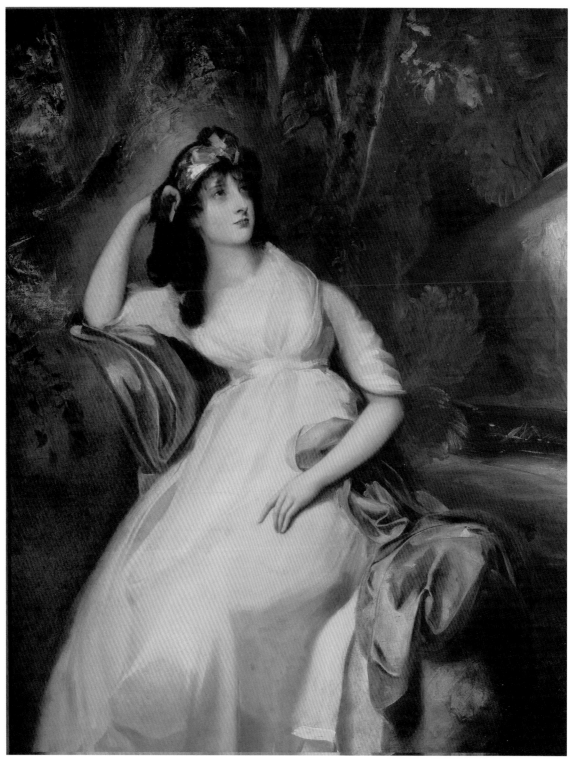

Plate 17 Portrait of Sally Siddons by Sir Thomas Lawrence, c.1795. Private Collection. Fine Art Images/Heritage Images/ Getty Images.

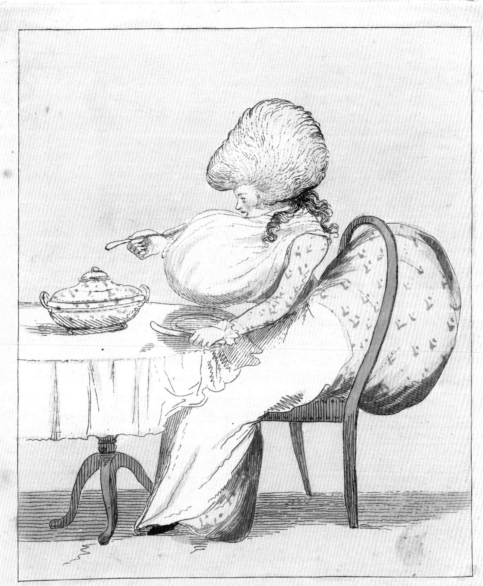

THE INCONVENIENCE OF DRESS

Rage for Dress —— Bewitching passion!
Who'd not starve to lead the Fashion?
Starve! where's the Beaux so very dull,
To think they'll starve with crops so full?
Published 19.ᵗʰ May 1786, by S. W. Fores, at the Caricature Warehouse, N.º 3 Piccadilly.

Plate 18 Caricaturizing the pigeon-breasted fashions. George Townly Stubbs, *The Inconvenience of Dress* (London: S.W. Fores, 1786). Image number: lwlpr05984. Courtesy of The Lewis Walpole Library, Yale University.

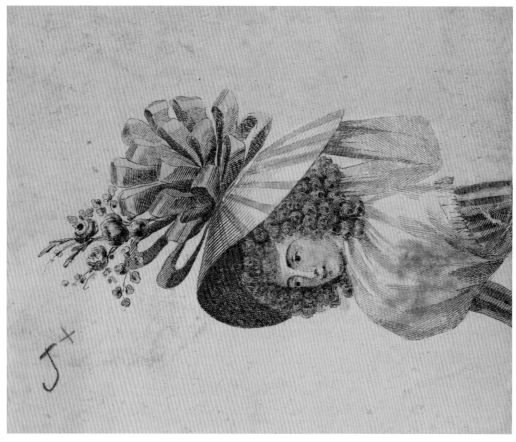

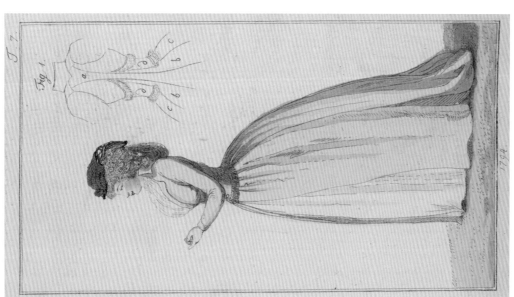

Plate 19 1790s fashions. Left: Hand-colored engraving, France, 1794. Right: Hand-colored engraving showing a woman wearing an elaborate hat and hairstyle. France c.1790. Museum number: E.21620-1957. © Victoria and Albert Museum.

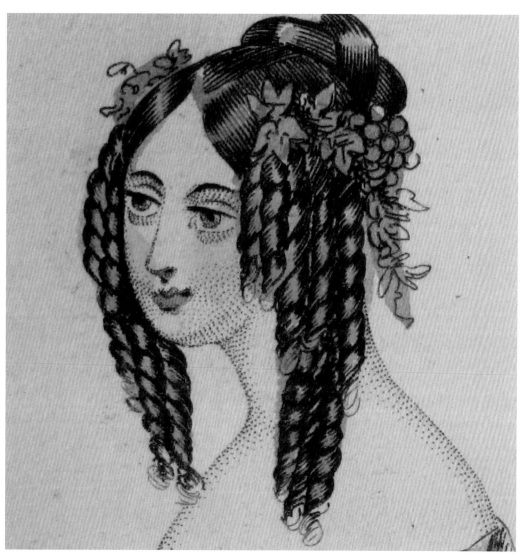

Plate 20 Windows of the Soul. Fashion Plate from *The New Monthly Belle Assemblée*, Vol. XXIV (London: Joseph Rogerson, 1846). Image provided by Louisiana State University Special Collections.

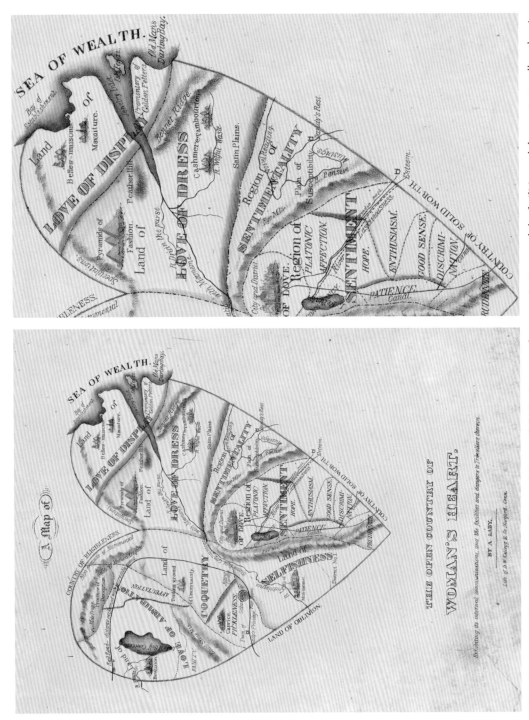

Plate 21 A map of the open country of woman's heart exhibiting its internal communications, and the facilities and dangers to travellers therein. By a lady. (Hartford: Lith. of D. W. Kellogg & Co. Hartford, Conn., between 1833 and 1842). Courtesy, American Antiquarian Society.

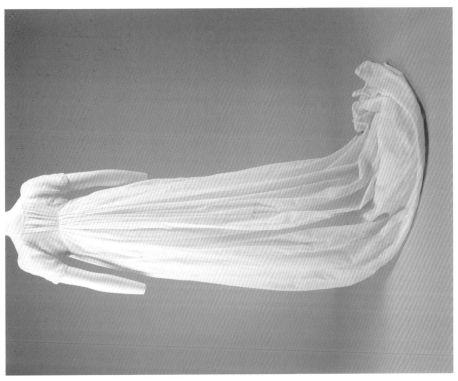

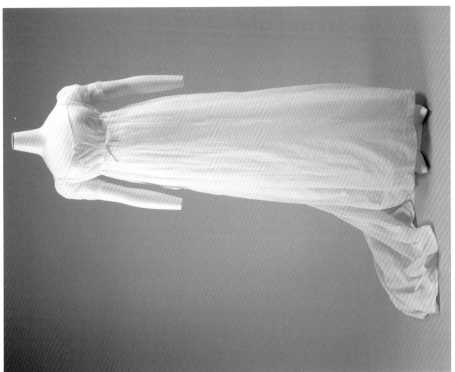

Plate 22 English example of neoclassical dress with train (front and back), c.1803. Accession number: 1983.401.1. Courtesy of the Metropolitan Museum of Art, New York.

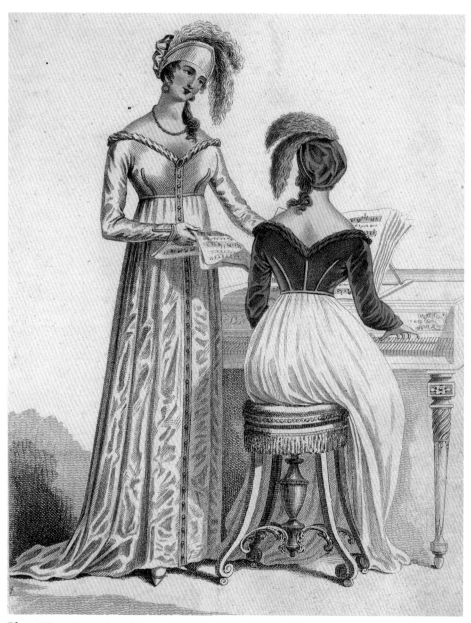

Plate 23 Fashion plate illustrating the highlighting of the décolletage and posterior furrow. "Evening Full Dress 1810," *La Belle Assemblée,* Vol. I (London: J. Bell, 1810.) Casey Fashion Plates, Los Angeles Public Library.

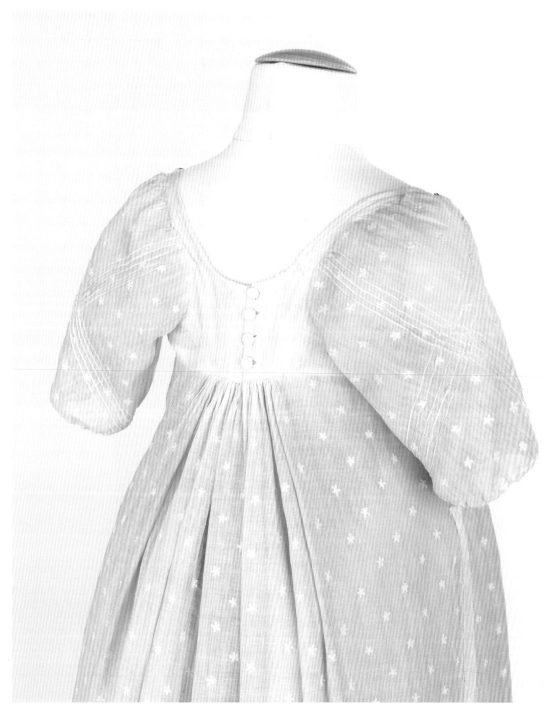

Plate 24 Dress (1809) illustrating the low back that would have showcased the backbones. Evening Dress 1809 (French). Accession number: 2009.300.1806. Brooklyn Museum Costume Collection at The Metropolitan Museum of Art, Gift of the Brooklyn Museum, 2009; Gift of Theodora Wilbour, 1947.

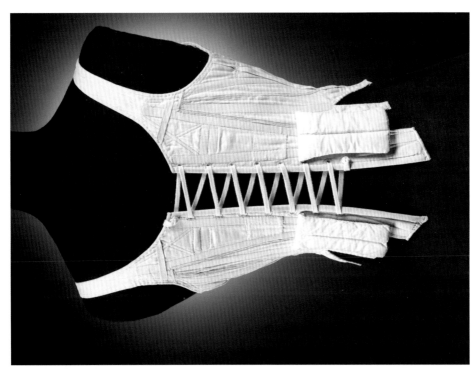

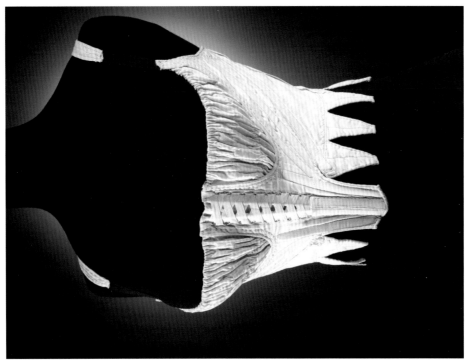

Plate 25 Short diaphragm-length pair of stays c.1790. Stays, Britain, 1795–1805. Cotton, linen, whalebone (baleen), trimmed with silk ribbon. Museum number: T.237-1983. © Victoria and Albert Museum, London.

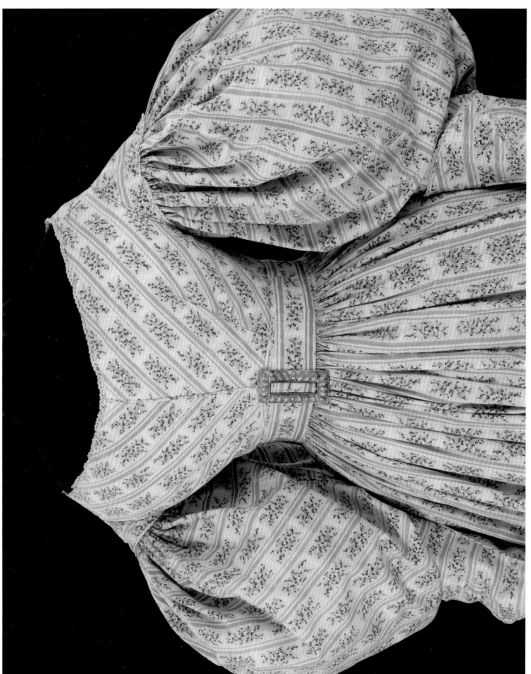

Plate 26 Day Dress (c.1830–1834) with exaggerated gigot sleeves and proportionately smaller waist that led to women being compared to "wasps," "bottle spiders," or "ants". Example of a day dress (c.1830–1834), British. Museum number: T.1688A-1915. © Victoria and Albert Museum, London.

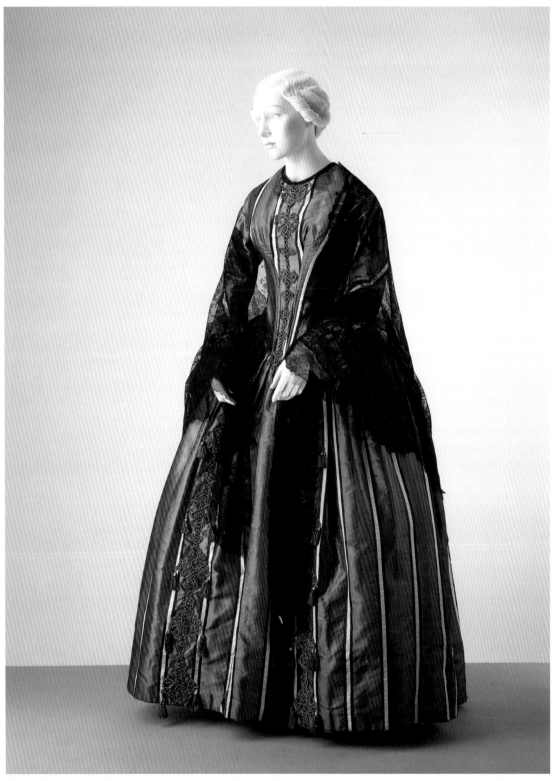

Plate 27 Example of Sentimental Dress (1840s). Dress of British origin (c.1845–1850). Museum number: T.856-1919. © Victoria and Albert Museum, London.

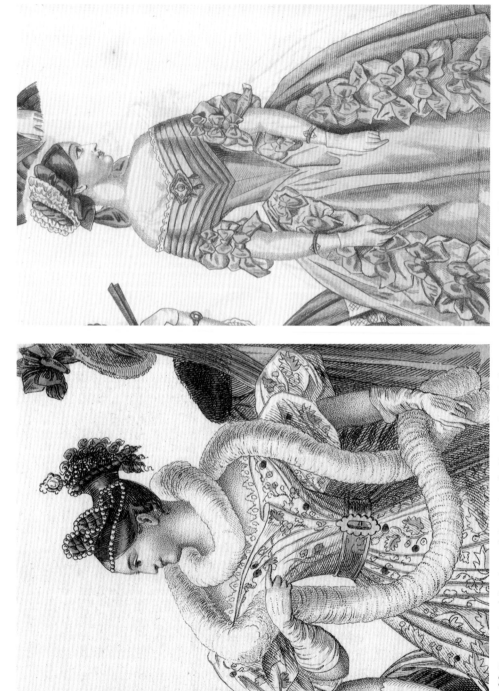

Plate 28 Romantic and Sentimental decoration for Evening Dress. Left: Romantic Dress, *La Belle Assemblée, Vol. XV* (London: Edward Bull, 1832), Casey Fashion Plates, Los Angeles Public Library. Right: Sentimental Dress, *The World of Fashion, Monthly Magazine of the Courts of London and Paris, Vol. XXV, No. 286* (London, 1848). Cambridge University Library.

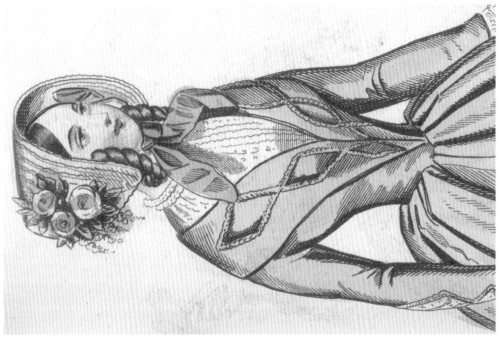

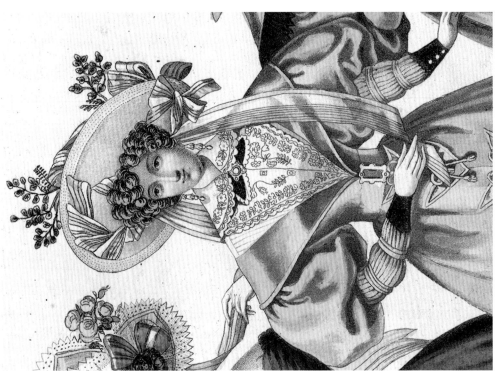

Plate 29 Romantic and Sentimental decoration for Day Wear. Left: Romantic Dress, *La Belle Assemblée*, Vol. XI (London: Whittaker, Treacher, and Co., 1830), Casey Fashion Plates, Los Angeles Public Library. Right: Sentimental Dress, *The New Monthly Belle Assemblée*, Vol. XXIII (London: Published at Norfolk Street, 1845). Cambridge University Library.

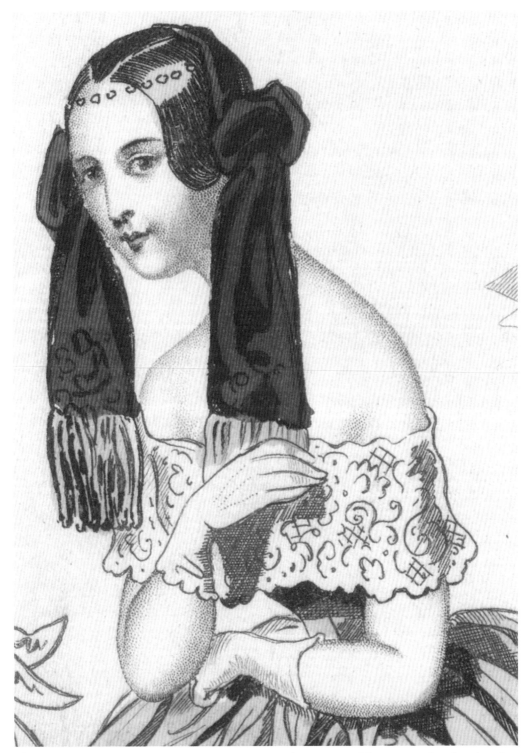

Plate 30 Stooping posture reminiscent of consumption. *The Magazine of the Beau Monde*, Vol. 11 (London: 1842), Cambridge University Library.

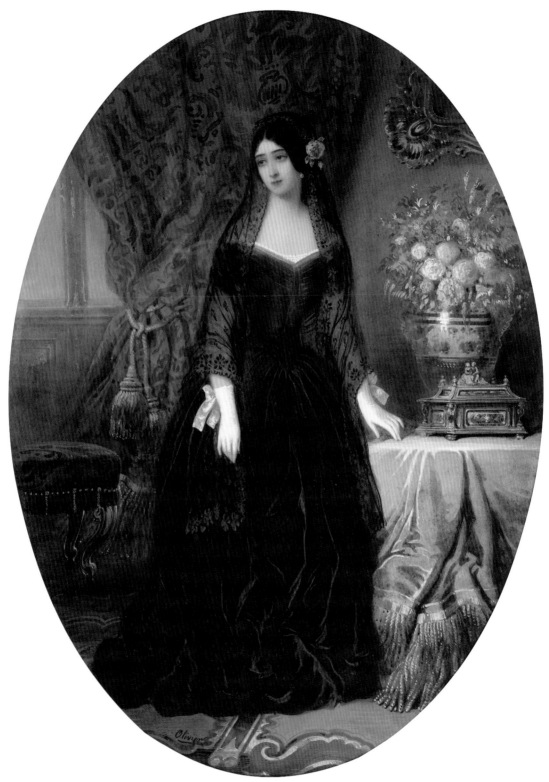

Plate 31 Marie Duplessis. Jean-Charles Olivier, Portrait of Marie Duplessis (1824–1847), *La Dame aux Camélias*, c.1840. Photo by Fine Art Images/Heritage Images/Getty Images.

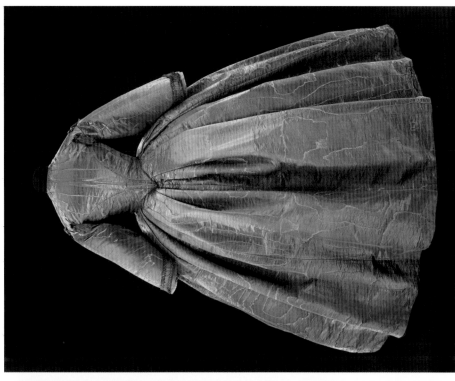

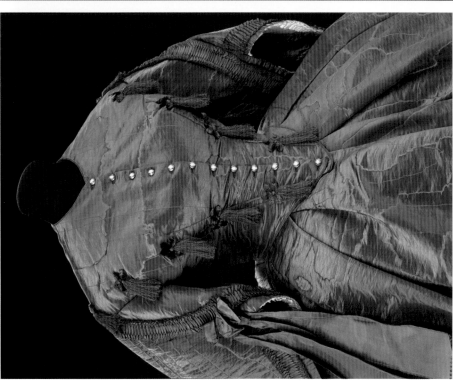

Plate 32 Dress (c.1853–1862). Example of a dress, of British origin, demonstrating move away from elongated tubercular shape, emulative of consumption, and towards a more robust frame (c.1853–1862). Museum number: T.908&A-1964. © Victoria and Albert Museum, London.

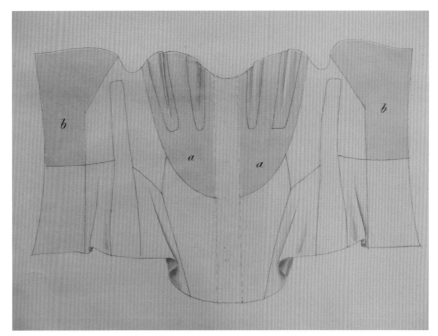

Plate 33 "Hygean or Corporiform Corset," Patented by Roxy Caplin's husband Jean Francois Isidore Caplin (1849). The dark pink sections, which focused on the lungs, were intended to be "readily adapted to the natural form of the body." "Hygean or Corporiform Corset," Jean Francois Isidore Caplin, Useful Registered Design Number: 1995, August 15, 1849. Courtesy of the National Archives, UK.

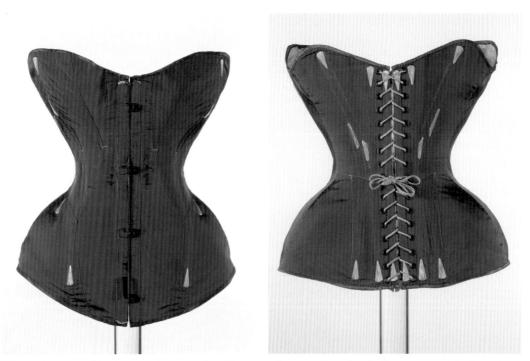

Plate 34 Front and back views of a new style of "Reformed" corset. Blue ribbed silk corset, made by Roxy Anne Caplin, which may have been the display model exhibited at the Great Exhibition in 1851. Corset, c.1851. Photo by Museum of London/Heritage Images/Getty Images.

beauty" to consumption by immediately quoting the following poem: "Behold that fragile form of delicate-transparent beauty/ Whose light blue eyes and hectic cheeks are lit by the bale fires of decline."[29]

For Burke, feminine beauty "almost always carries with it an idea of weakness and imperfection."[30] He argued that there was a conscious participation by women in constructing this connection as they learned "to lisp, to totter in their walk to counterfeit weakness, and even sickness . . . [because] Beauty in distress is much the most affecting beauty."[31] Burke was participating in a wider discourse on refinement and delicacy, one that medical practitioners also helped perpetuate. For instance, John Leake described consumption as a "flattering malady," one that "seizes the young and most beautiful of the Female Sex; for such from their natural delicacy of frame, are more particularly subject to its malignant power."[32]

Despite this, contemporary sources certainly blamed Burke for the flowering of disease chic. In 1811, *La Belle Assemblée* published a tirade against the notion that illness was attractive and asked, "when then is all this distressing sensibility . . . become so universal in the female world?"

May we charge this dereliction from nature on Mr. Burke's celebrated Essay on the Sublime and Beautiful? Did the rising of that brilliant star of genius paralyse [sic] the female mind? Could the fair reader not withstand the temptation of his assertions, when he tells them that they follow nature in the improvement of beauty, when they learn to lisp, to totter in their walk, to be amiably weak, and lovely in distress?

The author likened the affectation of illness to a disease itself, touting "its contagious influence" and stating it "continues to extend itself far and wide among those who cannot be accused of having had communication with the devastating source . . . the misapprehension of his notions may have contributed very largely to transform the genuine glow of healthful beauty into sickly languishment and affective debility, by encouraging habits ruinous to the constitution."[33] Burke's strongly gendered classifications were extended during the nineteenth century to include a standard of femininity that was defined by beauty and delicate debility, particularly in the middle and upper classes.[34]

In 1813, the author of the satire *The Age We Live In* articulated the growing tension over the relative importance of health versus beauty, writing "I scarcely know which is the worst, whether to have one's health or one's beauty injured, for I am sure the former is of very little consequence in this world without the latter. Indeed, I cannot fancy a more distressing situation than that of knowing yourself to be the ugliest person in the room."[35] This privileging of aesthetics over corporeal soundness was an important aspect of the debates over fashionable life and by the nineteenth century the ideal qualities espoused for women came to embody a great number of the predisposing causes for consumption. As a result, the delicate constitution of the female provided an excellent basis for creating a metaphor of tubercular beauty. This was not simply a literary creation; medical writers also helped to articulate and construct this relationship.[36]

By the early nineteenth century, health and activity were deemed vulgar, while languid and listless ladies sporting pale complexions were all the rage.[37] Evidence of the continued acceptance of this type of beauty can be gleaned from the satire "Scenes of the Ton, No. 1. *Bringing out Daughters*" (1829), where one mother remarks on the shortcomings of the other's daughter. "But I think Miss Bella's countenance is somewhat too sanguine and healthy, I mean fresh and ruddy, for the ton. A genteel paleness and lassitude in a *debutante* is a necessary qualification. There is an agreeable placid languor, which is a strong line of demarcation from vulgarity."[38] Fortunately, Bella's affliction of good health could be readily cured by "a month's round of visiting."

There is nothing like a winter in London for imparting that air of ton which, as you observe, is so essential to people of birth! Nothing can be more horrid than to see a milkmaid's flush amid a town rout.

The redness of the rose is out of place, where the languid delicacy of the lily is the prevailing object of admiration, as Lady Betty Cockletop[39] used to observe in her elegant way. What a creature of alabaster she was! . . . I never saw so beautiful a specimen of the complexion adapted for people of respectability.[40]

Life in London and the follies of fashionable life provided an enormous number of contributory hazards for developing consumption. Society robbed a woman of rest and placed demands upon her system, the consequence of which could be illness and even death. In 1825, Mrs. William Parkes lamented, "You have known young women, once healthy and vigorous, become feeble, drooping, and spiritless, when their early habits have been broken through, and when, by joining the circles of fashion, they have turned the hours of rest into the seasons for gaiety and amusement. Late and irregular hours of going to bed are much against the preservation of health."[41]

Since health was out of style, if an illness did not occur naturally, a number of ladies affected the trappings of sickness. *The World of Fashion* touched on this phenomenon in 1832, detailing the antics of one Parisian lady.

There are some people who cannot live unless they are ill; this may appear paradoxical, but it is strictly true. A celebrated French physician was called to attend upon a Lady of distinction whose disease had baffled all the skill of all the medical world in Paris. She admitted to her new attendant that she ate well, drank well, and slept well; that she had indeed every appearance of being in perfect health. "Very well then" said Monsieur, "you have only to follow my directions, and I will soon remove every appearance of health, I assure you![42]

So widespread and accepted was the rage for illness that it was even used as part of the debate over the passage of the First Reform Act. *Tait's Edinburgh Magazine* mentioned it as evidence that the bill was a necessity to break the hold of "people of fashion." "Who ever heard of a 'woman of fashion' wearing the hue of health upon her cheeks? Why it would be the death of her pretensions."[43] As the appearance of poor health became increasingly popular, one of the illnesses chosen as a model for emulation was consumption. How did the fashion for illness translate into a link between beauty and tuberculosis and why choose consumption as the model? The answer may lie in the established connections between the hallmarks of beauty and the physical characteristics imparted by the disease and used as diagnostic markers. Beauty was believed to be one of the significant signs of a hereditary predisposition to tuberculosis; moreover, once established, the symptoms were also thought to increase the attractiveness of the sufferer.[44]

The Art of Beauty (1825) addressed the tricky and convoluted relationship between health and beauty in general, and the role of tuberculosis in particular. This was the first thorough account on the subject of beauty in England and enjoyed widespread popularity with women of the middle and upper classes.[45] Although the work made an explicit point that beauty arose from a state of health (taking issue with Burke's assertion that beauty was "delicate, and easily injured"), it exploded this connection in the case of tuberculosis, through one of its most characteristic symptoms, the hectic fever.

Health is said to be an invariable association with beauty; it would follow, that we could not tell whether a lady was healthy or not, unless her face was beautiful. Nay, there are some diseases, hectic fever, for instance, which greatly improves [sic] the beauty of particular complexions . . . in such cases, even the physician, who knows it as the indication of fatal disease, cannot force himself to think that the face is not beautiful,—is not improved in beauty.[46]

Medical explanations of the disease only increased the popularity of the idea of consumptive beauty. A delicate physical appearance was not only seen as a product of consumption, due to the acceptance of hereditary explanations, it was often employed as a marker identifying those most vulnerable to the disease. In 1799, the *Medical and Physical Journal* certainly purported that genuine consumption arose from "peculiar circumstances of constitution" that swept "away whole families, particularly females" marked "by beauty."[47]

Observation and experience led medical investigators to conclude that individuals bearing certain characteristics were more likely to suffer from consumption than others who lacked those qualities. These "suspect" physical traits meshed with the idea of a predisposition to create a litmus test for tuberculosis. Due to the difficulties of diagnosis, as well as a lack of obviously visible symptoms, individuals were often not even aware they were afflicted until the disease's final stages. However, over time the patient manifested the anatomical alterations characteristic of *habitus phthisicus*.[48] As a result, many saw certain physical attributes, beauty among them, as an indication of those individuals most vulnerable to the disease, rather than simply as the product of the illness. Thus, beauty was often employed as a diagnostic marker and was a significant sign of hereditary predisposition. For instance, in 1801 *The Monthly Magazine*'s "Accounts of Diseases in London" stressed a connection between a consumptive countenance and "a physiognomy that is in general, especially in females, more than commonly interesting and attractive." It went on to assert that "Beauty is allied to phthisis" and "The qualities which it is delightful to contemplate, it is not always desirable to possess! Those exquisite charms … touch … on the confine of disease."[49] The difference between predisposition and active disease seemed to be a matter of degree and gradually the litany of what denoted a predisposition came to be the same as the numerous purported causes of phthisis.

Consumption seemed to enhance its victim by amplifying those qualities already established as attractive. For instance, the idea that white skin, red cheeks and lips denoted beauty was a notion of longstanding dominance in advice and instruction manuals.[50] These same qualities were also characteristic hallmarks of the consumptive disease process, which caused a pallor and hectic flush upon the cheeks. Medical references to the symptoms of the disease consistently describe the body as slight, thin, delicate, and slender in make, with a narrow chest, projecting clavicles, and shoulder blades that gave the appearance of wings.[51] This torso was accompanied by slight limbs and a flattened abdomen that contracted as the disease progressed. The complexion, designated as fine and delicate—marked by a clear, smooth, soft, nearly transparent skin that was pale in color—possessing an almost brilliant whiteness that was only relieved by the "bloom of the rose," the result of the low-grade hectic fever. The pale translucent complexion was criss-crossed by the blue of the veins running just below the surface and the face was complemented by white teeth. The eyes sported dilated pupils, fringed with dark luxurious eyelashes, while the whole of the figure was crowned by glossy flowing hair.[52] The descriptions of the ideal feminine form in the nineteenth century tended to bear a striking similarity to those provided in the case of consumption. The recurring accounts of these symptoms provide a glimpse as to why the disease beautified as it destroyed.

The eyes and complexion provided two of the main ways in which tuberculosis and beauty were linked. Eyes had long been a pivotal component of beauty; large expressive eyes were particularly prized as they provided access to emotion.[53] The "Criticism on Female Beauty" argued that "The finest eyes are those that unite sense and sweetness. The colour of the eye is a very secondary matter. Black eyes are thought the brightest, blue the most feminine, grey the keenest. It depends entirely on the spirit within."[54] Thickly lashed eyes with large, dilated pupils were both attractive and well-established symptoms of consumption. *The Family Oracle of Health* attested in 1824: "A large pupil, though it is certainly one of the highest marks of beauty, is also a sure token of a weak, and perhaps a consumptive constitution; so much so, that whatever renders the body delicate, will seldom fail to dilate and enlarge the pupil, and make the eyes beautifully languid."[55] The author of this medical treatise went on to provide a method of achieving this look if one did not possess the consumptive constitution.[56]

We cannot with safety recommend any practical method of enlarging the pupils of the eyes founded on this principle. There is, however, a certain drug called extract of belladonna which has a most powerful

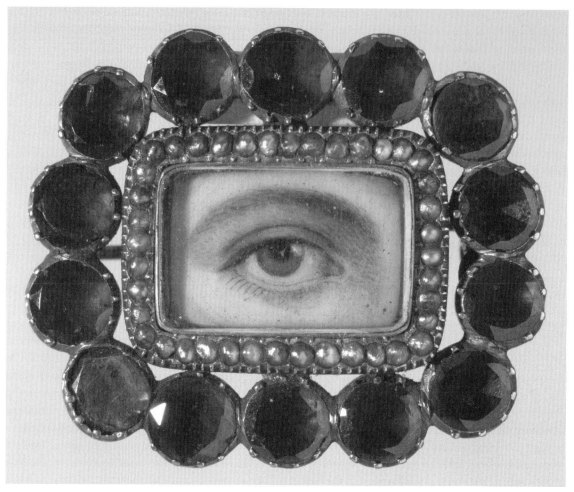

Figure 7.2 Capturing the Window to the Soul. Eye Miniature, England, early nineteenth century (painted), Museum number: P.57-1977. ©Victoria and Albert Museum, London.

effect in enlarging the pupil. A very little of it rubbed on the eye-lids will in a short time enlarge the pupil to a wonderful degree, and the effect will continue for some hours.[57]

The assertions about the beauty of the eye and consumption were supported in other sources, including *The Art of Beauty*.

A large pupil has, in most ages and countries, been considered as a mark of beauty ... A large pupil, however, although it is esteemed a mark of beauty, is, at the same time, one of the strongest indications of a weak habit of body and a delicate constitution. It is very common in those liable to consumption.[58]

The framing of the eye was significant and eyelashes played a role in enhancing the beauty and once again, there was a link to tuberculosis. One work detailing the markers for the hereditary consumptive constitution stated that the most consistent indicator was "that the pupils of the eyes are uncommonly large and full, to which some physicians add, that the eye-lashes are long and glossy."[59] There were a variety of ways an individual could achieve this look that occurred normally in a person suffering from consumption. Popular works of advice promoted an endless list of methods to darken lashes, including rubbing them with elderberries or a concoction made from resin and mastic, with solutions that used black frankincense, or lampblack.[60]

The complexion, however, remained the most significant aspect of beauty, as well as an important indicator of health in women. In 1807, "On the Beauty of Skin" discussed the connection:

> The beauty of the skin contributes in so astonishing a manner to beauty in general, that many woman [sic] who are deemed very handsome, possess no other advantages than that of a beautiful skin ... A white skin, slightly tinged with carnation, soft and smooth to the touch, is what we commonly call a fine skin ... in our climate, carnation may be regarded as the true thermometer of the state of health ... Thus a fresh and blooming tint, rosy lips, a lively and sparking eye, are indications of good health.[61]

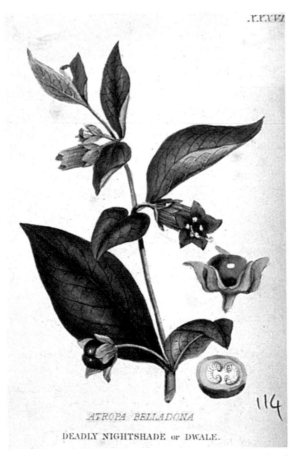

Figure 7.3 Deadly Nightshade (*Atropa belladonna*). Colored reproduction of a wood engraving by J. Johnstone (Glasgow: Blackie & Son). Wellcome Library, London. Copyrighted work available under Creative Commons Attribution only licence CC BY 4.0 http://creativecommons.org/licenses/by/4.0/

Yet once again, the protestations that beauty could only be found in health fell apart when it came to consumption.[62] For the smooth white complexion, sparkling eyes, rosy lips and cheeks, were also the signs of a hereditary predisposition to the disease. *The Modern Practice of Physic* (1805) listed the indicators for consumption as: "a fine, clear, and smooth skin, large veins, delicate complexion, high-coloured lips . . . white, and transparent teeth."[63] The quality and beauty of the complexion rested on its level of whiteness. "The Ladies Toilette" insisted "Whiteness is one of the qualities which it is requisite for the skin to possess, before it can be called beautiful."[64] This whiteness was a distinguishing feature of consumption, as John Armstrong stated in 1818:

> The first changes which indicate the approach to phthisis are to be found in the skin. The colour of the cheeks always becomes paler and more delicate than before . . . A beautiful bloom will be spread for a moment over some part of the cheeks, and then receding it will leave a remarkable palidity, almost approaching whiteness . . . and the superficial veins may be observed running in different parts of the skin, somewhat like blue lines through white marble . . . and an expression of interest, and even of beauty is not unfrequently thrown over the whole countenance, most remarkable in persons whose faces had been previously plain.[65]

In 1831, *The Atheneum* argued: "In some hereditary cases, particularly in females of a fair and delicate complexion, the skin assumes a semi-transparent appearance . . . Poets ought not to describe the hands of their imaginary mistresses as transparent, except when they are conducting them . . . to their graves. 'Tis a bad sign of a young lady's health when you can see through her hand as easily as her heart; and, instead of a parson, you should call in a physician."[66]

The prominence and distinction of the veins provided yet another link between attractiveness and consumption, one detailed in various literary works, like "The Harvest-Home" (1824):

> Gently supported by pillows, there lay the dying maiden . . . Wasted almost to a shadow, and sinking under the pressure of a mortal sickness, she was still lovely; but her beauty was of now a strange, unearthly character. Too delicately fair for this life, she seemed like an inhabitant of the aerial world. The motion of the blood was almost visible in the small blue veins wandering across her pale marble forehead; and a light emanated from her mild eyes, full of a pure, lofty, and spiritual meaning.[67]

The importance of contrast and role of the veins, can be found in an 1806 piece on painting, which addressed the aesthetics of the circulatory system in the portraiture of women. The author wrote the veins "in women . . . appear merely as faint blue lines in the transparent skin," and although he expressed indecision about including them, stated "In natural colouring, their effect is a faint tinge of blue, which gives a delicacy to the white, and mingles with the prevailing carnation."[68] The artist may have had doubts about highlighting the veins, but it appears that fashionable women did not possess the same qualms, as cosmetic enhancement was at various times employed to achieve this look. *The Mirror of the Graces* (1811) condemned the practice and railed against women drawing "the meandering vein through the fictitious alabaster with as fictitious a dye."[69]

The smile was yet another critical link between tuberculosis and beauty, as phthisis was also believed to whiten the teeth. Colin Jones has addressed the growing importance of the smile in the aesthetics of sensibility during the eighteenth century and has argued "a pleasing smile was . . . becoming a significant commodity."[70] Jones also asserts that "from the middle decades of the century, the cult of sensibility evident in fiction, drama, and painting revalorized the smile as a marker of inner and outward beauty and as an emblem of identity."[71] By the turn of the century a beautiful smile was a desirable and highly sought-after facet of beauty. In 1780,

Medical Commentaries articulated "the marks of a predisposition to phthisis" stating that "sound teeth" were a significant sign and "that of those who are carried off by this disease, the greater number will be found never to have had a carious tooth."[72] *The Physician's Advice for the Prevention and Cure of Consumption* articulated "white transparent and sound teeth" as a characteristic commonly associated with those predisposed to the illness.[73] A wide variety of tooth powders were available commercially, and an even greater number of recipes that could be compounded at home were in circulation. These were published in a number of recipe books and in the periodical literature of the nineteenth century. These substances were advertised as essential to achieving healthy, gleaming, white teeth.[74] Colin Jones has even argued that the use of rouge was as much for the lips as cheeks, as "ruby red lips set off and showcased lovely white teeth."[75]

White teeth, white skin, rosy cheeks, and lips—all highly desirable qualities—were also all evidence of tuberculosis. *The Art of Beauty* demonstrated a conscious acceptance that consumptive illness was one sure path to beauty, but also recognized less deadly ways to achieve this goal seeking to find a balance between beauty and health.

> Leaving diseases altogether out of the question we can recommend training to our fair readers as the only certain and infallible means ever discovered for improving the brightness of the eyes, and the clearness and transparency of the complexion . . . the superfluous rosy colour of the face; which we may remark, is not so much a sign of high health, as it is too commonly supposed, but is closely allied to inflammatory diseases, and sudden death in consequence. Save us, say we, from rosy cheeks and fatal inflammations.[76]

Beyond the "natural" beauty conferred by consumption, there was a growing element of emulation associated with the disease during the nineteenth century, as beauty practices were co-opted into the rage for illness. The turn of the century brought with it an alteration in the accepted color for the complexion. The brilliantly red faces that had been popular during the eighteenth century had been supplanted by the pale and pallid white by 1807.[77] That same year, one writer stated "that it is so much the fashion to look pale, that . . . first rates use a sort of lotion to promote that interesting and sickly shade of the lily."[78] There was also a more "fallible means" for attaining the consumptive look—cosmetics—however, their improper use was thought to bring about the disease. Again, balance seemed to be the key. The periodical literature and publications dealing with the toilet and beauty continually reiterated that "the complexion which is considered the most beautiful is a pale carnation, in which neither the white nor the red can be said to predominate."[79] This delicate balance of color was accomplished naturally in consumption. Cosmetics had diverged from the artificial, heavily contrived look popular in the previous century and moved instead towards a restrained subtlety intended to mimic nature. *The Art of Beauty* called paint "the sheet anchor of the fair sex."[80] Six years later, *The Servant's Guide and Family Manual* stated, "A good selection of Cosmetics is important for the completeness of a lady's toilette. Whether the use of paints, washes, &c. be judicious, is not for us to determine; but in giving the following receipts, we have endeavoured to distinguish those which are the most objectionable."[81]

There was also a recognition of the limitations of cosmetics—that they could not create what was not already present but could "only assist nature."[82] The use of white paints seems to have raised the most ire, as the application of metallic oxides, advertised as "pearl white" and wielded to give a very white complexion, were roundly condemned. *A New System of Domestic Economy* (1827) called for the use of soap and water or buttermilk to improve the skin. Despite these pleas, metallic oxides remained a popular staple of the lady's dressing table. When used to achieve a pale complexion, they were also thought to bring about the consumptive illness that naturally provided the fair pallor. *The Art of Beauty* argued that white paints, made from extracts of bismuth, lead, or tin, were capable of penetrating "through the pores of the skin, acting, by degrees, on the

... lungs, and inducing diseases."[83] While John Murray's *A Treatise on Pulmonary Consumption* vehemently asserted that "the *chemicals* of the toilet ... very materially assist the messenger of death."[84] Beyond a death from consumption, additional possible consequences included the risk of severe public embarrassment. For instance, one author provided a few hints to the unwary suitor to allow him to determine whether or not "his fair one's lillies and roses are really her own or not!" The work suggested that the gentleman take the object of his affection to "Harrowgate" [sic] where the waters acted "powerfully upon all the metallic oxides ... If the fair one's face retains its pristine beauty after half a dozen ablutions, he may consider the article as genuine and unadulterated, and free from all the terrors of 'Death in the Pot'—but if the dame or damsel begin to look blue, or turn black, he will at once perceive that beauty, like London porter, may be doctored for the market."[85] By the beginning of Queen Victoria's reign, the connection between the use of cosmetics and the incidence of consumption was firmly established and although artificial aids remained available, by the latter 1830s, their employment became increasingly secretive.[86] Despite the rejection of cosmetics as an acceptable avenue for achieving aesthetic perfection, the emulation of consumptive beauty not only continued but even grew.

Sentimental Beauty

The early Victorian ideas of beauty were heavily influenced by sentimentalism which advocated the idea that emotional authenticity was not revealed through overt demonstration but rather was confirmed through subtle exterior signs and subdued behavior.[87] The notion of sensibility was central to the ideology of sentimentalism and reflected the ability of the nervous system to accept sensation and convey the body's will. Sensibility defined not only personal feelings and emotions but also the physical manifestations of those sentiments. Even a woman's complexion offered insight. Pallor and blushes, for instance, were taken as evidence of the intensity of sensibility and transparency of emotion. This involuntary openness was seen as one of the finest attributes a woman could possess.[88]

Sentimental ideology further elevated the power of disease with the notion that a woman's true character could not be revealed unless she was fighting illness. Already evidence of this attitude existed early in the nineteenth century, as many conjectured that illness revealed a woman's personality, earnestness, genuineness, and the most fundamental truths about her.[89] Thomas Gisborne, a member of the Clapham sect, argued in his 1806 *An Enquiry into the Duties of the Female Sex*, "With respect to supporting the languor and the acuteness of disease, the weight of testimony is wholly on the side of the weaker sex." Women, he went on, exhibited "the highest patterns of firmness, composure, and resignation under tedious and painful trials."[90] Further evidence of the importance of suffering to the character of women can be seen in the descriptions of Miss Gwatkin, while she "gradually sunk under a pulmonary consumption" in 1814. The author wrote, "Amidst the ravages which disease made upon her bodily frame, 'the ornament of a meek and quiet spirit' suffered no decay; but became more conspicuous."[91]

By the early Victorian era, suffering and illness were considered important functions of female life. Mrs. Sarah Stickney Ellis addressed the role of sickness in her work *The Women of England* (1839), even making specific mention of "the hectic flush of beauty" when addressing the need for awareness of the abbreviated time an individual had on earth.[92]

> Neither is it necessary that the idea should be invested with melancholy, and associated with depression. It is but looking at the truth. And let us deceive ourselves as we may, the green church-yard with its freshly covered graves—the passing-bell—the slowly-moving hearse—the shutters closed upon the

apartment where the sound of merriment was lately heard—the visitations of disease within our homes—even the hectic flush of beauty—all remind us that the portion of time allotted for the exercise of kindly feeling towards our fellow-creatures, is fleeting fast away.[93]

In *The Daughters of England* (1843), Mrs. Ellis admonished her reader to "make the best use of the advantages of illness," which were both physical and spiritual.[94] She also directly addressed the position of disease in female life: "there is a strength and a beauty in her character, when labouring under bodily affliction, of which the heroism of fiction affords but a feeble imitation. Wherever woman is the most flattered, courted, and indulged, she is the least admirable; but in seasons of trial her highest excellences shine forth."[95] Charlotte Brontë wrote in similar terms of the character of her sisters, Emily and Anne, while they suffered from consumption. In a letter on January 18, 1849, she stated, "Anne is very patient in her illness, as patient as Emily was unflinching. I recall one sister and look at the other with a sort of reverence as well as affection—under the test of suffering neither has faltered."[96]

For the sentimentalist, the exterior revealed the character beneath, and beauty was now "both moral and personal."[97] This belief in an association between the exterior form and interior disposition was evident in an 1834 article in the *London Journal*, which asserted that "The more we consider beauty, the more we recognize its dependence on sentiment . . . O Sentiment! Beauty is but the outward and visible sign of thee."[98] These notions were reinforced by medical investigators who stated that "Goodness and beauty in woman will accordingly be found to bear a strict relation to each other; and the latter will be seen always to be the external sign of the former."[99] The phrenologist George Combe provided a biological basis for the significance of the external, arguing that "If the countenance beams with intelligence and goodness, this is an indication that the moral and intellectual regions of the brain predominate; and the individual . . . is one of nature's nobility."[100]

The physical symptoms of consumption could now be rationalized as reflecting the victim's moral virtue, and consumptive women were increasingly presented as too good and beautiful to live. For instance, *Clinical Lectures on Pulmonary Consumption* argued:

We may often observe in families, that the members in whom the hereditary tendency is most apt to betray itself, are those characterized by refinement of feeling, and delicacy of sentiment. Selfishness and hardness of character . . . less frequently present themselves in persons susceptible of this form of disease. The common expression, "Too good to live," may so far have a foundation, and the poet may be justified in his exclamation—"The good die first."[101]

Because true beauty came from within, the body of a beautiful woman was charming because it revealed the soul.[102] *The Englishwoman's Magazine and Christian Mother's Miscellany* (1846) argued the case: "The influence of beauty must be acknowledged to be very extensive and powerful; but surely it is so, because that beauty is considered as the index of the heart."[103]

This relationship between the internal character and external beauty led to a proliferation of directions for perfecting the hearts and minds of women. For instance, *The Ladies Hand-book of the Toilet* of 1843, stated "That internal state of purity, or impurity, is depicted in legible characters upon the external countenance, and . . . the fair one, who would become really beautiful, must make the cultivation of her mind . . . her first and principal care."[104] While *The Ladies Science of Etiquette* (1844) argued that since "the face is the index of the mind . . . That a proper and somewhat careful attention to the preservation of personal beauty is not only advisable, but a positive duty."[105] With all these moral and social overtones, it is unsurprising that the aesthetics of the countenance assumed a growing importance. The face, considered the most transparent part of the

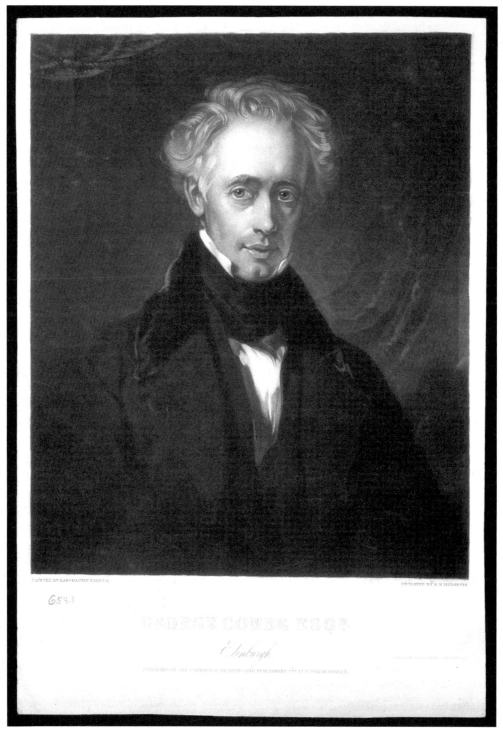

Figure 7.4 George Combe. Mezzotint by R. M. Hodgetts after Sir D. Macnee. Wellcome Library, London. Copyrighted work available under Creative Commons Attribution only licence CC BY 4.0 http://creativecommons.org/licenses/by/4.0/

body, and "the index of the mind," permitted access to the woman's feelings, as revealed in her smile, her complexion, and, even in her eyes.[106] Consumption then, which provided exterior beauty as a result of an inherent internal constitution, tightened the bonds between the internal workings of the body and the exterior manifestations of those circumstances.

This sentimental fixation on the external as a moral quality reinforced the association of consumption and beauty in both the popular imagination and in the medical profession. Henry Gilbert's medical treatise *Pulmonary Consumption* (1842) even resorted to the poet's hand to describe its symptoms and allude to their significance in creating beauty in a woman.

> With step as noiseless as the summer air,
> Who comes in beautiful decay? Her eyes
> Dissolving with a feverish glow of light;
> > and on
> > Her cheeks a rosy tint, as if the tip
> Of beauty's finger faintly press'd it there:
> > Alas! Consumption is her name[107]

In 1849, Charlotte Brontë acknowledged the dominance of the belief in a connection between consumption and beauty stating, "Consumption, I am aware, is a flattering malady."[108] This beauty, attached to tuberculosis by both popular mythology and by medicine, provided one more avenue of correspondence between the illness and sentimentalism.

The transparency of the skin and whiteness of the complexion, both significant aspects of the consumptive symptomology, became ever more important as an explicit aspect of beauty. Transparency took on a spiritual or character-defining quality that grew in significance, particularly in the latter part of the 1830s and the 1840s. However, the connection was already in evidence in the 1820s and 1830s, as *The Art of Beauty* referred to it in defining the characteristics of a beautiful complexion: "A smooth, soft, and transparent skin, is no less indispensable to the perfection of beauty, than elegance of figure."[109] The author went on to associate "A pure, delicate and transparent complexion" with descriptions "of lillies [sic] gemmed with dew, and roses breathing their balm in the freshness of a summer morning."[110] These roses, the work acknowledged, combined with the sought-after transparent complexion in consumption. The hectic flush of the disease, confined "to a small bright spot on the top of the cheek emulated the rose's bloom," which the author dubbed "the hue that haunts it to the tomb … This may occur in every variety of complexions; but it is … more common in those who have a very fine transparent skin, very light colored hair, blue eyes, and a weak constitution. It is usually the token of a fatal disease, particularly consumption."[111] This hectic flush was termed one of the "marks of confirmed consumption" according to *The Family Oracle of Health*, which went on to describe the physical alterations that accompanied it, using the same terminology as *The Art of Beauty*: "the cheek assumes the rose's bloom, the hue that haunts it to the tomb. The sad dejected look of the countenance of the first stage now brightens into a sepulchral smile."[112]

The whiteness of the complexion was the most commonly mentioned aspect of tuberculosis connected to prettiness and was also an important component in achieving sentimental transparency. Alexander Walker maintained that pale and transparent skin allowed the influence of emotion to shine through and asserted "So greatly, indeed does whiteness contribute to beauty, that many women deemed beautiful by us, have little other right to that epithet except what they derive from a beautiful skin."[113] These notions were also found in toilet manuals, like *Female Beauty* (1837) which asserted, "Whiteness is the most essential quality of the skin."[114] As such, a white complexion became a central concern of the lady's toilet, as well as a defining marker of both attractiveness and consumption. James Clark applied this view to the ravages of the disease.

The character of the constitution is still more clearly indicated by the countenance. The eyes, particularly the pupils, are generally large, the eye-lashes long; and there is usually a placid expression, often great beauty of countenance, especially in persons of a fair, florid complexion.[115]

The face and particularly in the eyes, as Clark mentions, illustrated the woman's feelings. Since, in the sentimental tradition, the eyes were styled "windows of the soul" and were thought to "speak" because they revealed the emotions and character as "the seat at once of intellect and love" they also enhanced the beauty of the consumptive.[116] Large pupils, in particular (see Plate 20), persisted as a defining characteristic of comeliness,

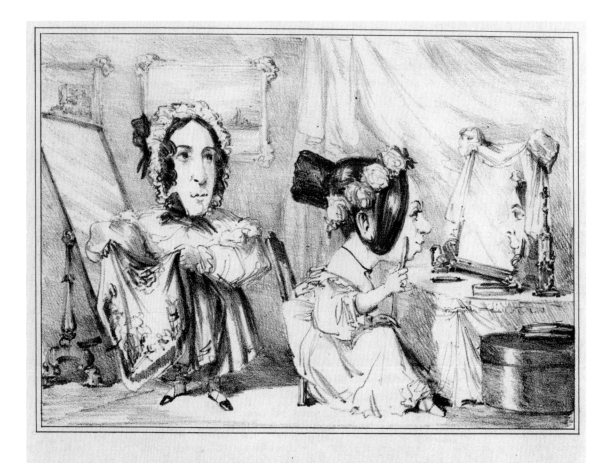

DONT MAKE IT ANY REDDER M'EM,

ELSE THEY WILL THINK YOU PAINT.

Published for the Proprietor by S. Knights, Sweetings Alley, Cornhill.

Standidge & C.º Litho London.

Figure 7.5 Don't make it any Redder M'em, Else they will think you paint. Lithograph. (London: Published for the proprietor by S. Knights, 1845?) Image number: lwlpr14169. Courtesy of The Lewis Walpole Library, Yale University.

and it was readily acknowledged that this "mark of beauty" was "rarely connected with robust or general health, and is in some instances a decided indication of bodily weakness."[117]

There was an inherent tension, however, between sentimentalist views that what was observed upon the exterior was a pure representation of what lay in the heart of the woman, and the desires of women to use make-up and other devices to enhance their beauty and imitate the consumptive look. For to create something that did not already exist, could be interpreted as an attempt to compensate for a deficiency in the underlying character and the element of deception inherent in the use of cosmetics was a growing point of concern. There were numerous diatribes against artifice in both dress and the toilette as *The Young Woman's Own Book* in 1840 called it "both unsuccessful and sinful."[118] Instead, sentimentalists argued that the key to beauty lay in the cultivation of desirable qualities rather than in cheap imitation. Before the onslaught of such criticism, the use of make-up became ever more furtive and by the 1840s the obvious use of cosmetic enhancements was no longer acceptable.[119] As a result, cosmetics were either applied with a light hand or not at all and their use was certainly not admitted to. Many women heeded the call of *The Art of Dress* (1839), which decried the use of cosmetics and instead called for ladies to "keep your complexion clear and beautiful, pure and clean, by simple soap and water!"[120] Make-up went underground—still present but never proclaimed and manuals concerned with the subject started to provide beauty recipes based on socially desirable characteristics.

Mrs. King's *The Toilet* (1838), for example, listed innocence as the best white paint and modesty as the best rouge. *The Ladies Gazette of Fashion* (1848) put out "A Recipe for a Lady's Dress" that stated: "Let chastity be your white, modesty your vermillion . . . virtue your robes, and conscious integrity the finish of your dress."[121] Despite these admonitions, the centrality of the complexion in beauty meant that cosmetics remained an important but controversial element of the ladies' toilette. There was therefore a focus on an increased

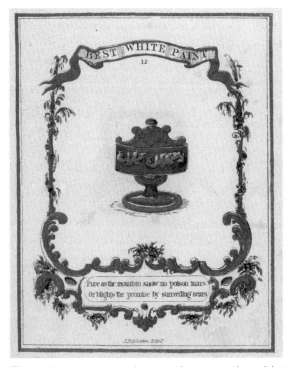 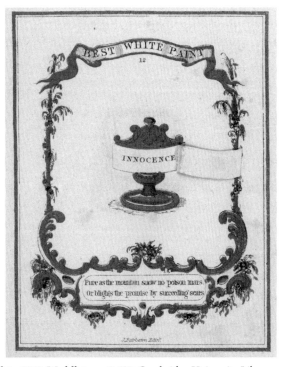

Figure 7.6 Innocence is the Best White Paint. *The Lady's Toilet* c.1845. Waddleton.e.9.628, Cambridge University Library.

discretion in their use.[122] Magazines remained filled with advertisements for items to beautify the face, the form, and the figure. Purveyors of cosmetics continued to do a brisk trade in toilet waters and other preparations, as well as rice and pearl powder, which were used to subtly achieve the consumptive complexion, while books of the toilet continued to offer recipes for home preparation.[123] Yet at the same time, the outcry against the overt use of cosmetic enhancements was coupled with the notion that beauty was something natural to a woman of virtue. As a result, tuberculosis, with its ability to enhance female beauty without deception or artifice, would by implication be the exterior manifestation of the virtuous character as well as one way of naturally achieving beauty.

Ironically the disease also furnished one symptom that demanded the use of pretense and trickery. It was believed that during the course of tubercular illness, "The hair loses its strength, so that it cannot be kept in order as before. You observe this particularly in females. There appears to be a softness of the hair, which will not allow it to remain in the way in which it has been placed."[124] These sorts of deficiencies were mitigated through a combination of less intricate hairdressing and augmentation by hairpieces. The elaborate large coiffures, like the Apollo knot typical of the Romantic style of the 1830s, were supplanted by a softer sentimental style in which the hair typically parted down the middle, framed the face with a cluster of ringlets, or was held back in a soft knot or bun at the rear. Nevertheless, false means were resorted to in an effort to make up for the deficiencies created by disease, as the ringlets that framed the countenance were often not genuine, but rather composed from artificial clusters of hair attached to hidden bands. Thus, hairpieces were used to provide the look of simplicity and artless charm.

The cultural expectations that surrounded consumption were articulated in literature, medical treatises, and those works concerned with defining fashion and the female role, all of which overflowed with examples that connected the disease to beauty. These works reveal a shared consciousness that tuberculosis was indeed attractive and, as a result, contemporary patterns of representation were modeled upon this precept. Despite these positive representations, the hallmarks of tubercular beauty all told "The direful tale of an enemy at work within; not the less dangerous because decking his intended prey with delusive and dangerous attractions." Consumption, then, was a "death adorned in the brilliant masquerade garb of beauty."[125]

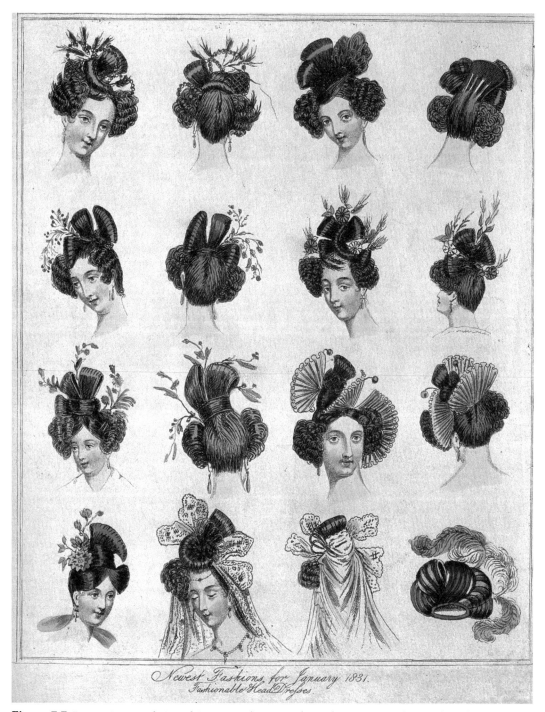

Newest Fashions for January 1831.
Fashionable Head Dresses.

Figure 7.7 Romantic 1830s hair and Sentimental 1840s styles with instructions for attaching false hair. Left: Women wearing the newest fashionable head-dresses of 1831. Overleaf: Women wearing fashionable dresses, hairpieces, and accessories, and a diagram explaining how hairpieces are attached to natural hair. c.1840. Wellcome Library, London. Copyrighted work available under Creative Commons Attribution only licence CC BY 4.0 http:// creativecommons.org/licenses/by/4.0/

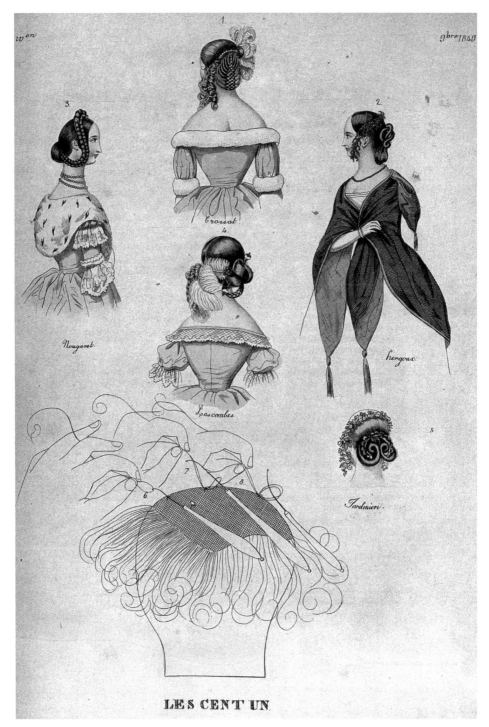

Figure 7.7 *Continued*

CHAPTER 8
THE AGONY OF CONCEIT: CLOTHING AND CONSUMPTION

In the early nineteenth century, enthusiasm for all of the twists and turns of fashion was considered an innate weakness of a woman's character, one outside of her control.[1] Women were fashion victims, not just by choice but due to their physiology, and a slavish devotion to fashion was beyond a woman's power to restrain fully.[2] *La Belle Assemblée* tackled this issue on numerous occasions, as when it stated, in 1806, that "Some moralists have censured attention to dress; but very unjustly. It is perfectly useless to censure a propensity inherent in the nature of the fair sex."[3] This sentiment was reiterated time and again; although, over the course of the nineteenth century the love of fashion was replaced by the love of "variety" in dress as the female weakness—a much more complicated issue. Mrs. William Parkes wrote in 1825,

> A woman's wardrobe may be divided into two parts,—the ornamental and the useful. In the first I include all the various articles which are affected by fashion; everything, in fact, of external dress. In these a good economist will avoid a superabundance. She will endeavour to check that feminine weakness—the love of variety, which so frequently displays itself by an ever-varying costume, and will confine the ornamental part of her wardrobe into as narrow bounds as the extent of her general style of living and visiting will permit.[4]

Like nervous sensibility and the predisposition to consumption, a devotion to fashion was yet another biologically determined facet of the nineteenth-century woman. (See Plate 21.) Not surprisingly, then, clothing has played a prominent role in the mythology and rhetoric of tuberculosis, both as prescription against and as originator of the malady. The specifics of how clothing functioned as a causative agent of tuberculosis fluctuated alongside the fashions, as did the admonitions with respect to preventing the sickness.

Too little, too much, too tight, too loose, all of these descriptors were employed at one time or another to decry the pernicious effects of fashion on health. Despite the alterations in style from 1780 to 1850, there was a great deal of continuity in the objections and the most common criticisms related to protection from the elements and the pressures applied by clothing upon the body. It was often argued that contemporary fashions caused tuberculosis by failing to protect their wearers from the vagaries of the English climate or because they pressed upon the lungs and consequently created consumption. There was also a consistent element of imitation of several different physical symptoms of consumption; however, the substance of the complaints against dress and the modes of emulation changed alongside the fashions themselves.

Classical Consumptive and the Dangers of Fashionable Life

In the latter part of the eighteenth century, fashions began to shift radically away from the extravagance and artifice that had marked the earlier portion of the century, turning instead toward a fashioned simplicity.[5] England felt the influence of the move toward informality and a more "natural" shape by the mid-1780s, with the introduction of the chemise dress.[6] Fashion in the last decades of the eighteenth century continued to simplify and there was a movement "towards a more natural, minimalist aesthetic."[7] By 1800, the classical lines were firmly established, and a distinctive silhouette identified with French fashionables made a determined assault on England. As neoclassical styles were adopted, waistlines rose and necklines dropped; however, the dresses embraced in England remained more modest than their French counterparts. Beyond an adherence to classical lines, these fashions also reflected the classical attitude that clothing should reveal rather than conceal the beauty of the body it covered. Women's fashions achieved this aim in a number of ways. One was through the use of thin sheer fabrics, laid over a bare minimum of underclothing, all of which served to emphasize and allude to the bare body. Extensive portions of the anatomy were exposed, including the bosom, back, shoulders, and arms. The legs, however, remained covered, with a hint of their shape given by the clinging nature of the fabric of the skirt. Women's gowns during this period were constructed of soft, diaphanous, even transparent fabrics (like muslin and gauze), which draped nicely, embracing and revealing the "natural" shape beneath.[8] One ladies' magazine detailed the style in 1811: "over this strangely manufactured figure, a scanty petticoat, and as scanty a gown is put. The latter resembles a bolster slip more than a garment; and not content with the closeness of its adherence round the body, it is cut away at the breast and back, to shew the bosom and shoulders naked; and the sleeves are snipped off."[9]

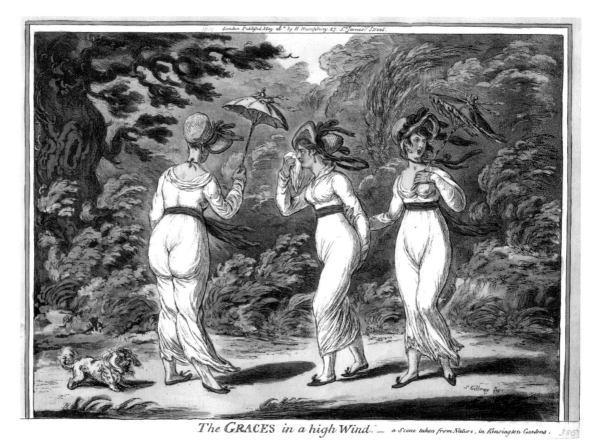

Figure 8.1 "The Graces in a High Wind" by James Gillray, published by H. Humphrey, May 26, 1810. 1868,0808.7943. ©The Trustees of the British Museum.

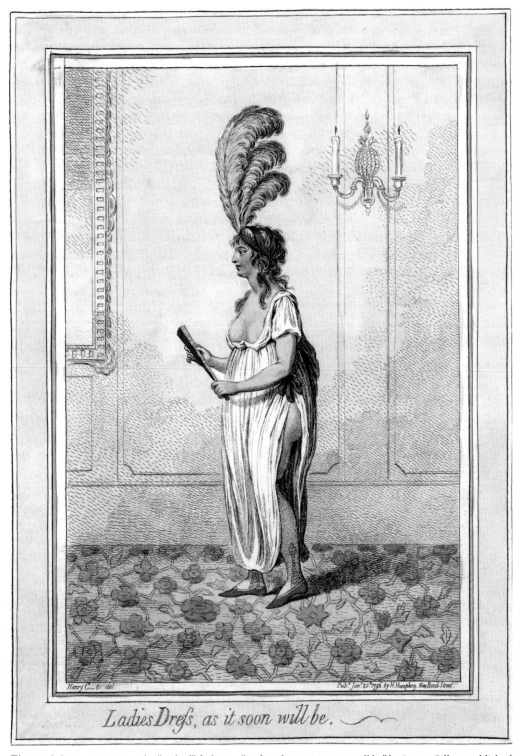

Ladies Dress, as it soon will be.

Figure 8.2 Caricaturizing the "Naked" fashions. "Ladies dress, as it soon will be" by James Gillray, published by Hannah Humphrey, January 20, 1796. J.3.85. ©The Trustees of the British Museum.

While the female silhouette depended upon undergarments, the style of these garments changed. Unsurprisingly, new types of this attire were developed to accommodate the sleek shape, particularly when women's skirts narrowed around 1810. Some innovations included "smooth knitted drawers"[10] and invisible petticoats, which placed "the odious and vulgar article which formerly supplied its [the petticoat's] place, entirely on the shelf."[11] In 1807, *La Belle Assemblée* advertised Mrs. Robershaw's "much approved" invisible petticoats, claiming they provided a slimmer silhouette, as they would "add less to size than cambric muslin."[12] In the same year, one gentleman complained of the "undress" made possible by these advances, writing, "As by means of modern invisible petticoats and transparent drapery, there were exposures below as well as above."[13] Charlotte Burney wrote of her experience with the new fashions in inclement weather, stating "the wind was so intolerable that we dared not walk about . . . lest our light French clothing should give way & no shade be left to our complete perfections."[14] These same problems were satirized by James Gillray in his 1810 "The Graces in a High Wind."

The scanty nature of both dress and undergarments was lamented and lampooned from the very beginning of the neoclassical trend and women were rebuked for their naked fashions, which were thought to have consequences for both health and decency.[15] In 1785, *The European Magazine and London Review* bemoaned the sad state of affairs arguing the "modern habits of fashionable life," particularly female dress meant "that health, ease, and beauty, are hardly to be found to be genuine among the sex." Even worse, "The caprice of fashion . . . hurry the unfortunate fair to sickness or the grave." This was a concern not just for the current generation, but for future ones as well as "there is reason to dread that generations yet unborn will be heirs to the morbid effects of imprudent dress."[16]

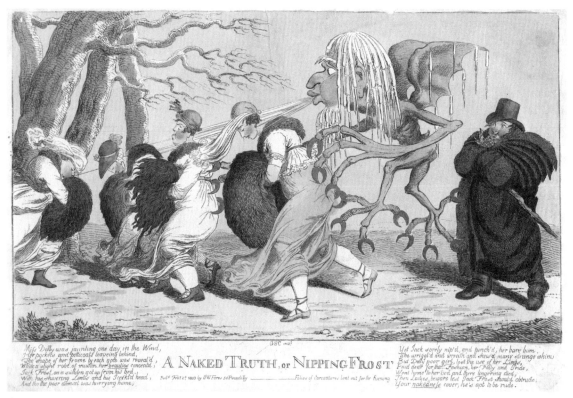

Figure 8.3 "A Naked Truth or Nipping Frost" (1803), by Charles Williams, published by S. W. Fores. Image: lwlpr10384. Courtesy of The Lewis Walpole Library, Yale University.

Caricaturists and journalists alike berated women for their dearth of clothing.[17] In a nod to the political climate, as well as to the importance of the constitution in health, *The Times* stated, "If the present fashion of nudity continues its career, the Milliners must give way to the carvers, and the most elegant *fig-leaves* will be all the mode ... If the fashion for *nakedness* should continue much longer, our healthiest fashionables will be glad to rob Abbé SYEYES's pigeon-holes of a new Constitution."[18] Concern over the damage to the "constitution" and the unsuitableness of such fashions in the cold, variable climate of England were often ignored. As one young lady bemoaned in 1792: "Short sleeves are to be worn this winter ... The stays are all to be cut down, & worn as low ... I hate short sleeves in winter, but it will very soon become a singularity to wear long ones."[19]

The exposure to cold became one of the most lamented anxieties over the new styles, the result of the large expanse of flesh on display as well as the insufficiency of the thin fabrics called for in neoclassical dress.[20] The climate, and the inadequacies of clothing to withstand its fluctuations, reoccurred as themes in both the literature of fashion and in treatises on tuberculosis. In 1799, the *Essay on Pulmonary Consumption* argued that "Our ladies, however, would undoubtedly save themselves some suffering by ceasing to expose themselves, half-undressed, to the fogs and frosts of our island."[21] In 1804, according to *The Fashionable World Displayed*, ladies were sure to fall into consumption: with their "limbs ... stripped, and the bosom laid bare."[22] Caricaturists, social commentators, and medical professionals all took up the author's complaint. "A Naked Truth or Nipping Frost," illustrated the problem of fashionable attire, as Miss Dolly paid the price for leaving off her petticoats when Jack Frost "sorely nip'd, and pinch'd, her bare bum." Unfortunately, the poor girl "Paid Dear for the Fashion, her Folly and Pride/ Went home to her bed and there lingering died.' The lesson was clear, 'Ladies, beware lest Jack Frost should obtrude/ Your nakedness cover, he's apt to be rude."[23] These fashions provided ample fodder for satire and even made an appearance in George Coleman's comedy *The Gentleman* (1806), where he remarked "An English gentlewoman, of the year eighteen hundred, emulates an English oak; which is ... beautiful, but bare, in the depth of December."[24]

Thin fabrics and exposed limbs, backs, and décolletage provided a recipe for disaster when combined with the vagaries of the English weather. As one medical author complained, "The baneful custom, however, of accommodating our dress to the almanack and the fashion, rather than the vicissitudes of the weather, in this inconstant climate, must necessarily be productive of many disagreeable consequences."[25] Pre-eminent among those consequences was consumption. These fashions caused problems when it came to preserving the constitution and thereby preventing tuberculosis. *A Treatise on Medical Police, and on Diet, Regimen* articulated the problem of the constitution, stating "With regard to dress in general, it may be observed, that the very sparing quantity of it used by many of the fair sex ... is very inexcusable, being highly destructive even to the strongest constitution."[26] John Armstrong also made the tubercular connection clear, complaining that the majority of consumptive cases came particularly from "the insufficient protection which the dress of females affords."[27]

The clinging thin gowns of the classical style did not provide the same protection as their predecessors had, and there was also an accompanying reduction in the number of petticoats.[28] As *La Belle Assemblée* remarked, "our climate is a terrible enemy to that airy elegant style of dress so well adapted to the light nymph-like figure of our fair country women."[29] Despite the exaggerated reports of caricaturists and social commentators, women garbed in thin neoclassical materials turned to a variety of garments for warmth. To ward off the cold, women could choose from an assortment of fashionable items including enveloping shawls, cloaks, and stoles or more tailored garments like the spencer and the redingote.[30] The fashion for the "India shawl" continued long after the waning of neoclassical dress and certainly made an appearance in the evocative description of Eliza Hebert who "was wasted almost to a shadow,—attenuated to nearly ethereal delicacy and transparency. She was dressed in a plain white muslin gown, and lying on an Indian shawl, in which she had been enveloped for the purpose of being brought down from her bedchamber. Her small foot and ankle were concealed beneath white silk stockings, and satin slippers– through which it might be seen how they were shrunk from the full dimensions of health."[31] In this instance the shawl provided warmth and a fashionable frame to the shrunken consumptive body.

The use of these sort of outer coverings remained insufficient however, for medical investigators, particularly for those women who were already exhibiting a constitutional delicacy. Physicians focused their objections to the scanty fashions not on outerwear, but on the adaption of the undergarments to the weather and the absence of fleecy hosiery and flannel. For instance, John Armstrong stated that most phthisical cases occurred "in patients who had been careless about their clothing" and that those who were exempt from the illness owed their continued health "to the constant use of a general covering of flannel or of fleecy hosiery."[32] To this he added the importance of guarding against the fluctuations in temperature, particularly for "females, whose natural delicacy renders them less competent to resist the vicissitudes of the atmosphere."[33] In these women, maintaining a constancy of temperature, through appropriate clothing, was key.

James Saunders' *Treatise on Pulmonary Consumption* reiterated the well-established connection between the symptoms of consumption and climate:

> Emaciation makes evident progress; cold air, dampness, wet feet, or cold any how applied, produces an uncommon degree of chilliness, attended always with an instantaneous paleness and sharpening of the features … the face becomes pale … except that an inconstant redness occasionally enlivens the countenance.[34]

Wet feet provided yet another link between fashion and tuberculosis and the problem became an important point for comment, as the flowing fashions were often worn with thin shoes or sandals. In 1806, John Reid granted the feet a pivotal role in the disease process of tuberculosis, arguing "by a careful preservation from chill in the feet … susceptibility to consumption will be considerably diminished."[35] Descriptions of the trends the following year showed a demonstrable lack of concern over the state of the feet remarking, "Muslins are usually worn very clear, and the petticoat so short, as to exhibit the ankle through, which is laced in the sandal style, ornamented with the open-wove stocking."[36]

In 1807, in the *Monthly Magazine*, a father expressed his alarm over the effect that the new dress styles would have upon his daughter, who was already exhibiting signs of consumption, but also acknowledged his

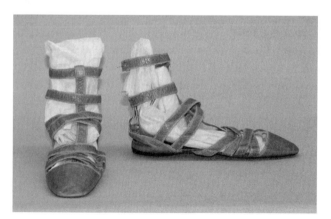 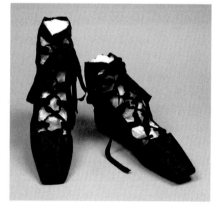

Figure 8.4 Early nineteenth-century sandals. Left: Shoes, 1806–1815, E. Pattison (British), Gerson and Judith Leiber Foundation Gift, 2001 (2001.576a, b) ©Metropolitan Museum of Art. Right: Pair of woman's "Grecian Sandals", c.1818. England. Council Fund (M.2000.10.2a–c). LACMA Image Library.

failure to get her to dress more appropriately for both the weather and her constitution. She was "far from being strong," he wrote, "and has at times a little hectic cough." However, whenever he attempted to intervene in her choice of dress, out of fear for her health, she affected "a liveliness and flow of spirits, and assures me she is better, though I can perceive all the time, that it is a forced effort, merely assumed to prevent me from actually forbidding what she knows I wish her to avoid."[37] Despite these admonitions, fashion seems to have trumped the fear of phthisis. As William Burdon explained in 1820, "Such is the domination of fashion over the female sex, that tho' the lightness of their dress perpetually exposes them to the attacks of consumption . . . they had rather submit to the chance of these most dreadful calamities, than deviate in a single article from the strictest law of fashion."[38]

Inadequate protection was not the only concern, indeed there was even a direct link made between consumption and a prominent component of the neoclassical look—the dress train—which was blamed for causing the disease. (See Plate 22.) In 1806, *La Belle Assemblée* attacked the "enormous length of our fashionable women's trains."[39] The author stated, "The trains, such as they now are, are hurtful to public salubrity." How could something as seemingly innocuous as a train be blamed for harming the public good? The answer lay in the enormous clouds of dust created as ladies strolled down the lanes of Green Park and St. James's. The article addressed the consequences, asking what rendered "the air breathed there so fatal to delicate lungs, and causes so many colds, sore throats, and consumptions? The trains,—the unfortunate trains. The greater part of mankind go there to exhale the pure and uncontaminated air, but return suffocated." These trains, according to the author, also were a hazard indoors: "In winter, at all our balls, and routs, the evil is increased rather than diminished . . . it is impossible to describe the consequences which must result from a carpet badly brushed, or an ill chalked floor. Sometimes, to oblige the ladies to take up these instruments of death, we have seen mischievous coxcombs set their foot on that part which lay on the ground. The lady, wishing to disengage her train, seizes its undulations, and cautiously shaking it, a cloud of dust arises from its folds, and obliges the unwary coxcomb to retire immediately for fear of suffocation. For pity's sake, ladies . . . consider the delicacy of our lungs."[40]

Yet alongside these diatribes over the pathological consequences of these fashions, there was a simultaneous explosion of literature that connected consumption with clothing in a more positive manner. Authors of poetry and fiction also articulated a certain ideal of the beautiful female, one dominated by a model of a languorous, pale, and graceful feminine beauty that was in keeping with certain aspects of consumption.[41] For instance, in 1809 an author in *La Belle Assemblée* provided a description of Juliana, who "possess[ed] the very soul of sensibility." Her physical appearance was characterized by a pale countenance and willowy conformation, and her dress was evocative of consumption.

> Her person is in a great degree the index of her mind; with a pale and interesting countenance is united a figure of sylph-like symmetry . . . It is impossible to produce a more striking contrast than this romantic yet interesting girl . . . the apparent delicacy, and retiring yet graceful simplicity.[42]

Edward Ball's melodrama *The Black Robber* provided a similar description of the "sylph-like Julia" as she tumbled into consumption. Julia assumed "an appearance almost celestial . . . But alas! Each succeeding day was far from bringing health to her faded cheek, true the rose's glow beamed brightly there, but it was only the hectic colouring of consumption."[43]

Beyond the silhouette of consumption, marked by "a figure of sylph-like symmetry" and "delicacy," dress also highlighted certain features of the disease process. One of the most prominent examples was the fashion for displaying the backbones, an affectation that would have heightened the visibility of consumption by accentuating its wing-backed symptom. References to exposed backbones litter the fashion journals of the period. (See Plate 23.) *La Belle Assemblée* referenced this practice in 1806 stating, "The Parisian ladies wear the back of their gowns lower than ever . . . but our English belles have very politically advanced theirs within these last three weeks. Surely the compressed shoulders, and consequently distorted back, must exhibit a most uninteresting spectacle."[44] These "compressed shoulders" and "distorted back" were eerily reminiscent of the consumptive form where, as John Reid described, "the clavicles and shoulder-blades are thrust out from their proper position, and made to assume in some measure the form of wings . . . just raised from the body and about to expand for flight."[45]

Fashion continued to emphasize the physical consequences of consumption and, despite repeated complaints, the uncovered back and exposed shoulder blades remained an integral part of female dress for more than a decade. (See Plate 24.) In 1818, *The Lady's Magazine* stated that "many of our would-be-fashionable damsels exhibit themselves as walking deformities, with a hump on their backs . . . [and] appear like snails carrying their houses."[46] In the same year, *A Picture of the Changes of Fashion* claimed that "The disgusting and frightful fashion of shewing the back bones is disappearing."[47] Such an assertion may have been premature as in 1820 *La Belle Assemblée* once again reprimanded the fashionable about the spectacle, stating "I am surprised to see the British ladies . . . make so ample a display of bare backs."[48] Modish women "stooped to conquer" the social satirist Felix M'Donogh claimed, and he lamented the feminine style for "the fashionable hump upon [the] back."[49] His caricature censured the "high shoulders, and often a stoop in walking" accorded as part of the consumptive constitution.[50] The popularity of this consumptive look led him to complain in 1820 that fashions exhibited "a strange practical paradox of dress and undress, poor, meagre, thin creatures were sewed up in niggardly covering, which set one shivering to look at it; and the chest was so exposed with hollow collar bones, distinct ribs, and ill-covered shoulder-blades, that a surgeon might have studied osteology from these living anatomies."[51]

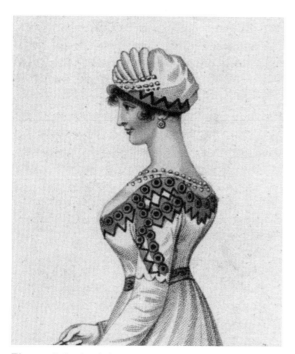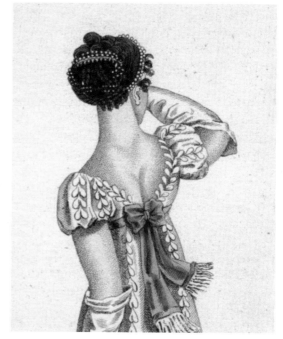

Figure 8.5 The fashionable hump and prominent shoulder blades reminiscent of the winged-back appearance of consumption. Left: "Evening Full Dress," *La Belle Assemblée* (London: 1811), Casey Fashion Plate Collection, Los Angeles Public Library. Right: "Parisien Ball Dress 1811," *La Belle Assemblée* (London: 1811), Casey Fashion Plate Collection, Los Angeles Public Library.

However much the styles changed, to remain fashionable, women necessarily needed to do things that not only threatened their health but were actually believed to create tuberculosis. As a result, the preoccupation with climate continued even after the neoclassical style was supplanted. The association between women's fashion and consumption continued to grow in the 1820s and 1830s, and the clothing itself increased in importance in the discussions of causation, to the point of being given primacy in explanations of the disease. As an example, *The Ladies Pocket Magazine* in 1829 stated, "It is not our intention to enter into any general remarks upon the nature of that fatal disease. In very many cases the origin of a consumption is an ordinary cold; and that cold is frequently taken through the want of a proper attention to clothing, particularly in females."[52] The same sentiment was expressed in *A Practical Manual for the Preservation of Health and of the Prevention of Diseases* (1824), which asserted, "Many patients, especially females, fall into consumptive complaints from the want of attention to this particular."[53]

The protests against the pernicious effects of certain fashions continued to revolve around a number of the same themes addressed in the preceding decades, including the role played by excessive exposure and inadequate warmth on both the initiation and progress of tuberculosis. For Sir Arthur Clarke "women, according to present fashion, dress warmly, and over the whole of the person in the morning, but strip their shoulders, and adopt light dresses, in the evening. Thus circumstanced, when after the exercise of dancing they rush into draughts of cold air, they frequently lay the foundations of diseases which embitter and shorten existence."[54] *La Belle Assemblée* also commented on the inadequacy of fashionable clothes in protecting the wearer from the effects of the climate. This insufficiency was due in part, according to an 1827 article, to the refusal of fashionable ladies to ruin the line of a gown by adopting appropriate outerwear when attending evening social events. The lack of warm clothing, it claimed, contributed to the declining health of many a young woman. The mischief occurred when, "at the now chilly hour of nine, they [fashionable ladies] may have quitted their warm dwellings, and have risked the exposure of the susceptible chest, from the fear of deranging the trimmings on their dress."[55] Fashion writers were joined by medical authors in continuing to link scanty clothing to consumption, as seen in *The Modern Practice of Physic* (1828).

> Various causes have indeed been assigned for the increasing prevalence at the present time of this distressing disease in the United Kingdom … there is great reason to suspect that the warmth and closeness of our apartments, together with the present scanty, light, and flimsy attire of our modish females, very much increase the liability to this complaint.[56]

The Pocket Medical Guide (1834) similarly maintained, "Sudden changes in temperature produce hurtful effects on the body, under various circumstances. Passing into the open air from a hot and crowded ball-room, is a very common mode in which the exposure takes place. How many coughs and consumptions take their origins in such circumstances!"[57]

Fashion did not function in a vacuum and already in 1823 *The Ladies Monthly Museum* had expanded the issue beyond insufficient clothing, admonishing its reader that "the enjoyment of health, is a duty, inasmuch as on the possession of health depends the proper performance of our various parts in the grand drama of life … While conforming to the rules of fashion and of pleasure, health is never allowed to urge its plea."[58] The journalist went on to complain:

> In vain reason argues against the costume that fashion recommends, or the hours that dissipation enjoins. The young and lovely woman of fashion breathes the infected air of crowded rooms night after night, instead of seeking the salutary repose the constitution of their nature requires; and in return sinks

into feverish slumbers during those hours when the inartificial beauty of humbler life, is catching health from the pure air of the young day. This course has consigned thousands to an early grave.[59]

These sorts of criticisms occurred over and over again, seemingly to no avail, as fashionable pursuits were thought to combine with exposure to cold to produce consumption.[60]

Fashionable life was articulated, not just as a cause of consumption, but also as one of the main reasons for the high incidence among the upper and middle classes. *The London Medical Gazette* complained in 1833 that:

[T]he utmost attention should be paid to clothing. A large number of females in this country fall into consumption chiefly through their own fault. The poorer classes cannot dress well, cannot be expected to take that care of themselves that they should, because they have not the means; but the rich and the middle classes do everything they can to fall into consumption.[61]

The author criticized, in particular, the insufficient attention to the variability of the environment by women who "will go from the hottest rooms without any thing about their feet; they take little sleep; have party after party every night; and then, at last, fall into a state of consumption: and neither themselves nor their friends will believe that this want of rest, and this extreme excitement, has been the cause of it; but I am quite sure it has."[62] Improper raiment continued to play an integral role in the dialogue surrounding consumption.

Consumptive Corsetry and Romantic Fashion

Just as too little clothing could bring about consumption, so could too much, or at least clothing that was too tight. As a result, corsets were the subject of much contention in both the debates surrounding fashion and those involving disease. It was widely believed that certain styles of clothing could harm the wearer either by impeding "the growth and functions of the body from inequalities of pressure, or by occasioning an improper exposure to irregularities in external temperature." These considerations were extremely important for those with a weak constitution, as mechanical force increased "constitutional sensibility" and led to "a concurrent degree of physical sensibility to the powers of heat and cold."[63] Wearing restrictive clothing, then, could escalate the effects of temperature variation upon the delicate constitution and ease the way for consumption to take hold. The issue of tightness was particularly pertinent with regard to corseting, as the practice was believed to create a tubercular diathesis by applying injurious pressure to the pulmonary system, leading to systemic illness.

The problem of restraint upon the torso had been a running theme during the eighteenth century, when the graceful female body was the product of heavy lacing and the practice was repeatedly condemned as being "in the highest degree prejudicial to health."[64] Even early in the eighteenth century, it was accorded a role in the etiology of consumption. Cheyne in discussing the case of Catherine Walpole's illness (which in the end proved to be consumption), wrote "There is plainly a Depression and falling in on that Side" which he suggested may have resulted from the use of "the Iron-Stayes."[65] Corsets and their connection to the development of consumption remained a recurring motif in the eighteenth and nineteenth centuries. In his 1757 work on the disease, Benjamin Richardson called corseting "slow suicide"[66] while in 1765, Dr. John Gregory explicitly linked the wearing of stays to the creation of consumption in women.[67] These sentiments were articulated by countless other medical and social commentators who saw the practice of corseting as ruining the constitution and producing disease.[68]

There has been a great deal of debate over whether or not women discarded stays at the turn of the century in an effort to achieve the neoclassical silhouette; however, numerous contemporary references suggest they

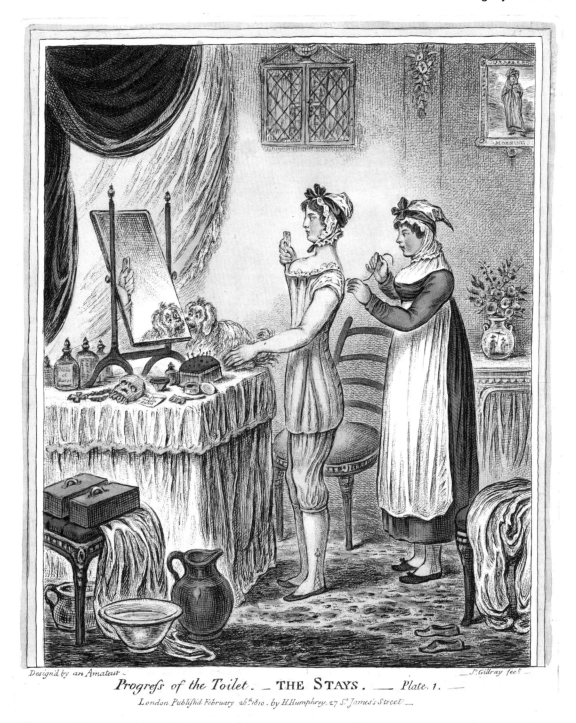

Designd by an Amateur.

Progress of the Toilet. — THE STAYS. — Plate 1. —

J. Gillray fect.

London Publish'd February 26th 1810. by H. Humphrey. 27 St James's Street —

Figure 8.6 "Progress of the Toilet—The Stays" (1810). Image number: lwlpr12221. Courtesy of The Lewis Walpole Library, Yale University.

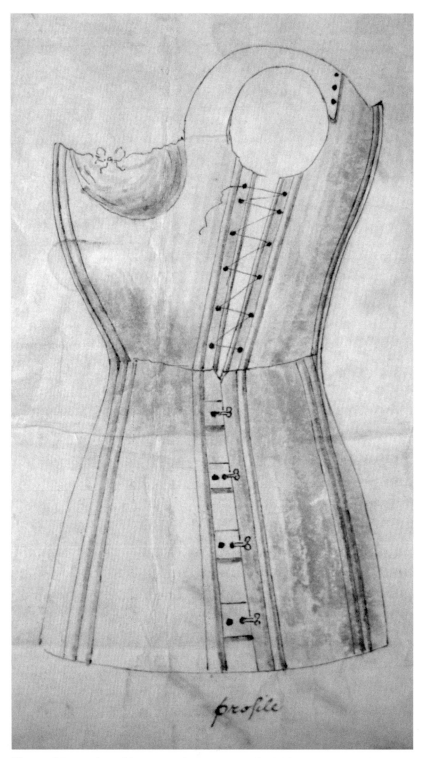

Figure 8.7 Martha Gibbon, Stays for Women and Children, patent number 2457, December 17, 1800. The National Archives, London, UK.

did not.[69] A number of items aided in the achievement of this figure, including a variety of shorter undergarments (see Plate 25); while caricatures, fashionable literature, and trade cards provide evidence that the long stay was also available for those women requiring extra support.[70] Most likely, the elongated corset was designed to help in controlling the outmoded bulge and aid in creating a fashionable figure, increasingly marked by thinness.[71] In 1800, Martha Gibbon took out a patent for the *Je Ne Sais Quoi* Stay which purported to slim the middle by preventing "any protuberance of the intestine,"[72] while an 1806 treatise on consumption bemoaned the "sickly and mis-shapen" form of females, the product of stay wearing, stating that "Very straight lacing and straining for a fine shape . . . hath made many a fine girl spit blood."[73]

The chorus of disapproval over the use of corsets grew louder near the end of the first decade of the nineteenth century when the item returned as a universal fixture of fashion. In 1809, John Roberton hoped in vain that the practice would remain absent, remarking:

> It is now many years since the barbarous custom of wearing on the body tight laced stays have [sic] been justly laid aside. It would appear, however, in some instances, that they are beginning again to be worn. I sincerely hope, however, that the custom will never be so common as it has been, for by indulging in it much disease was produced. The free expansion of the lungs was prevented . . . shortness of breath followed, and, in many, terminated in consumption.[74]

Roberton's hopes were dashed however, as both English and French journals continued to proclaim the re-ascendency of the corset.[75] By 1811, slenderness of the female frame was re-established as an integral part of female beauty.[76] In that same year *Mirror of the Graces* complained "the present mode of bracing . . . in what is called the long stays . . . With the tight pressure of steel and whalebone on the most susceptible parts of the frame . . . are the positive causes of consumptions."[77] While *La Belle Assemblée* argued that "the excessive compression" of the corset produced "diseases too frightful to name."[78] As styles moved away from the strictly neoclassical toward an ebullient Romantic style, the new fashions placed the emphasis on a progressively thinner waist instead of on the bosom.[79] Increasingly, the degree to which this slenderness was pursued became a cause for concern, and with it came further complaints over the use of stays as causing disease.

The power of the Romantic Movement, so synonymous with literature and the arts, became noticeable in fashion after 1820. Fashion historians have characteristically assigned the period from 1820 until around 1850 as the Romantic era in dress; however, they frequently break that period into two major epochs. For the purpose of this work, the term Romantic will be used to refer to the period from 1820 to the mid-1830s, and the term sentimental will be used to denote the period dating from around 1836 to 1850. The emphasis on feeling, fierce and exuberant emotion, and the revival of historical themes that characterized Romanticism all influenced clothing styles, particularly in women's fashions, in the earlier period. Elements of historic dress appeared in sleeve styles, neck ruffs, and certain types of embellishment, and fabric colors were often given fanciful designations like "Egyptian Earth" and "dust of ruins."[80] The influence of Romanticism was also evident in the effusive trimming that was particularly popular during the 1820s and the first half of the 1830s.[81] This excess decoration was the material manifestation of "the change in the feminine ideal from classical goddess to ornamented doll."[82] Aileen Ribeiro has also argued that the conventions of female beauty in the 1830s and 1840s tended toward the "doll-like."[83]

Dress remained of vital importance in defining women during the Romantic period. The author of the *Kalogynomia* (1821) argued "the woman who possesses a cultivated taste and a corresponding expression of countenance, will generally be tastefully dressed; and the vulgar woman, with features correspondingly rude, will easily be seen through the inappropriate mask in which her milliner or dress-maker may have invested her."[84] By 1825, the new silhouette was firmly established, defined by an increasingly widening skirt and progressively contracted waist. An ostensibly V-shaped bodice emerged, one with enlarged shoulders, made to appear even more so by expansive collars and rapidly growing sleeves, a trend that would continue until the mid-1830s. Headgear and hairstyles also increased in size and complexity and were elaborately decorated with artificial flowers, feathers, and jewelry.[85] As the waistline moved downwards toward its natural level, the back of the bodice, which had been rather narrow in the neoclassical presentation, began to flare, becoming ever wider with increasingly exposed décolletage. This alteration threw the upper portion of the torso and the throat into prominence and further heightened the impression of a sloped shoulder, which had emerged as an essential aspect of female attractiveness.[86] The over-exposed décolleté, regulated in the daytime by the use of fichus and cape-like pelerines, was presented in all its glory during the evening hours. Finally, the sense of smallness at the waist was enhanced by a contrast with the widening skirts and enormous sleeves. On top, the shoulder span also slowly expanded, as the upper portion of the sleeve continued to grow.[87] The gigot or leg-of-mutton sleeve swelled spectacularly from the shoulder line, narrowing as it moved toward the wrist.[88] It was

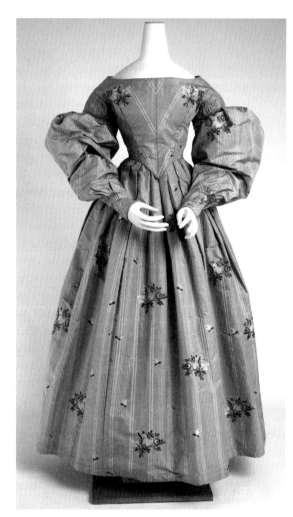
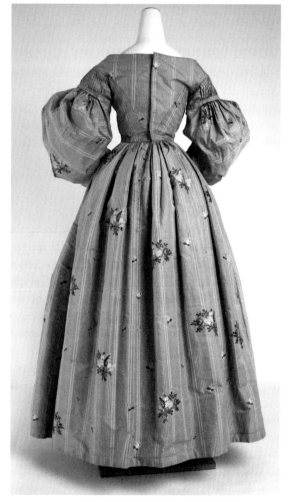

Figure 8.8 Romantic fashions. Dress c.1836 (British) Credit: Irene Lewisohn Bequest, 1966. Accession Number: C.I.66.35.1 ©Metropolitan Museum of Art, New York.

joined in 1829 by other enormous sleeve designs, including the evocatively named "Imbecile" and the less descriptive Donna Maria and Mameluke, all of which made the upper portion of the arm appear double the size of the waist. All of these fashions helped augment the image of the ethereal, languishing Romantic angel.

This angel, no longer clad in flowing drapery, achieved a look of delicacy and diminutiveness through corsets that were laced ever tighter, aided by a wide belt and buckle that further imprisoned her waist. (See Plate 26.) With the increased attention to the waist, the corset was now calculated to slim the bodylines, rather than artificially alter the natural shape, as its eighteenth-century predecessors had done. Corset dimensions became a hotly contested aspect of the toilet, particularly as the waist was subjected to ever more strenuous tight lacing in an effort to increase the contrast between the constructions both above and below. The extreme hourglass shape, the subject of the 1829 cartoon "Waist and Extravagance," was also the object of criticism in *The New Monthly Magazine* that same year, which complained that "The finest figure, thus encumbered … might be mistaken for two pillow-cases hanging on a stick, so small is the space into which the waist is compressed between these appendages."[89]

With the focus firmly on the waist, the body increasingly became an object to control through diet, exercise, and most importantly through constraint and physical manipulation. Innovative developments in the corset, in shape and construction, were in line with the renewed emphasis on the small waist. A stiffer but shorter corset developed, one that accentuated the waist while elevating the bust. The new style allowed both the bosom and hips to assume an increasingly rounded shape by virtue of gussets, inserted on both the top and bottom to accommodate these features. The new corset style also often had a wide busk,[90] encased in a sleeve of some sort in the center front of the corset.[91] The new corset shape diminished the size of the waist by pressing it into a circular rather than kidney shape, while at the same time accentuating the breast and hips. Additionally, the practice of pulling the corset laces extremely tight to further reduce the measurement and exaggerate the effect became increasingly popular. This practice could only be carried so far in the early 1820s, because stitched eyelet holes could only take so much stress before they ripped.[92] However, in 1828 the invention of metal eyelets, for use in the lacing of corsets, allowed for a considerable reduction in the size of the waist.[93]

Unease and debate over the practice of tight lacing continued throughout the 1830s, 1840s, and 1850s, as the injurious pressure associated with corseting became the primary complaint of those commenting on fashion and one of the main presumed causes of consumption. As the corsets tightened, so too did the link with tuberculosis. As one author lamented, "Yet, to follow the fashion of a smaller waist than Nature has designed the person,—'The stays of deadly steel, in whose embrace. The tyrant fashion tortures injured grace,' are resorted to, and females are laced to such a degree of tightness, that if the fashion lasted long their health, if not life, must soon fall sacrifice."[94] Undue pressure upon the organs of respiration was thought to result in phthisis, and the new style of corset, along with the practice of tight lacing, became one of the major causes articulated to explain the incidence of consumption in women. Not only did the look remain fashionable, but the waist also continued to diminish in size and in the 1840s would be joined by the torso as an object to be reduced.[95] In 1842, an article in *Fraser's Magazine* laid responsibility for the death of 31,090 English women from consumption at the door of the "unnatural and injurious practice of tight lacing."[96]

Physicians were outraged; caricaturists had yet more fodder for their cartoons; and journalists, social commentators, and even fashion writers decried the use of tightly laced corsets to no avail.[97] There were countless discussions of the consequences of corseting in both popular and medical literature, and many also included visual aids in the form of anatomical drawings in an effort to drive home the pernicious effects. These diagrams usually contrasted the unhealthy form of the tightly laced woman with the healthy natural form of the body.[98] Quite a few of these articles called for women to continue their emulation of the ancient Greeks,

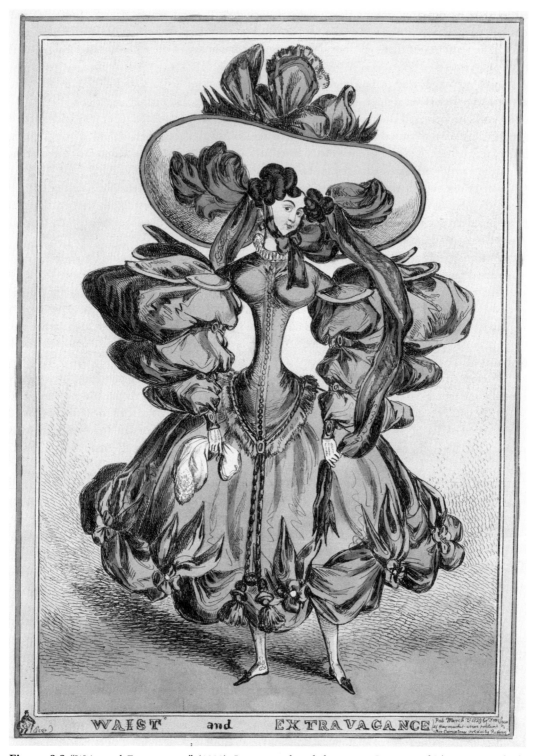

Figure 8.9 "Waist and Extravagance" (1829). Image number: lwlpr13285. Courtesy of The Lewis Walpole Library, Yale University.

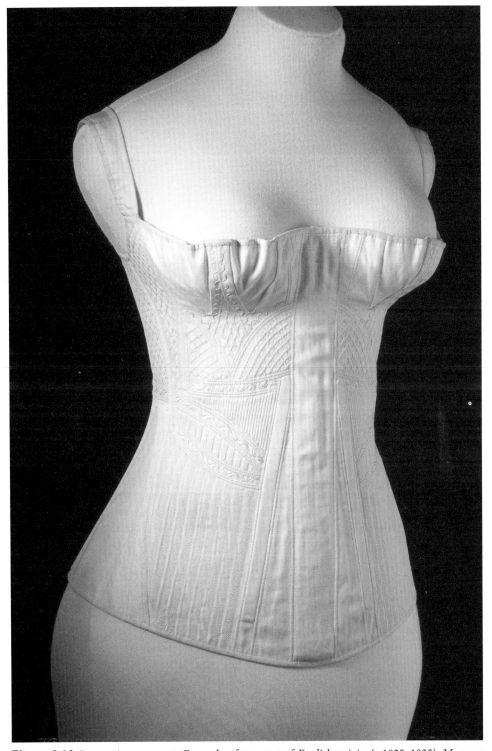

Figure 8.10 Romantic era corset. Example of a corset of English origin (c.1825–1835). Museum Number: T.57-1948. ©Victoria and Albert Museum, London.

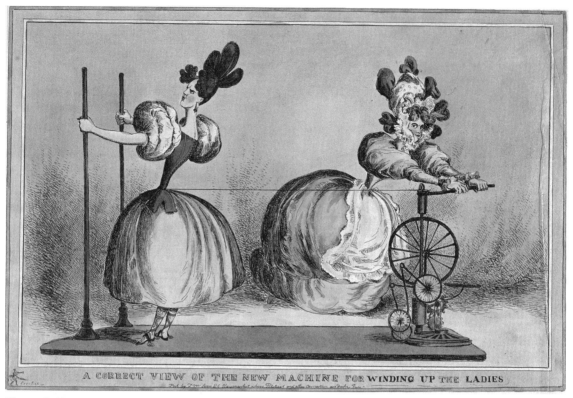

A CORRECT VIEW OF THE NEW MACHINE FOR WINDING UP THE LADIES

Figure 8.11 A woman is turning a wheel to make the young girl's waist smaller. Etching by W. Heath, c.1830. Wellcome Library, London. Copyrighted work available under Creative Commons Attribution only licence CC BY 4.0 http://creativecommons.org/licenses/by/4.0/

not in dress style as during the neoclassical period, but instead in the beauty of the Grecian form. In 1825, one author exhorted her readers to "follow the example of the elegant Greeks, the ease and beauty of whose forms are so much admired. They put no unnatural straps on their young ladies . . . and the effect was seen in their every limb, and their every motion."[99] In 1827, *La Belle Assemblée* echoed these assertions, exclaiming "It is monstrous, and excites only ridicule. Where is the easy well-rounded form, that might defy the chisel of the statuary to equal? Tortured into a waist like that of a wasp, with, apparently, round hips, formed of whalebone!"[100] The purported distortion caused by corseting was a vitally important link to tuberculosis, as "deformities of the chest" were "commonly ranked among the exciting causes of consumption."[101]

Despite the volume of writing against the use of the corset, many diatribes on the subject accepted that women were unwilling to give up this crucial part of their wardrobe, upon which everything else rested. Authors acknowledged the difficulty in persuading women to surrender their corsets, but some still hoped to persuade them to prevent the ruination of the succeeding generation. Thus an 1825 article argued "that it would be vain to attempt to dissuade ladies from the use of this pernicious article of dress; but, however much they may disregard themselves, they ought, certainly, to reject for their children, whatever shall be hurtful to them."[102] Further complicating the issue was a widely held belief that corsets were essential to maintaining not just a slender waist but also a straight spine, for instance the *Art of Beauty* stated: "Unfortunately, the idea that the bodies of girls require support during their growth has, by time and custom, become so firmly rooted in the minds of most mothers, that no persuasion will influence them to give up the practice."[103]

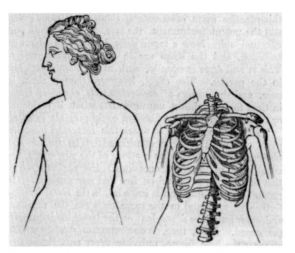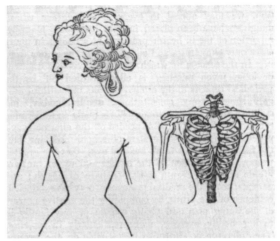

Figure 8.12 Figures represent the statue of the Venus de Medici, and the natural skeleton is contrasted with the shape of the "modern boarding-school miss" and her remodeled skeleton. *The Penny Magazine of The Society for the Diffusion of Useful Knowledge* (London: Charles Knight, 1833). 80. L900.b.69.1, Cambridge University Library.

The conundrum of corsets remained a serious issue of not only fashion but also medicine, as the garment was considered both the creator and corrector of deformity.[104] As early as 1801, Charles Pears acknowledged a beneficial role for corsets in the consumptive disease process. He combined the belief in the favorable effects of support with the idea that consumption ceased during pregnancy to assign corsets a role in treating the disease, reasoning:

> Phthisis is suspended during pregnancy; probably from the elevation and pressure of the uterus, producing a degree of rest to the lungs . . . If so, it might be beneficially imitated by bandage . . . as well as from the support that is derived from the use of stays thus medically employed with advantage.[105]

Additionally, corsets were accorded the power to correct spinal deformity and as such prevent the tuberculosis associated with this condition. There were a variety of patents and devices built upon the corset that claimed to correct the malformations of the spine and chest that could be productive of disease. Inventions including the "Gardner Stays for Support," patented in 1822, and nearly twenty years later the "Kingdon Apparatus for the Support of the Human Body" were billed as able to correct malformations of the body. These devices, like the corsets themselves, became more complex and tighter over time.

Beyond the promotion of devices, based upon the corset, to correct deformities, there also developed an industry that sought to make safer versions in an effort to deal with the reality of fashion and a society that could not, and would not, do without the corset. Staymakers constructed a variety of garments they claimed would provide the fashionable silhouette without producing consumption, for example, those designed to allow a freer motion of the chest, like John Mills' "Elastic Stays for Women and Children," patented in 1815. Mills introduced "a flexible or elastic portion in those parts of the stays best calculated to give relief to the wearer while at the same time preserving that stability and support usually given to the body by the common adoption of whalebone steel and other hard or inflexible materials."[106] He even developed a pregnancy option. In 1825, *The Art of Beauty* took up the quest for "healthy corsets," calling for the elastic sorts of garments Mills had patented.

If stays, however, are worn, and it should be done with great caution, we must altogether prohibit the use of whalebone or steel as decidedly injurious. The materials should all be elastic, so as to yield to every movement without compressing any part of the body.[107]

Many staymakers answered the call; one of the most famous was Mrs. Bell, the wife to the editor of *La Belle Assemblée*. In 1831, the magazine, understandably, lauded her for utilizing India rubber in her stays.

Mrs. Bell's house has long been unrivalled for the elegance of its corsets, which boast those advantages so rarely united, of strengthening and supporting the frame, and adding singular grace to the shape. A recent discovery enables Mrs. Bell to extend these advantages still farther, by substituting India rubber for elastic wires.[108]

Despite these innovations, corsets continued to receive blame from the medical community for causing many cases of consumption and were one of the primary reasons articulated to explain why women were more predisposed to the disease than men.

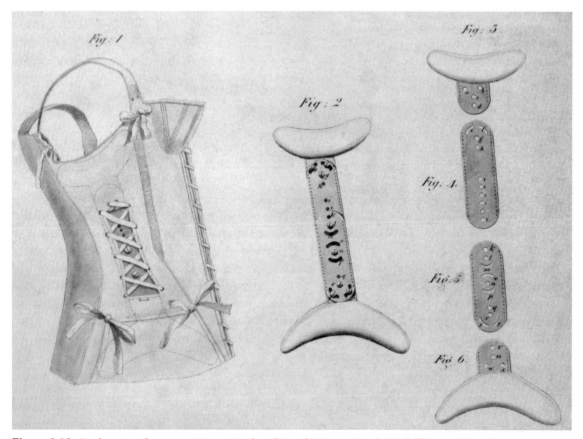

Figure 8.13 Gardner stays for support. Denny Gardner, "Stays for Supporting the Body," Patented June 13, 1822. Courtesy of The National Archives, London, UK.

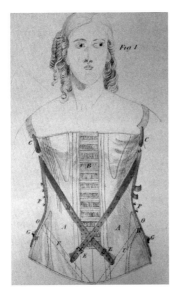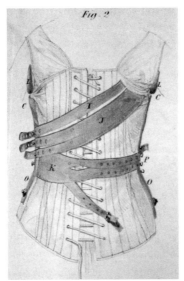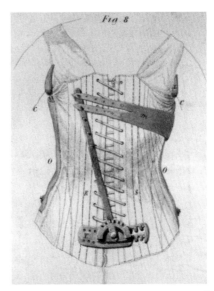

Figure 8.14 Richard Kingdon, "Apparatus for the Support of the Human Body," patented February 25, 1840. Courtesy of The National Archives, London, UK.

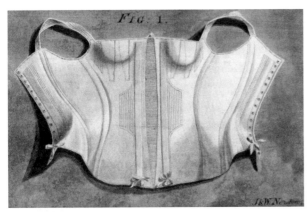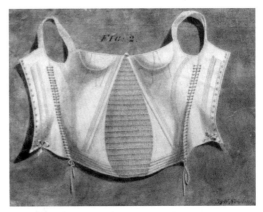

Figure 8.15 Elastic stays for women and children (1815). Left: Stays for young growing persons or adults of a sound constitution. Right: Pregnancy stays. John Mills, "Elastic Stays for Women and Children." Courtesy of The National Archives, London, UK.

Even as corsets were accused of creating disease, they also emulated certain features of tuberculosis. In 1829, "The Pernicious and Often Fatal Effects of the Compression of the Female Waist By the Use of Corsets" tackled the current fashions. The author remarked:

We know that as often as the waist is lengthened to its natural limits, this tendency to abridge its diameter appears . . . Corsets are employed to modify the shape, to render the chest as small below, and as broad above, as possible, and to increase the elevation, fullness, and prominence of the bosom . . . The natural form of the thorax, in short, is just the reverse of the fashionable shape of the waist. The latter is narrow below and wide above; the former is narrow above and wide below.[109]

The physical shape imparted by the fashionable corset, the "narrow below and wide above," emulated the conformation that was the product of tuberculosis. Width at the top was provided by the shoulders and from the widening of the upper back. As Francis Ramadge asserted in 1834, the conformation present during consumption included,

> . . . the projection of the shoulder-blades (which has been noticed as resembling wings) while at the same time the chest is narrowed in its lateral, as well as transverse diameter, in consequence of the increased convexity of the ribs which has a greater inclination downwards, and which thus likewise admits of the nearer approach of the sternum towards the back. On the upper and anterior part of the chest, the intercostal spaces appear widened and depressed, and the belly is at the same time flat and retracted.[110]

During the 1830s there was yet another shift in fashion that would increase the appearance of imitating consumption, one that began in the latter part of the decade and conformed to the emerging ideas of sentimentalism. These were primarily concerned with three major areas: etiquette, dress, and social ritual.[111] The shift toward the sentimental style of clothing began during the 1830s and was firmly on track by the end of the decade. The female silhouette was demonstrably changing, and clothing started to lose its Romantic exuberance in favor of a restrained and decorous silhouette. As the bodices simplified and became increasingly close fitting they produced sloping lines that focused down and created a drooping appearance.[112]

The Romantic fashions of the 1820s and early 1830s had been distinguished by full sleeves, wide shoulders, and flared skirts. By contrast, the fashions of the 1840s were timorous, diffident, and reserved. Sentimentalism even influenced color choice, favoring browns and dark greens, which combined with the structure of clothing to impart a subdued appearance.[113] The bodice was pulled tight to the body by virtue of heavily laced corseting and by its construction. The pointed waist enhanced the appearance of thinness, while the open décolleté highlighted the rounded shoulders all of which emphasized "the sensitive, graceful and feminine features" of the 1840s woman.[114] In sentimental dress, the waist was narrower than it had been in the previous decade and the focus was increasingly on a slimming of the torso as a whole.

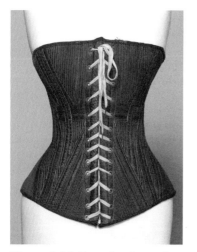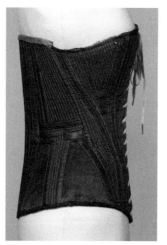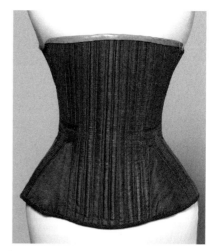

Figure 8.16 Example of a sentimental style of corset (c.1840–1850). This front lacing style of corset tilted the hips forward, and compressed the torso and pushed the shoulder blades up enhancing the hunched appearance. Accession Number: 1972.7. Courtesy of the Manchester Art Gallery.

As a result, the corset remained an indispensable and acknowledged component of style and was the essential instrument for achieving the slim lines and long, tight waist called for by fashion.[115] *The Magazine of the Beau Monde* complained in 1836 that women had set a new standard for beauty, one marked by a waist that "tapers rapidly below the arms, and is not above two-thirds of the natural girth."[116] Although already established in the 1830s, the new corset style altered again during the 1840s in an effort to accommodate the changing outer layers of female dress.[117] The corsets, like the bodices, lengthened in keeping with the emerging sentimental shape and did not appreciably shorten again until the 1860s.[118] The consternation over the practice of tight lacing increased with the development of a new style of lacing in 1843, known as *a la paresseuse* or lazy style. This technique allowed a more precise control over the lacing itself, permitting even tighter lacing of the corset at the waist, much to the disgust of various commentators.[119]

The practice of tight lacing intensified the debates surrounding clothing and consumption, as the fashions were accorded even greater agency in creating tuberculosis. Hence, Esther Copley wrote in 1840:

> So preposterous and fantastic are the disguises of the human form which modern fashion has exhibited, that her votaries … while individually priding themselves on their elegance and taste, they have very commonly appeared, in the eyes of an indifferent spectator, to be running a race for the acquisition of deformity.[120]

Medical tracts and the writings of moral instructionists were filled with diatribes against the evils of tight lacing and cited it as a cause of pulmonary consumption. Despite voluminous writings against the use of the corset, young women continued to garb themselves in clothing thought to be ruinous to their health, much to the frustration of Dr. Francis Cook who angrily wrote in 1842, "The compression to which the dress of young females subjects the chest, is a most frequent cause of pulmonary disease. It is however, vain to expect, that the

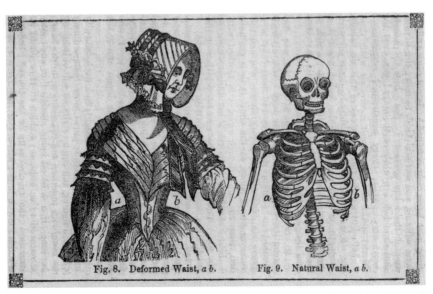

Fig. 8. Deformed Waist, *a b.*   Fig. 9. Natural Waist, *a b.*

Figure 8.17 Contrast of the "Deformed" corsetted waist versus that of the "Natural" uncorsetted waist. *Health Made Easy for Young People* (London: Darton & Clark, 1845), 56. 8300.e.13. Cambridge University Library

warning voice of the physician will be listened to in preference to the dictates of fashion."[121] *Health Made Easy for Young People* (1845) also asserted that consumption would be the inevitable result for those women whose chests were "bound up, 'to make them look pretty,' and considered the practice 'Monstrous!'"[122] The arguments of physicians notwithstanding, it was acknowledged that, "One of the greatest ideal evils in a figure, in the eye of a young lady of the present day, is that of a thick waist."[123] Nearly a decade later, in 1848, the sentiment remained the same when *Blackwood's Lady's Magazine* stated, "The beauty of the female figure consists in being gently serpentine."[124] Despite the proliferation of anti-corset works, not only did the practice continue, but sentimental dress as a whole was accorded positive qualities. For example, in 1848 *The World of Fashion* remarked that: "The female attire of the present day is, perhaps, in as satisfactory a state as the advocates of nature and simplicity can desire … The dress is one calculated to bring out the natural beauties of the person."[125]

Tubercular and Tight the Sentimental Way

The sentimental ideal of beauty, took the appearance of the woman as a whole to be an expression of her character, and clothing played a significant role in the fashioning of this character. Designed to showcase the sensibility that shone from the countenance of the early Victorian woman, sentimental dress enhanced rather than detracted from the face. The fashionable woman's form was slender; her face was pale and free of cosmetics, while her dress was relatively inconspicuous. *The Young Lady's Friend* in 1837 directly connected dress to the character of its wearer. "Such various qualities of mind are called into action in connexion with dress … and the more Christian principles prevail … the more truly will dress be an indication of the character."[126] Fashion, thus, progressively became a form of moral self-improvement, a way of enhancing one's personal qualities, or at least displaying them.

The constrictive forms of sentimental dress during the 1840s were not an effort to disguise or distort a woman's body, although they did; instead the dress was designed to reveal the feelings of the woman who wore it. The overall effect of sentimental dress in the 1840s was one of decorous, modest, and meek passivity, mirroring the prescribed ideal for the Victorian woman. (See Plate 27.) As such, these fashions were historically and culturally specific, demonstrating the influence of the rhetoric of respectability and Christian morality.[127] During the 1840s the place of feelings and sentiment was elevated, taking precedence over corporeal soundness, as the fashionable woman was increasingly constrained by her clothing. In the ideals laid down by writers like Mrs. Ellis, it was clear what was expected of women: softness, delicacy, weakness, and modesty, combined with a small waist and curving shoulders.[128] Similarly, in his 1845 work on consumption, Alfred Beaumont Maddock described those possessing the hectic constitution as having "a narrow or pointed chest, high prominent shoulders, long thin neck, and generally slender frame."[129] While, Mrs. Merrifield in her *Dress as a Fine Art* acknowledged these features as integral to beauty in the female.[130] On the whole, the early Victorian woman was less dynamic, in both body and demeanor, than English women had been in the earlier decades of the century, as the emphasis turned toward the articulation of moral character through a graceful demeanor, poses, and attitudes.[131] As one author remarked, "Graceful movement, an unaffected elegance of demeanour, is to the figure what sense and sweetness are to the eyes. It is the soul looking out. It is what a poet has called the 'thought of the body.'"[132]

The main effect of this type of costume upon a woman's deportment was a limitation of movement; furthermore, the shoulders narrowed and dress imparted a drooping appearance, as the body seemed to be pulled downwards.[133] The extended bodice was ornamented in a manner that heightened the appearance of length. For instance, the pleated fabric overlays that had been a feature of decoration in the 1830s were being applied by the 1840s on an exaggerated diagonal, in an effort to highlight and narrow the shoulders and emphasize and elongate the pointed waist.[134] (See Plates 28 and 29.) The heavy corseting made the upper body appear delicate, thin, and weak, in a manner reminiscent of the consumptive torso. The fashion plates from the period illustrate the changes in female costume and in the overall appearance, showing the hair close to the head, the bonnet drawn close, and the heavy corseting to make the upper torso appear delicate, thin, and weak.[135] The sentimental image conferred by the new clothing was wilted and almost lifeless, and the overall demeanor was dreamy and tender.[136]

The trend toward delicacy intensified over the decade, with the application of even tighter sleeves, and a consequent narrowing of the shoulder line. As one author asserted, "Delicacy is, indeed, the point of honour in woman . . . A delicate woman, too, will be more loved, as well as more respected, than any other."[137] Thus, as Douglas A. Russell has argued, "the ideal for woman had changed in a little over a decade from a gay butterfly to a domesticated doll."[138] The bodices simplified and became increasingly close fitting, producing sloping lines that focused downward.[139] The sentimental woman appeared long and willowy, with a sloping narrow shoulder line and a slender waist. The armhole was now very low off the shoulders and was set with tight fitting sleeves, cut on the cross, which prohibited the wearer from lifting her arm above a right angle.[140] The

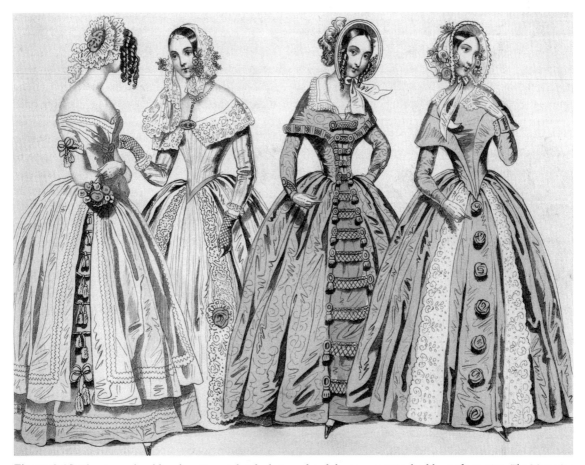

Figure 8.18 The stoop-shouldered sentimental style that emulated the consumptive bodily conformation. *The Magazine of the Beau Monde*, Vol. 11 (London: 1842). T434:6.b.6.1-. Cambridge University Library.

drop-shouldered style also forced a round-shouldered conformation and in doing so, emulated the physical silhouette of the consumptive female, by imposing a stooped posture natural in the case of consumption, and one believed to produce the illness.

Sentimental dress also emphasized delicacy and restricted gesture and movement, just as the debilitating effects of the disease did. *Commentaries Principally on Those Diseases of Females Which are Constitutional* made particular mention of the overall demeanor and posture thought to denote the early symptoms of consumption. (See Plate 30.) "There is a degree of feebleness and stooping observed in the gait, very early in the disease; and this remains little augmented."[141] As the illness progressed, "The mode of walking is peculiar, being attended by stooping, weakness and caution."[142] In 1830, Marshall Hall described those with the illness as having "a peculiar appearance of the countenance, a peculiar mode of walking, and a peculiar attitude and manner in general, all denoting debility and great disease"[143] Stooping was presented as both the architect and indicator of consumption, and women's education was one target of blame. *A Physician's Advice for the Prevention and Cure of Consumption* thus argued:

> In connection with the present system of conducting the education of young females in the higher classes, it is right to mention, that an inactive sedentary mode of life appears to dispose to the formation of tubercles, and the recurrence of consumption; first, by debilitating the system in general; and secondly, by the habit of stooping, hurting the lungs in the same manner with malformation of the chest.[144]

Similarly, Henry Deshon claimed in 1847, "The sickly school girl, with her pallid countenance and stooping gait, would seem to predict her fate—pulmonary disease."[145] His *Cold and Consumption* also lamented a young schoolgirl "stooping over her writing desk" as productive of the illness.[146]

All of this was seen as a cause of consumption. Women were also considered more susceptible to tuberculosis than men due to their upbringing. A woman's role in society was articulated as a predetermining factor in the development of the disease. Doctors, such as John Tricker Conquest, expressed their disgust over the type of upbringing guaranteed to bring about illness. In *Letters to a Mother on the Management of Herself and Her Children in Health and Disease* (1848), Conquest wrote:

> Nature is turned off as a dunce, and girls must sit up 'like ladies' and eat 'like ladies'; and instead of trundling the hoop, and playing with bat and ball, and shuttlecock, and skipping, they must sacrifice the inestimable blessing of vigorous health to mental acquisitions and (falsely called) 'lady-like habits.' That horrid word 'lady-like', haunts the poor girls of the middle and higher classes through years which should be devoted to physical education, and leaves them, at last, the prey of deformity and disease . . . Fashion is the war cry of tyranny.[147]

When the idea of illness as character-illuminating is combined with sentimental culture as a whole, it is easy to see how consumption could invade the popular ideals of beauty and fashion.

Over the period from 1780 to 1850 tuberculosis was consistently intertwined with the contemporary discourses on fashion. The focus of the rhetoric tended to be on the role that fashion played in creating the disease. The neoclassical styles that typified the period from 1780 to around 1820 were primarily connected to consumption through its inadequacies in providing protection from the climate. Cold, damp, and even dust particles were believed to find a path to creating tuberculosis through their interaction with female dress. The concern over fashion and climate remained influential over the whole period. As corsets became an increasingly important part of female dress in the 1830s and 1840s it also became the primary focus of the criticisms as the concern over the pressures applied by the clothing continued to intensify as the fashions became ever tighter. The connections between consumption and clothing throughout the period moved beyond the ability of fashion to cause the disease and also consistently displayed elements of emulation as the fashions, to varying degrees, either highlighted the consequences of tuberculosis or actually imitated the symptoms of the illness.

EPILOGUE: THE END OF CONSUMPTIVE CHIC

Although contemporary authors viewed woman's prescribed place in society and the prominence of fashion in that role as important factors affecting female health, the paradox created by the demand for "simplicity" in sentimental clothing could not be ignored for long. As a result, by the 1850s the debate over the artificiality of fashion and its biological consequences made inroads in the attitudes toward consumption and aided in changing female fashion. Sanitary reform, plus social concerns, combined to transform tuberculosis in the latter half of the nineteenth century from a condition presented as conferring beauty and intelligence into a biological evil that was the product of social conditions that could and should be changed and controlled.

The full-blown consumptive look that typified the sentimental clothing of the 1840s shifted in the 1850s, and as Valerie Steele asserted, "the rather insipid simplicity of 1840s styles gave way in the 1850s to a revived worldliness as the somewhat drooping silhouette became more ample and brilliant again."[1] In the succeeding decade there was a new acceptance of feminine vivacity.[2] The ailing and delicate sentimental woman was replaced entirely, by the 1860s and 1870s, with the return to a fashion for "healthy" women.[3] Alongside this move toward healthy beauty there was a parallel shift in the interpretation of consumption and its meaning for women. As the grip of the consumptive ideology on the British population began to wane, that accompanied a shift in the perception of the disease and a loss of respectability, fashion no longer followed the dictates of disease. This repudiation of consumptive chic was not only rooted in the social/sanitary reforms, but also was the product of the changing rhetoric of the disease in literature, that began in the latter part of the 1840s.[4]

While a romanticized consumptive mythology remained, the object of the discourse shifted away from respectable females toward a model of fallen womanhood. The publication of the popular *La Dame aux Camélias* by Alexandre Dumas fils in 1848 illustrated the change. The work was published in 1856 in English with the title *The Lady with the Camelias*.[5] But even before its translation, the English would have been familiar with the tale as it was reviewed[6] and remarked upon repeatedly in the periodical literature often in discussions of the gossip from Paris, as in the case of *Blackwood's Edinburgh Magazine* writing on the work, "The great success of the year, the only marked and decided one, has been *La Dame aux Camelias*, "The Lady with the Camelias," which, after running a hundred nights or more in the spring, has been revived this autumn with scarcely less success."[7] The story was inspired by the life of (Alphonsine) Marie Duplessis (1824–1847), a courtesan who had what she described as "one of those diseases that never relent. I shall not live as long as others, I have promised myself to live more quickly."[8] (See Plate 31.) She died of consumption at the age of twenty-three after a brief and celebrated career as the toast of the Parisian demi-monde.[9] Duplessis was so famous that when, after her death, her possessions were auctioned off at a public sale, it even attracted the attention of Charles Dickens, who attended.[10]

Dumas fils transformed the relationship between consumption and femininity. Although he portrayed the wasting associated with the disease as an enhancement to female beauty and character, he also highlighted the redemptive nature of the affliction. He continued the association between the disease and strong passion, particularly that of love, but privileged a connection between the suffering caused by the disease and the concept of absolution for moral transgressions. Such redemptive suffering became the major focus of the literary works that utilized tuberculosis as a literary device in the mid-nineteenth century. Dumas's work, first performed at the Théâtre de Vaudeville in 1852, was reviewed by Théophile Gauthier. Gauthier wrote of Marguerite, "As she begins to be troubled and then filled with real love, she becomes humble, shy, tender- and ill. She is consumed not only by love for Armand but also by the disease that consumed her body. Now the courtesan is stripped away and she becomes an innocent young girl!"[11] In her illness, the fallen woman, Marguerite, achieved a form of purity. The torment created by consumption and the tragedy of the youthful death "represented the impossibility of innocent love in a wretched world," making the "consumptive courtesan a motif for Woman herself—seductively simple, desirable yet doomed."[12]

Dumas began a trend of works in which a fallen woman could obtain spiritual salvation through the hardship of consumption, and as such they mark the transfer of the concept of redemptive suffering from the arena of respectable womanhood. Although the notion of moral achievement through suffering, which had been part of the duty of Victorian women, remained the same, the subject of the discourse changed. As a result, reputable women increasingly distanced themselves from the consumptive ideology. Novels, like Henri Murger's *Scenes de la Vie de Boheme* (1851), removed consumption from the sphere of genteel womanhood and placed it firmly with the fallen woman. Murger's Francine was also a young vivacious consumptive whose face manifested "a saintly glow as if she had died of beauty."[13]

Other factors may have aided the shift away from respectable to fallen womanhood in the rhetoric surrounding consumption. These included the increasing visibility of the disease among the poverty-stricken and the beginning of the acceptance of a contagion theory for tuberculosis toward the end of the 1840s.[14] However, the idea that the disease was passed from one person to another remained inadequate to account for why not everyone caught a disease, something that the hereditary constitution explanation had been able to do. As a result, the contagion theory had difficulty supplanting the popular miasma scheme, which advocated the view that disease was spread not through personal contact, but rather emanated from appalling environmental conditions that produced bad air, the disease trigger.[15] The proliferation of the disease in the overcrowded slums of industrial England, the growing awareness of this circumstance, and the flourishing of works that identified the disease with moral transgressions, all helped alter the ideology surrounding consumption. Once these associations were established, consumption could no longer be rationalized as an acceptable identifier for respectable women, and by the end of the 1840s the disease had become tainted by poverty and promiscuity, connections that continued through to the end of the century and beyond.

The demotion of consumption from the ranks of the respectable, and the increased visibility of the disease amongst the poor, corresponded with a movement for dress reform. Clothing was just one more aspect of society that drew the attention of reforming individuals and organizations during the second half of the nineteenth century.[16] Espousing the same complaints about women's dress that had been made over and over again, since the eighteenth century, these reformers were finally able to make headway. They focused their concern on what they saw as the adverse mental and physical consequences of fashionable dress— among which consumption figured prominently—problems for which the undergarments in particular were blamed.[17]

Despite the routinely professed belief in the connection between health and beauty, tuberculosis had up to this point been exempted from this association, a special exception that disappeared in the 1850s.[18] This shift was evident in Thomas Chandler Haliburton's *Nature and Human Nature*, in which he described one young woman in the following terms: "Her eyes had no more expression than a China-aster, and her face was so deadly pale, it made the rouge she had put on look like the hectic of a dying consumption. Her ugly was out in full bloom, I tell *you*."[19] The abandonment of consumption as fashionable and the espousal of health in its place were reflected in the styles of the period, as bodices shortened and the torso widened. The sleeves also widened, achieving a cone shape with the introduction of the pagoda sleeve.[20] (See Plate 32.) Although the bodice remained tightly fitted over corsets, the degree of tight lacing lessened with the advent of the crinoline and the enormous width it imparted on the skirt, which made all waists seem smaller in comparison.[21] One periodical even went so far as to declare in 1851, "Tight-lacing has completely gone out of fashion amongst ladies in the higher and middle classes, who have discovered that undue compression is destructive of both grace and symmetry. It is amongst young females of the humbler classes that the practice is now most prevalent."[22]

There were alterations in the appearance of the corset that corresponded with the changing emphasis on the female body in the 1850s. In a move away from the narrow almost "consumptive" torso, rational reform in the construction and design of the corset combined with technological innovation to alter the form of that garment. In the latter part of the 1840s, corsets began to be shaped by the joining of separate pieces rather than created from a single piece of fabric augmented with gussets. This style became increasingly popular until it was supplanted in the latter part of the 1860s by the steam-molded corset.[23] During the 1850s and 1860s, the corsets and bodices shortened, moving away from the willowy sylph-like silhouette of the 1840s

Roxy A. Caplin was at the forefront of dress reform in England. She was among those who sought to rationalize, rather than eradicate, all the undergarments that provided shape to women's fashion. Dress reformers, like Caplin, argued that clothing should instead be re-imagined through an alteration in the shape of underwear and in retaining the outer complexity of fashionable dress, these reformers achieved a balance that was at last acceptable to many women. In helping to alter the industry that provided these garments, they effected real change in the shape of women's fashion.[24] Caplin orchestrated the first successful large-scale push for healthy corsets, exhibiting some of her new corset designs at the Great Exhibition of 1851, and was the only British corsetiere to win a medal. Interestingly, Caplin entered her designs for "Hygeianic corsets" in the Philosophical, Musical, Horological, and Surgical Instruments division.[25] Caplin's new style of corset reflected her desire to "make corsets for the body to be fitted to," rather than fitting "the corset to the body."[26] The garment maintained a small waist, around nineteen inches, but allowed a freer movement of the torso, thereby relieving the pressure thought productive of consumption. The effect was to move visibly away from that narrow consumptive look. (See Plates 33 and 34.) Caplin followed her success at the Great Exhibition with a book in 1856 entitled *Health and Beauty; or Corsets and Clothing, Constructed in Accordance with the Physiological Laws of the Human Body*. In it she admonished everyone to:

> Adhere to their own profession; for it is evident to us that the Doctor knows no more about stay-making than we do of Sanscrit . . . It never seems to have occurred to the Doctor that ladies must and will wear stays, in spite of all the medical men of Europe. The strong and perfect feel the benefit of using them, and to the weak and delicate or imperfect, they are absolutely indispensable; but when we say this, we mean corsets properly constructed; for if the construction be imperfect, the mistake will be equally as bad.[27]

These sorts of technological innovations in both the cut and construction of female clothing, combined with a measured re-evaluation of what constituted respectable femininity, further loosened the ties between respectable women and tuberculosis.

Gradually, consumption lost its positive associations among the more prosperous classes and was increasingly relegated to the world of the working class and the poor. This shift would lead to a stigmatization of the illness and a change in the coping strategies employed by society at large. Thus, the mythology and stable of imagery that developed around consumption, which provided structure for an individual's experience, was shifting by the mid-century. These notions also supplied rationalizations for the perceived relationships between one's susceptibility to pulmonary consumption and the distinct social roles and character of the afflicted individual. These representations were informed by social differences and supported by accepted notions of behavior and beliefs surrounding deviance.[28] By the 1860s, the disease was presented almost exclusively as the product of harmful or inappropriate behaviors, which had direct and serious consequences for both the individual and society at large. Consumption was no longer simply an individual illness, but one that had an unavoidable effect on the productivity and competitiveness of the community as a whole.

CONCLUDING THE FASHION

One of the primary concerns of medical investigation has been to supply acceptable explanations to the public for the various diseases with which it is afflicted, while creating inclusive unitary theories of illness that encompass all possible aspects of the disease process. Over the course of the nineteenth and twentieth centuries, as researchers identified a definitive, single cause for each infectious disease, as a result of the advances that accompanied germ theory and microbiology, multi-causal approaches waned in popularity. In the antibiotic age, the model simplified: a bacterium, virus, etc., causes an illness, a chemotherapeutic agent was administered, and the patient was subsequently cured. A single cause, once addressed and eradicated, effectively removed the disease. This simplicity is no longer a defining feature of twenty-first century medicine however, for the proliferation of chronic and systemic illnesses as well as new investigations into infectious disease, has once again made unfashionable the notion that a complicated illness could have a simple cause. Today's medicine has once more established a role for external causative explanations in the case of those illnesses that cannot be easily eliminated by medication. Echoing earlier theories of illness, there is once more a role for the influence of an individual's lifestyle and environment in the case of illnesses like Type II diabetes, heart disease, or cancer. Once again, notions of illness cross the boundaries between medicine and society, as they did in the eighteenth and nineteenth centuries when the association between tuberculosis, society, and the sick individual was a fluid relationship, whose terms were constantly being renegotiated, changing, and adapting to new social conventions and emerging medical information.

Social analysis of the causes and course of a number of diseases became an important component of the public health movement during the nineteenth century, and the interpretation of health along class lines remained a prominent theme in the discourse of disease. In the first part of the nineteenth century, consumption in the working class was seen as the product of the deleterious influence of a range of vices, including fornication and alcoholism; however, in the middle and upper classes it was presented as the product of delicate sensibilities and social refinement. These class distinctions were not just a result of material and social disparity. They were seemingly confirmed by the perception of physiological divergence, with members of the upper classes being touted as possessing a more refined nervous system than those of the lower classes. Middle- and upper-class women in particular were presented as being more likely to develop pulmonary consumption because of their weakened and innately fragile constitutions. This was an idea that also fit well with hereditary notions of the disease, since the refinement which characterized both the illness and the nervous constitution of the upper orders could be passed on to the children. In the late eighteenth and early nineteenth centuries, the hereditary constitution, the environment, and any other strains provided by lifestyle, continued as prominent themes in the working knowledge of tuberculosis. There was an acceptance by physicians, and society alike, of an association between the illness and the sophisticated lifestyle pursued by members of the middle and upper classes. Notions about disease were shaped by social definitions of those illnesses believed to be products of "civilization."

These ideas were critically important in intertwining consumption with beauty and fashion from 1780–1850. Evangelicalism and Romanticism also proved influential in creating positive representations of tuberculosis. Romantic ideology helped strengthen the connections between consumption and the best and brightest members of society, those intelligent, delicate individuals who seemed so prominent in the ranks of its victims. As a consequence, there developed a prototype for the consumptive disease process and death, one that encompassed evangelical notions of resignation and submission to Divine will with a Romantic ideology that saw the victims of tuberculosis as unable to withstand the buffeting of the wider world due to nervous debility and creative genius.

The cultural construction of the disease was refashioned in the 1830s and 1840s under the influence of sentimentalism, when it was increasingly interpreted as a function of the weakness and delicacy of the female victim, and meaning was assigned to the disease experience based upon gender. The separate spheres ideology mingled with a growing medical literature that saw tuberculosis as linked to women through the actions of the increased quantity of nervous sensibility accorded them in contemporary biological theory. By the early Victorian period sensibility and, by virtue of its association with that quality, tuberculosis, had become explicitly feminine. The harsh reality of the consumptive disease process did not fit neatly into the altered reality promoted by Romanticism and sentimentalism. As a result, the illness was rationalized in an effort to cope with its devastating effects. The Romanticized notions and sentimental rhetoric applied to the disease, provided a way of imposing order on an aspect of their lives that middle- and upper-class English people had little other control over. Increasingly, women were the focus of a discourse that not only set acceptable behaviors but also reinforced and legitimated these functions through the medical and physiological sciences. Observed biological differences were extended into social expectations and saw femininity, in part, as a function of excess sensibility. These biological ideas were then transformed into a code of propriety, sensibility, and physical delicacy, all of which presented women as balanced on the edge of disease, and, by implication, tuberculosis. These concepts were employed to construct persistent representations of consumption as a disease that was not only denoted by beauty but was also one that could confer that quality upon its victim.

During the first half of the nineteenth century, the disease not only infused popular ideals of beauty, but the belief that tuberculosis was a disease characterized by attractive aesthetics became a dominant theme. Beauty was thought to be one of the noteworthy symptoms of the hereditary predisposition to tuberculosis; moreover, once the disease was established, the symptoms were also believed to increase the attractiveness of its victim as its effects became visible in the complexion, eyes, and even the smile. This beauty was denoted by thin frames, long swan-like necks, large dilated eyes, luxurious eyelashes, white teeth, and pale complexions accented by blue veins and rosy cheeks. As the notions of sentimentalism gained purchase, beauty was taken to be the reflection of the internal character of a woman. As a result, tuberculosis also came to confirm the character of the sufferer through its ability to confer beauty. Increasingly, the acquisition of beauty was believed to occur through the cultivation of those qualities believed to be desirable in women (modesty, innocence, goodness, nurturance, delicacy) rather than in the cheap imitation found in cosmetic aids. Under the influence of sentimental rhetoric, the use of make-up became more furtive and once cosmetic aid was eschewed, tuberculosis's role in creating beauty naturally increased the links between that condition and positive aesthetics. The cultural expectations that surrounded consumption were articulated in literature, medical treatises, and those works concerned with defining fashion and the female role, all of which overflowed with examples that connected the disease to beauty and reveal a shared consciousness that tuberculosis was indeed attractive.

The relationship between tuberculosis and attractiveness also played out in the rhetoric and practice surrounding the fashions of the day. Not only did these ideas reflect attitudes about beauty, health, and the female role, but clothing actually played an active role in defining contemporary notions about the relationships between beauty and disease. Clothing was not only assigned a reflective function but it also was given an active role in both the emulation of the illness and in creating consumption. From 1780 to 1850, consumption appeared repeatedly in the contemporary discourses surrounding fashion, and the focus of the discussions of clothing and the disease tended to accord female fashions agency in creating the illness. As the clothing moved from the willowy neoclassical to the ornamented Romantic and eventually to the subdued sentimental style of dress, the role of fashion as a cause of consumption also altered. The insubstantial nature of the neoclassical fashions were thought unequal to the task of protecting their wearers from the English climate. The environment, in the form of damp, cold, and even dust, interacted with neoclassical clothing to cause consumption. The concern over climate and fashion persisted even after the style waned. With the move toward Romantic styles, the corset became the main link between fashion and the disease, an association that continued to intensify as corsets tightened with the move toward sentimental styles.

The connections between tuberculosis and dress moved beyond the ability to cause the disease and also encompassed an imitation of some of the physical signs of the illness. The clothing, to a varying degree depending on the style, either highlighted certain symptoms of tuberculosis (like the wing-back present in neoclassical fashion) or actively imitated certain manifestations of the illness (like the stoop shoulder seen in sentimental dress). In the 1850s the power of consumptive beauty and fashion began to wane. The interpretation of the disease in women altered due to the influence of sanitary reform and the changing rhetoric of the disease in literature, which had shifted toward a model of fallen womanhood.

During the second half of the nineteenth century, the notions that dominated the lower-class interpretation of the disease—the ones that saw tuberculosis as the result of moral and hygienic shortcomings, complicated by filthy and crowded living and working conditions—gained purchase and were increasingly applied at all levels of society. This approach to tuberculosis gradually became the dominant image of the illness, particularly with the growing focus on public health in the middle of the nineteenth century. The introduction and eventual acceptance of the germ theory of disease would make this hygienic model, with its moral undertones, the sole explanation for tuberculosis, and so would impart an unsavory element to the illness. Health was now privileged as a desirable goal in the face of mounting social concerns and fears over biological degeneracy.

NOTES

Introduction

1. Hugh Belsey, *Gainsborough's Beautiful Mrs. Graham* (Edinburgh: National Gallery of Scotland, 2003), 27.

2. Belsey, *Gainsborough's Beautiful Mrs. Graham*, 31–32, 35; E. Maxtone Graham, *The Beautiful Mrs. Graham and the Cathcart Circle* (London: Nisbet & Co. Ltd, 1927), 248–249.

3. Lynedoch MS. 3591, National Library of Scotland.

4. Belsey, *Gainsborough's Beautiful Mrs. Graham*, 32, 35.

5. Belsey, *Gainsborough's Beautiful Mrs. Graham*, 43.

6. Graham, *The Beautiful Mrs. Graham*, 128; Belsey, *Gainsborough's Beautiful Mrs. Graham*, 281–282.

7. Graham, *The Beautiful Mrs. Graham*, 284.

8. Wednesday June 20, 1792, Lynedoch MS 16046, National Library of Scotland.

9. Tuesday June 26, 1792, Lynedoch MS 16046, National Library of Scotland.

10. Tuesday July 17, 1792, Lynedoch MS 16046, National Library of Scotland.

11. Belsey, *Gainsborough's Beautiful Mrs. Graham*, 46.

12. The dress remains in private hands and cannot be viewed, however Hugh Belsey states "This simple gown was preserved by Thomas Graham as a treasured relic of Mary Graham until his own death in 1843 and has remained in the family ever since. The cut and length of the dress suggest that Mary was . . . very slender, her figure having become skeletal as she wasted away from pulmonary tuberculosis." Belsey, *Gainsborough's Beautiful Mrs. Graham*, 42.

13. Donald L. Spieglburg, ed., *New Topics in Tuberculosis Research* (New York: Nova Science Publishers, Inc., 2007), 3.

14. C. Herzlich and Janine Pierret, *Illness and Self in Society* (Baltimore: The Johns Hopkins University Press, 1982), xi.

15. Herzlich and Pierret, *Illness and Self in Society*, xi.

16. Susan Sontag, *Illness as Metaphor and Aids and Its Metaphors* (New York: Doubleday, 1990), 28–32; Clark Lawlor, *Consumption and Literature: The Making of the Romantic Disease* (New York: Palgrave Macmillan, 2006), 3.

17. Arthur Caplan, "The Concept of Health, Illness and Disease," *Companion Encyclopedia of the History of Medicine*, Vol. 1 (London: Routledge, 2001), 240–241. For Foucault, the artificiality of civilization diminished health and multiplied the incidence of disease while simultaneously altering its identity. Foucault contended "as one improves one's conditions of life, and as the social network tightens its grip around individuals, health seems to diminish by degrees" Michel Foucault, *The Birth of the Clinic: An Archaeology of Medical Perception* (New York: Vintage Books, 1994), 16–17.

18. Rene Dubos and Jean Dubos, *The White Plague: Tuberculosis, Man, and Society* (New Brunswick: Rutgers University Press, 1987), 3.

19. Selman A. Waksman, *The Conquest of Tuberculosis* (Berkeley: University of California Press, 1964), 8.

20. Henry C. Deshon, *Cold and Consumption* (London: Henry Renshaw, 1847), 31.

21. Waksman, *The Conquest of Tuberculosis*, 8.

22. Henry Ancell, *A Treatise on Tuberculosis* (London: Longman, Brown, Green & Longmans, 1852), xxiv.

23. Thomas Dormandy, *The White Death: A History of Tuberculosis* (London: Hambledon and London Ltd., 1998), 9.

24. Most notably, Rene and Jean Dubos's *The White Plague* (1952) argued that public health measures and sanitary reform in England were responsible for the decline in mortality observed in the second half of the nineteenth century. *The White Plague* remains one of the most influential works on the subject, in part because it located tuberculosis in its

social context rather than simply enumerating exclusively scientific advances and the work focused primarily on the link between poverty and the disease. Thomas McKeown's *The Modern Rise of Population* (London: Edward Arnold, 1976) asserted that the decline in mortality from tuberculosis was the product of better nutritional standards in England. McKeown's thesis remains hotly contested and there is continued reappraisal of its validity and the empirical evidence upon which it rests. For instance, Simon Szreter echoes the Duboses' assertion that sanitary intervention was critical in creating the decline in Britain's mortality rates. Upon a careful assessment of McKeown's evidence, Szreter claims, "the epidemiological evidence collected by the registrar general and analyzed by McKeown did not in fact show a definite downturn in the national incidence of respiratory tuberculosis until after 1867." Simon Szreter, *Health and Wealth: Studies in History and Policy* (Rochester: University of Rochester Press, 2007), 113. For more information on the debates over mortality also see Anne Hardy, "Diagnosis, Death, and Diet: The Case of London, 1750–1909," *The Journal of Interdisciplinary History*, Vol. 18, No. 3 (1988); Andrea Rusnock, *Vital Accounts: Quantifying Health and Population in Eighteenth-Century England and France*; Graham Mooney and Simon Szretzer "Urbanization, mortality and the Standard of Living Debate: new estimates of the expectation of life at birth in nineteenth-century British Cities," *Economic History Review*, XL (1998), 84–112. E. A. Wrigley and R. S. Schofiled, *The Population History of England 1541–1871* (Cambridge: Harvard University Press, 1981); Anne Hardy, *The Epidemic Streets: Infectious Disease and the Rise of Preventative Medicine, 1856–1900* (Oxford: Clarendon Press, 1993).

25. These books include Sheila M. Rothman's *Living in the Shadow of Death: Tuberculosis and the Social Experience of Illness in American History* (1994), Katherine Ott's *Fevered Lives: Tuberculosis in American Culture since 1870* (1996), Barbara Bates's *Bargaining for Life: a Social History of Tuberculosis 1876–1938* (1994), and Georgina D. Feldberg's *Disease and Class: Tuberculosis and the Shaping of Modern North American Society* (1995).

26. "Tuberculosis into the 2010s: Is the Glass Half Full?" *Contagious and Infectious Diseases* (2009: 49, 574–583), 574.

27. XDR-TB is defined as a "disease caused by bacteria that are resistant to at least isoniazid and rifampin—both first-line TB drugs, resistance to which defines multidrug-resistant TB (MDR-TB)—plus resistance to any fluoroquinolones and resistance to at least 1 second-line injectable drug (amikacin, capreomycin, or kanamycin)." Although this is the base definition many of the XDR-TB strains are resistant to most other second-line drug and as such are untreatable. "Extensively Drug-Resistant Tuberculosis: Are We Learning from History or Repeating it?" *Contagious and Infectious Diseases* (2007: 45, 338–342), 338.

28. "The Challenge of New Drug Discovery for Tuberculosis," *Nature*, Vol. 469 (January 2011, pp. 483–490), 483–484.

29. "Extensively Drug-Resistant Tuberculosis: Are We Learning from History or Repeating it?" *Contagious and Infectious Diseases* (2007: 45, 338–342), 338.

30. "The Challenge of New Drug Discovery for Tuberculosis," *Nature*, Vol. 469 (January 2011, pps 483–490), 484.

31. For instance, see Lee B. Reichman and Janice Hopkins Tanne, *Timebomb: the global epidemic of multi-drug resistant tuberculosis* (New York: McGraw-Hill Professional, 2002); Matthew Gandy and Alimuddin Zuml, *The Return of the White Plague: Global poverty and the 'new' tuberculosis* (London: Verso, 2003); and Flurrin Condrau and Michael Worboys, *Tuberculosis Then and Now: Perspectives on the History of an Infectious Disease* (Montreal and Kingston: McGill-Queen's University Press, 2010).

Chapter 1

1. Gideon Harvey, *Morbus Anglicus: Or the Anatomy of Consumptions*, 2nd edn. (London: Printed by Thomas Johnson for Nathanael Brook, 1674), 2.

2. Lawlor, *Consumption and Literature*, 19.

3. Mark Caldwell, *The Last Crusade: The War on Consumption, 1862–1954* (New York: Athenaeum, 1988), 9.

4. F. B. Smith, *The Retreat of Tuberculosis 1850–1950* (London: Croom Helm, 1988), 4.

5. William Black, *A Comparative View of the Mortality of the Human Species* (London: C. Dilly, 1788), 170, 183.

6. John G. Mansford, *An Inquiry into the Influence of Situation on Pulmonary Consumption* (London: Longman, Hurst, Rees, Orme and Brown, 1818), 67.

7. Dubos and Dubos, *The White Plague*, 9.

8. Herzlich and Pierret, *Illness and Self in Society*, 24.

9. John M. Eyler, "Farr, William (1807–1883)." in *Oxford Dictionary of National Biography*, ed. H. C. G. Matthew and Brian Harrison (Oxford: OUP, 2004), http://www.oxforddnb.com/view/article/9185 [accessed June 5, 2008]; George Smith, *The Dictionary of National Biography*, Vol. VI (London: Oxford University Press, 1964), 1090.

10. Henry Gilbert, *Pulmonary Consumption: Its Prevention & Cure Established on the New Views of the Pathology of the Disease* (London: Henry Renshaw, 1842), 6.

11. Henry Gilbert, *Pulmonary Consumption*, 4–5.

12. Herzlich and Pierret, *Illness and Self in Society*, 24.

13. Quoted in Waksman, *The Conquest of Tuberculosis*, 20.

14. Stanley Joel Reiser, "The Science of Diagnosis: Diagnostic Technology," In *Companion Encyclopedia of the History of Medicine*, ed. W. F. Bynum and Roy Porter, Vol. 2 (London: Routledge, 2001), 826–827.

15. Lindsay Granshaw, "The Hospital," In *Companion Encyclopedia of the History of Medicine*, ed. W. F. Bynum and Roy Porter, Vol. 2 (London: Routledge, 2001), 1187.

16. Roy Porter, *The Greatest Benefit to Mankind*, 307.

17. The discovery of percussion by Leopold Auenbrugger (1722–1809) with its tapping of the chest and careful notation of the sounds produced opened an entirely new avenue of inquiry, by providing a window into the interior of the living body. However, his book and technique faded into obscurity until it was translated and popularized by Jean Nicholas Corvisart (1755–1820). Lyle S. Cummins, *Tuberculosis in History From the 17th Century to our own Times* (London: Baillière, Tindall and Cox, 1949), 94–96, 100–102.

18. Laennec and other devotees of the stethoscope were able to detect a variety of illnesses by differentiating between abnormal and normal respiration sounds. Roy Porter, *The Greatest Benefit to Mankind*, 307–309.

19. Cummins, *Tuberculosis in History From the 17th Century to our own Times*, 121.

20. Porter, *The Greatest Benefit to Mankind*, 311.

21. John Hastings, *Pulmonary Consumption, Successfully Treated with Naphtha* (London: John Churchill, 1843), 4.

22. Porter, *The Greatest Benefit to Mankind*, 311.

23. Barrow, *Researches on Pulmonary Phthisis, From the French of G.H. Bayle*, 3–4.

24. Gabriel Andral (1797–1876) was a French physician, who emphasized the purulent, inflammatory, and "secretory" manner of the changes in consumption. Porter, *The Greatest Benefit to Mankind*, 337, and Anton Sebastian, *A Dictionary of the History of Medicine* (New York: The Parthenon Publishing Group, Inc., 1999), 47.

25. Pierre Charles Alexandre Louis (1787–1872), was a Parisian physician and expert in tuberculosis and typhoid. Porter, *The Greatest Benefit to Mankind*, 337; Anton Sebastian, *A Dictionary of the History of Medicine*, 47; John Galbraith Simmons, *Doctors & Discoveries: Lives that Created Today's Medicine from Hippocrates to the Present* (Boston: Houghton Mifflin Company, 2002), 75.

26. Carswell (1793–1857) was hired by Professor John Thomson, while studying medicine at the University of Glasgow, to gather information in France and illustrate the findings for a course on morbid anatomy Thomson was developing. Upon returning to Britain, Carswell received the first chair of pathological anatomy, created in 1828 by the University of London in a jump ahead of the French; however, the position soon became a victim of the more established disciplines of practical and normal anatomy. Carswell's disillusionment with the lack of support, combined with his resulting difficulty in making a living, led him to leave the position. Andrew Hull, "Carswell, Sir Robert (1793–1857)," in *Oxford Dictionary of National Biography*, ed. H. C. G. Matthew and Brian Harrison (Oxford: OUP, 2004), http://www.oxforddnb.com/view/article/4778 [accessed June 5, 2008]; Edward K. Hass, "Morbid Appearances: The Anatomy of Pathology in the Early 19th century," *Journal of Interdisciplinary History*, Vol. 20, No. 1(Summer 1989), 139.

27. Localized concepts of disease sought to specify the seat of illness at the level of individual tissues or organs while taking into account more generalized pathological alterations, systemic changes, and symptomology.

28. Robert Hull, *A Few Suggestions on Consumption* (London: Churchill, 1849), 2.

29. Scrofula, often termed the king's evil, was a form of non-pulmonary tuberculosis characterized by an inflammation of the lymph nodes, and was accompanied by unsightly swellings caused by tubercles at the neck and under the skin in other areas of the body. Scrofula often resulted in ulceration of the skin due to the persistent and massive swelling.

30. Dubos and Dubos, *The White Plague*, 74.

31. James Sanders, *Treatise on Pulmonary Consumption* (London: Longman, Hurst, Rees, and Orme, 1808), v.

32. Henry M'Cormac, *On the Nature, Treatment and Prevention of Pulmonary Consumption* (London: Longman, Brown, Green and Longmans, and J. Churchill, 1855), 1.

Chapter 2

1. The idea that consumption was a contagious disease was a notion of long standing, Galen considered it both contagious and incurable. In 1546 Florentine physician Hyeronymus Fracastorius systematically argued for its contagious nature, making a distinction between contagious phthisis (which resulted from exposure to those already afflicted) and spontaneous phthisis (which was the result of some type of traumatic event). Waksman, *The Conquest of Tuberculosis*, 50. In the seventeenth century contagion was a widely-accepted part of consumption theory in southern Europe, and by the eighteenth century it was firmly entrenched, leading Italian physicians and anatomists, including Morgagni, to avoid dissecting the bodies of those who had expired from phthisis out of a fear of contracting the illness. Dubos and Dubos, *The White Plague*, 29.

2. Dubos and Dubos, *The White Plague*, 28.

3. Harvey, *Morbus Anglicus*, 2–3.

4. Harvey, *Morbus Anglicus*, 3.

5. Dubos and Dubos, *The White Plague*, 33.

6. England tended to follow the example of northern Europe, in part due to the similarity of climate.

7. Ancell, *A Treatise on Tuberculosis*, 481.

8. Porter, *The Greatest Benefit to Mankind*, 440.

9. John Reid, *A Treatise on the Origin, Progress, Prevention, and Treatment of Consumption* (London: R. Taylor & Co., 1806), 160–161.

10. Robert C. Olby, "Constitutional and Hereditary Disorders," In *Companion Encyclopedia of the History of Medicine*, ed. W. F. Bynum and Roy Porter, Vol. 1 (London: Routledge, 2001), 413.

11. Catherine Walpole (1703–1722) perished from the illness at age nineteen and Mary Viscountess Malpas (c.1706–1732) the wife of George James Lord Malpas (afterwards Earl of Cholmondeley) died at twenty-six of consumption.

12. Peter Cunningham, ed., *The Letters of Horace Walpole, Fourth Earl of Orford*, Vol.1 (Edinburgh: John Grant, 1906), xcix.

13. James Clark, *A Treatise on Pulmonary Consumption* (London: Sherwood, Gilbert and Piper, 1835), 2.

14. Waller, "The Illusion of an Explanation," 436.

15. Waller, "The Illusion of an Explanation," 443–444.

16. Thomas Reid, *An Essay on the Nature and Cure of Phthisis Pulmonalis* (London: T. Cadell, 1782), 2–3.

17. Dubos and Dubos, *The White Plague*, 36–38.

18. Charlotte Brontë to W. S. Williams, January 18, 1849, in Clement Shorter, *The Brontës: Life and Letters*, Vol. II (London: Hodder and Stoughton, 1908), 21.

19. August 18, [1836], In Emily Shore, *Journal of Emily Shore*, ed. Barbara Timm Gates (Charlottesville: University Press of Virginia, 1991), 146.

20. Dubos and Dubos, *The White Plague*, 42.

21. J. J. Furnivall, *On the Successful Treatment of Consumptive Disorders* (London: Whittaker & Co., 1835), 11.

22. M'Cormac, *On the Nature, Treatment and Prevention of Pulmonary Consumption*, 14.

23. Thomas Bartlett, *Consumption: Its Causes, Prevention and Cure* (London: Hippolyte Bailliere, 1855), 12.

24. Waller, "The Illusion of an Explanation," 421–422.

25. Erwin Ackerknecht argued that the hereditary constitutional approach gained popularity to address the difficulties that the anatomico-pathological approach faced in explaining systemic, expansive illnesses like tuberculosis, gout, and rheumatism. Olby, "Constitutional and Hereditary Disorders," 414. John C. Waller takes exception to Ackerknecht's thesis as insufficient, and echoes Charles Rosenberg, arguing that the concept of hereditary illness was "a by-product of a prior linkage forged between, on the one hand, the notion of incurable disease and, on the other, the ancient concept of the relatively unchanging individual constitution." For Waller, this conceptual linkage was the result of the medical profession's attempt to explain its powerlessness in the face of a variety of relentless chronic illnesses. Waller, "The Illusion of an Explanation," 414.

26. John Murray, *A Treatise on Pulmonary Consumption its Prevention and Remedy* (London: Whittaker, Treacher, and Arnot, 1830), 7.

27. Dubos and Dubos, *The White Plague*, xix.

28. Quoted in Waller, "The Illusion of an Explanation," 442.

29. Olby, "Constitutional and Hereditary Disorders," 413–414.

30. Clark, *A Treatise on Pulmonary Consumption*, 220–221.

31. *The Lancet*, Vol. XI, No. 183 (London, Saturday, March 3, 1826–7), 696.

32. James Sanders, *Treatise on Pulmonary Consumption* (London: Longman, Hurst, Rees, and Orme, 1808), 65.

33. "Domestic Occurrences," *The Gentleman's Magazine and Historical Chronicle,* Volume C, Part II (London: J. B. Nichols and Son, 1830), 461.

34. S. Hooll to Arthur Young on the death of his daughter Martha Ann (Bobbin) from consumption. In S. Hooll to Arthur Young, August 1797, Add 35127, folio 424, The British Library Department of Manuscripts, London, UK.

35. Black, *A Comparative View of the Mortality of the Human Species*, 176.

36. George Bodington, *An Essay on the Treatment and Cure of Pulmonary Consumption* (London: Orme, Brown, Green & Longmans, 1840), 1–2.

37. *The Magazine of Domestic Economy*, Vol. 6 (London: W. S. Orr & Co., 1841), 111.

38. Waksman, *The Conquest of Tuberculosis*, 56.

39. James Carmichael Smyth, *An Account of the Effects of Swinging Employed as a Remedy in the Pulmonary Consumption and Hectic Fever* (London: J. Johnson, 1787), 17 & 19.

40. Smyth, *An Account of the Effects of Swinging*, 20.

41. Sunday December 9, [1838], In Emily Shore, *Journal of Emily Shore*, 290.

42. Dubos and Dubos, *The White Plague*, 43. The prescription of sunshine and warm climes, which dated from Pliny and Galen, remained the most helpful and common advice well into the nineteenth century.

43. King George III to Lord Eldon, February 8, 1803, Eldon Family Papers, Add MS 82581, British Library Department of Manuscripts, London, UK.

44. John Armstrong, *Practical Illustrations of the Scarlet Fever, Measles, Pulmonary Consumption and Chronic Diseases* (London: Baldwin, Cradock, and Joy, 1818), 289–290.

45. Travel Diary of Emma Wilson (1828), UPC 158, 641x9, Norfolk Record Office, UK.

46. Clark was a friend as well as physician to Queen Victoria and her husband Prince Albert and was responsible for bringing Florence Nightingale to the attention of the Queen. R. A. L. Agnew, "Clark, Sir James, first baronet (1788–1870)," in *Oxford Dictionary of National Biography*, ed. H. C. G. Matthew and Brian Harrison (Oxford: OUP, 2004), http://www.oxforddnb.com/view/article/5463 [accessed June 22, 2006]; Helen Bynum, *Spitting Blood: The History of Tuberculosis* (Oxford: Oxford University Press, 2012), 82–83.

47. William Munk, *The Roll of the Royal College of Physicians of London*, Vol. III (London: Published by the College Pall Mall East, 1878), 224–225.

48. Bodington, *An Essay on the Treatment and Cure of Pulmonary Consumption*, iv

49. Bodington, *An Essay on the Treatment and Cure of Pulmonary Consumption*, iv.

50. Dubos and Dubos, *The White Plague*, 143–144; Bynum, *Spitting Blood*, 82–83.

51. Dubos and Dubos, *The White Plague*, 134 & 139.

52. *The London Medical Gazette*, Vol. III (London: Longman, Rees, Orme, Brown, and Green, 1829), 696.

53. "Tubercular Consumption," *The Lancet*, Vol. II (London: 1832), 423–424.

54. Dormandy, *The White Death*, 46.

55. Cupping was designed to draw infection and other deeply rooted toxins to the skin surface first by making a small slice in the skin then placing a glass cup possessing a slightly rounded lip that has first been heated to the incision site. As the glass cools the air contracts creating a vacuum that was to suck the pus, any necrotic tissue, and other toxins free of the patient's body.

56. Cod-liver oil became the chief therapeutic employed to restore the physically debilitated and as such was popular in the case of consumption, despite its revolting taste. Clinical trials to determine the beneficial effects of cod-liver oil were undertaken the Hospital for Consumption and Diseases at Brompton by Dr. C. J. Blasius Williams and Sir Peter Rose. Christopher F. Lindsey, "Williams, Charles James Blasius (1805–1889)," in *Oxford Dictionary of National Biography*, ed. H. C. G. Matthew and Brian Harrison (Oxford: OUP, 2004), http://www.oxforddnb.com/view/article/29489 [accessed September 18, 2008].

57. Anne Brontë routinely employed cod-liver oil in treating her consumption. Charlotte Brontë wrote of her sister's therapeutic regimen, "Mr. Wheelhouse ordered the blister to be put on again … She looks somewhat pale and sickly. She has had one dose of cod-liver oil; it smells and tastes like train oil." Five days later she stated, "She takes the cold-liver oil and carbonate of iron regularly; she finds them both nauseous, but especially the oil." Charlotte Brontë to Ellen Nussey, January 10, 1849 and January 15, 1849, in Shorter, *The Brontës*, 18.

58. Sir Alexander Crichton, *Practical Observations On the Treatment and Cure of Several Varieties of Pulmonary Consumption* (London: Lloyd and Son, 1823), 5.

59. Smith, *The Retreat of Tuberculosis 1850–1950*, 45.

60. John Baron, *An Enquiry Illustrating the Nature of Tuberculated Accretions of Serous Membranes* (London: Longman, Hurst, Rees, Orme, and Brown, 1819), 18.

61. Elizabeth Lomax, "Heredity or Acquired Disease? Early Nineteenth Century Debates on the Cause of Infantile Scrofula and Tuberculosis," *Journal of the History of Medicine and Allied Sciences* 32:4 (October 1977), 374.

Chapter 3

1. Thomas Bartlett, *Consumption: Its Causes, Prevention and Cure*, 2–3.

2. Clark Lawlor and Akihito Suzuki, "The Disease of the Self: Representing Consumption, 1700–1830," *Bulletin of the History of Medicine* (Vol. 74, No. 3, Fall 2000), 476.

3. In 1818 John Mansford addressed some concerns attendant to city life: "Amongst the causes of pulmonary consumption … is the breathing a dusty atmosphere: and I consider this a circumstance of so much importance in the choice of residence, that I cannot refrain from offering a few admonitory hints respecting it. Those who live in large cities, and in the vicinity of public roads, can never be said to breathe a pure air in dry and warm weather. The clouds of dust which are incessantly raised by the passing throng … become the sources of something more than mere inconvenience. I am persuaded that air … becomes when thus loaded, a powerful cause of irritation and subsequent disease in the lungs." Mansford, *An Inquiry into the Influence of Situation on Pulmonary Consumption*, 54–55.

4. Engels, *The Condition of the Working-Class in England in 1844*, translated by Florence Kelley Wischnewetzky (London: George Allen & Unwin, Ltd., 1892), 98–99.

5. The public's pulmonary organs were the parks of London. The article addressed the necessity of providing clean open spaces to temper disease. "The Lungs of London," *Blackwood's Edinburgh Magazine*, Vol. XLVI, (London: T. Cadell, 1839), 213.

6. Hull, *A Few Suggestions on Consumption*, 52.

7. Beddoes, *Essay on the Causes, Early Signs, and Prevention of Pulmonary Consumption*, 6.

8. In 1842, Henry Gilbert actually denied there was an increase in tuberculosis among the laboring classes: "As far as my own experience goes, I am disposed to think that the partial increase of consumption has chiefly occurred in the upper classes of society, and more especially among females; while among the lower classes the malady seems to have become less frequent. This may, perhaps, be accounted for by taking into consideration the greater comfort now enjoyed by laborers and the poor, which classes constitute so great a proportion of the population; while the rich, to gratify the morbid fancies of the age, indulge more and more in pernicious and unnatural luxuries, which gradually produce a tendency to disease. We see that this malady is not even heard among some nations, where the arts of refinement and the luxurious practices of civilized life have not as yet obtained a footing." Gilbert, *Pulmonary Consumption*, 22.

9. Hull, *A Few Suggestions on Consumption*, 53.

10. Beddoes, *Essay on the Causes, Early Signs, and Prevention of Pulmonary Consumption*, 125.

11. Beddoes, *Essay on the Causes, Early Signs, and Prevention of Pulmonary Consumption*, 64.

12. Dubos and Dubos, *The White Plague*, 197–198.

13. Charles Turner Thackrah, *The Effects of Arts, Trades, and Professions, and of Civic States and Habits of Living, on Health and Longevity*, 2nd edn. (London: Longman, Rees, Orme, Brown, Green, and Longman, 1832), 6.

14. This was one to the subscription balls orchestrated by the Tory White's club to celebrate the recovery of King George III from his illness.

15. Miss Lyddel the daughter of Henry George Liddell (1749–1791), 5th baronet of Ravensworth Castle, while Matthew Baillie (1761–1823) was a physician who specialized in thoracic and abdominal medicine who published *Morbid Anatomy of Some of the Most Important Parts of the Human Body* (1795). By 1799 his private practice was so large he stopped teaching and resigned from St. George's Hospital to focus on it. He was one of the physicians that attended George III's daughter Princess Amelia in the final stages of her consumption, and after her death became physician extraordinary to the king.

16. Hester Lynch Piozzi to Anna Maria Pemberton, June 1814, In Edward A. Bloom and Lillian D. Bloom, ed., *The Piozzi Letters: Correspondence of Hester Lynch Piozzi, 1748–1821 (formerly Mrs. Thrale)*, Vol. 5 1811–1816 (Cranbury, NJ: Associated University Presses, 1999), 278.

17. By a Physician, *The Manual for Invalids*, 2nd edn. (London: Edward Bull, 1829), 194.

18. "Cure of Phthisis Pulmonalis by Sugar of Lead combined with Opium and Cold Water," *The Medical Times*, Vol. XII (London: J. Angerstein Carfrae, 1845), 142.

19. Lawlor, *Consumption and Literature*, 19.

20. Roy Porter, "Diseases of Civilization," in *Companion Encyclopedia of the History of Medicine*, eds W. F. Bynum and Roy Porter, Vol. 1 (London: Routledge, 2001), 591.

21. Roy Porter, *The Greatest Benefit to Mankind*, 311; Dubos and Dubos, *The White Plague*, 127.

22. Barnes, *The Making of a Social Disease*, 29.

23. Robert Hull addressed the role of the passions in 1849: "The deposition of tubercle is wonderfully influenced by these [the passions of the mind]. Hilarity, joy, hope prevent, perhaps remove tubercular deposits. Gloom, fears, despondency lead to rapid and fatal mischief. The histories of young women, 'crossed in hopeless love,' furnish numberless cases of tubercular decline . . . Depression induces phthisis." Hull, *A Few Suggestions on Consumption*, 51.

24. Lawlor, *Consumption and Literature*, 52.

25. Some notable seventeenth- and eighteenth-century theorists of the nervous system include Thomas Willis, Albrecht von Haller, Robert Whytt, William Cullen, Alexander Monroe II, and John Brown. For more on discussions of the nerves and the influence of these theories see George S. Rousseau, "Nerves, Spirits, and Fibres: Towards Defining the Origins of Sensibility," *Studies in the Eighteenth Century*, R. F. Brissenden and J. C. Eade, eds (Toronto: University of Toronto Press, 1976); Clark Lawlor, "It is a Path I Have Prayed to Follow," in *Romanticism and Pleasure*, Thomas H. Schmid and Michelle Faubert, eds (New York: Palgrave Macmillan, 2010).

26. Peter Elmer, *The Healing Arts: Health, Disease and Society in Europe 1500–1800* (Manchester: Manchester University Press, 2004), 187.

27. William Cullen was an extremely powerful member of the Edinburgh medical school who published *First Lines of the Practice of Physic.* W. F. Bynum, "Nosology," in the *Companion Encyclopedia of the History of Medicine*, edited by W. F. Bynum and Roy Porter, Volume 1, pages 346–347 (London: Routledge, 2001), 346. Elmer, *The Healing Arts*, 167, 189; Roy Porter, ed., *The Cambridge Illustrated History of Medicine* (Cambridge: Cambridge University Press, 1996), 165.

28. Elmer, *The Healing Arts*, 189.

29. Bynum, "Nosology," 346–347.

30. Bynum, "Nosology," 347.

31. Porter, ed., *The Cambridge Illustrated History of Medicine*, 166.

32. From Dr. John Brown's Table of Excitement and Excitability, reproduced in John Rutherford Russell, *The History and Heroes of the Art of Medicine* (London: John Murray, 1861), 342–343.

33. Bynum, "Nosology," 347.

34. The literature on sensibility is vast, but some excellent guideposts are: G. J. Barker-Benfield, *The Culture of Sensibility: Sex and Society in Eighteenth-Century Britain* (Chicago: University of Chicago Press, 1992); Paul Goring, *The Rhetoric of Sensibility in Eighteenth-Century Culture* (Cambridge: Cambridge University Press, 2005); John Dwyer, *Virtuous Discourse: Sensibility and Community in Late Eighteenth-Century Scotland* (Edinburgh: John Donald Publishers, Ltd., 1987); John Mullan, *Sentiment and Sociability: The Language of Feeling in the Eighteenth Century* (Oxford: Oxford University Press, 1990); Markman Ellis, *The Politics of Sensibility: Race, Gender and Commerce in the Sentimental Novel* (Cambridge: Cambridge University Press, 2004); Chris Jones, *Radical Sensibility: Literature and Ideas in the 1790s* (London: Routledge, 1993); and Ann Jessie Van Sant, *Eighteenth-Century Sensibility and the Novel: The Senses in Social Context* (Cambridge: Cambridge University Press, 2004).

35. For instance, Paul Goring has investigated the ways in which fiction "promoted the performance of a language of a feeling, including a performance of weakness." Goring, *Rhetoric of Sensibility*, 14.

36. See Dana Rabin, *Identity, Crime, and Legal Responsibility in Eighteenth-Century England* (New York: Palgrave, 2004).

37. Iain McCalman, ed., *An Oxford Companion to the Romantic Age: British Culture 1776–1832* (Oxford: Oxford University Press, 1999), 102.

38. Porter, "Diseases of Civilization," 590.

39. Lawlor, *Consumption and Literature*, 49.

40. Lawlor, *Consumption and Literature,* 49–50

41. William White, *Observations on the Nature and Method of Cure of the Phthisis Pulmonalis,* edited by A. Hunter (York: Wilson, Spence, and Mawman, 1792), 22.

42. Porter, "Diseases of Civilization," 589.

43. This notion held well into the nineteenth century as Bodington argued, "those persons who are for the most part the freest from the attacks of consumption … are commonly but little troubled with nervous disorder; they are rather remarkable for an apparent obtuseness of nervous susceptibility." Bodington, *An Essay on the Treatment and Cure of Pulmonary Consumption*, 11.

44. Roy Porter, "Health Care in Enlightenment England: Knowledge, Power and the Market," in *Curing and Ensuring: Essays on Illness in Past Times*, Hans Binneveld and Rudolf Dekker eds (Rotterdam: Erasmus University, 1992), 96, 98–99; and Porter, "Diseases of Civilization," 589.

45. George Cheyne, *George Cheyne: The English Malady (1733),* Edited by Roy Porter, Tavistock Classics in the History of Psychiatry (London: Routledge, 1991), xi.

46. Cheyne, *George Cheyne*, xxxii.

47. Cheyne, *George Cheyne*, xxix.

48. Cheyne, *George Cheyne*, xxx.

49. Gout was particularly notorious as a disease of affluence and civilization, one associated with those of a certain status. See Roy Porter and G. S. Rousseau, *Gout: The Patrician Malady* (New Haven and London: Yale University Press, 1998).

50. The illness she referred to was most likely consumption, as her daughter had taken up riding "on a double horse," a popular treatment for tuberculosis. She did so "every other day, with Miss Wollonzoff, the Russian Ambassador's Daughter, a very charming girl, of about twelve years old—I have great hopes from it—but she looks like a Ghost still." Charlotte Burney to Fanny Burney, Aug. 17, 1790, Hill Street, Richmond, Eg 3693 Folio 63, The British Library Department of Manuscripts, London, UK.

51. Thackrah, *The Effects of Arts, Trades, and Professions*, 164.

52. Bodington, *An Essay on the Treatment and Cure of Pulmonary Consumption*, 10.

53. Bodington, *An Essay on the Treatment and Cure of Pulmonary Consumption*, 10–11.

54. J. S. Campbell, *Observations on Tuberculous Consumption* (London: H. Bailliere, 1841), 231.

55. Campbell, *Observations on Tuberculous Consumption*, 231.

56. These notions were extended to the nation as a whole, as it was believed that commercial success, along with intellectual and artistic accomplishment, and religious and political liberty set up conditions that made the population ripe for nervous disorders. This curse, or perhaps blessing, was a symbol of a nation's prosperity and wealth. In this idea consumption was a common illness because Britain was a prosperous nation and as its upper and middle classes were the most affluent it followed they were most likely to develop an illness of indulgence.

57. Herzlich and Pierret, *Illness and Self in Society*, 31.

58. Porter, "Diseases of Civilization," 592.

Chapter 4

1. Evangelicalism was a complex multifaceted phenomenon, typified by a string of unstructured and independent revivals in a number of geographical locations. By the mid-nineteenth century, evangelicalism made religion the language and the heart of the culture of the middle class. The role of the individual was central to this culture, as was the notion that salvation could only be achieved through intense struggle, and disease was one venue for that struggle to occur and the Christian to shine. Religion provided a reference structure for the classification of illness and evangelicalism played an important role in the conceptions surrounding consumption. Lenore Davidoff and Catherine Hall, *Family Fortunes: Men and Women of the English Middle Class, 1780–1850* (Chicago: The University of Chicago Press, 1987), 25, 83; and Boyd Hilton, *The Age of Atonement: The Influence of Evangelicalism on Social and Economic Thought, 1785–1865* (Oxford: Clarendon Press, 1997), 7, 10.

2. The achievement of a good death had been orchestrated through the *ars moriendi*, a highly influential set of rituals that surrounded Christian death during the early modern period. It addressed the necessity of preparation and provided instruction on how to die well. In general, these texts provided guidance for the final moment, addressing the preparedness of the soul, and the practical actions necessary for the management of the deathbed. Consumption figured prominently in the literature, as a death from this illness was treated as a blessing. The idea that consumption was a relatively painless way to die, combined to make it seem an ideal exit. Pain could mar the deathbed performance: it could make its victim ill tempered, impair the mental faculties, or push an individual into blasphemy or angry raving. The time it allowed for preparation, the perception of a relative absence of pain, and the lack of overt physical deformity all combined to elevate consumption in the *ars moriendi* tradition. Richard Wunderli and Gerald Broce, "The Final Moment Before Death." (*Sixteenth Century Journal*, Vol.20. 1989), 263; Ralph Houlbrooke, ed., *Death, Ritual, and Bereavement* (London: Routledge, 1989), 46, 48; Eamon Duffy, *The Stripping of the Altars: Traditional Religion in England 1400–1580* (New Haven: Yale University Press, 1992), 315; David Cressy, *Birth, Marriage, & Death: Ritual, Religion, and the Life-Cycle in Tudor and Stuart England*, (Oxford: Oxford University Press, 1999), 386; and Lawlor, *Consumption and Literature*, 35.

Notes

3. Tucker, ed., *A Companion to Victorian Literature and Culture* (Malden, MA: Blackwell Publishing, 1999), 114.

4. Pat Jalland has argued the Annales School and Ariès were too liberal in applying to all of Britain a narrow and unconventional approach, particularly as Ariès' work rested primarily upon the works, letters, and accounts left by the Brontës. Instead Jalland, based her work on extensive study of the private papers, correspondence, diaries, memorials, etc. of fifty different families over a century to characterize death in nineteenth-century Britain as a good evangelical death. Pat Jalland, *Death in the Victorian Family* (Oxford: Oxford University Press, 1996), 8–9.

5. Hilton, *The Age of Atonement*, 3.

6. Hilton, *The Age of Atonement*, 11.

7. Doddridge was a well-known and respected religious educator who promoted evangelical Christianity both in England and abroad. Isabel Rivers, "Doddridge, Philip (1702–1751)," in *Oxford Dictionary of National Biography*, ed. H. C. G. Matthew and Brian Harrison (Oxford: OUP, 2004); online edn, ed. Lawrence Goldman, January 2006, http://www.oxforddnb.com/view/article/7746 [accessed January 12, 2009].

8. January 4, 1736, In *The Correspondence and Diary of Philip Doddridge, D.D. edited by John Doddridge Humphreys*, Vol. V (London: Henry Colburn and Richard Bentley, 1831), 361–362.

9. January 4, 1736, In *The Correspondence and Diary of Philip Doddridge, D.D. edited by John Doddridge Humphreys*, Vol. V (London: Henry Colburn and Richard Bentley, 1831), 361–362.

10. S. Hooll to Arthur Young on the death of his daughter Martha Ann (Bobbin) Young from consumption. S. Hooll to Arthur Young, August 1797, Add MS 35127, Folio 424, The British Library Department of Manuscripts, London, UK.

11. June 29 [1836], *Journal of Emily Shore*, ed. Barbara Timm Gates (Charlottesville: University Press of Virginia, 1991), 140–141.

12. July 5 [1836], *Journal of Emily Shore*, 142.

13. December 15, [1836], *Journal of Emily Shore*, 170–171.

14. December 25, 1837, *Journal of Emily Shore*, 232.

15. December 25, 1837, *Journal of Emily Shore*, 232.

16. Emily Shore succumbed to consumption at Funchal, Madeira on July 7, 1839 and was laid to rest in the Strangers' cemetery where she first acknowledged the possibility of her mortality from the disease.

17. December 24 [1838], *Journal of Emily Shore*, 300–301.

18. November 6, 1836, *Diary of Thomas Foster Barham* (1818–1866), MS 5779, Wellcome Library, London, UK, 19.

19. November 6, 1836, *Diary of Thomas Foster Barham* (1818–1866), MS 5779, Wellcome Library, London, UK, 19.

20. November 6, 1836, *Diary of Thomas Foster Barham* (1818–1866), MS 5779, Wellcome Library, London, UK, 19–20.

21. *The Literary Gazette and Journal of Belles Lettres, Arts, Sciences, &c.* (London: James Moyes, 1831), 88.

22. *The Literary Gazette*, 88.

23. Hilton, *The Age of Atonement*, 11.

24. Peter C. Jupp and Clare Gittings, eds, *Death in England: An Illustrated History* (New Brunswick: Rutgers University Press, 2000), 235.

25. Herzlich and Pierret, *Illness and Self in Society*, 97, 100.

26. Jupp and Gittings, *Death in England*, 210.

27. What is termed "Romanticism" is a more or less arbitrary grouping of chronically overlapping groups of writers and artists with a partially shared sensibility. In England, the movement is generally viewed as beginning around the outbreak of the French Revolution in 1789 or with the publication of William Wordsworth's and Samuel Taylor Coleridge's *Lyrical Ballads* (1798) and continuing through the 1830s. The first generation of Romantics in England was typified by Wordsworth, Blake, and Coleridge and the second generation is commonly associated with Shelley, Keats, and Byron. The term Romanticism is a literary construct and the Romantic writers were designated by their contemporaries in England as belonging to various schools. For instance, Wordsworth and Coleridge were designated as belonging to the "Lake School" (because they all lived in the Lake District of England); while Keats was lumped in

the "Cockney School" (a disparaging term applied to Keats for what was seen as his plebian lower-class rhyming); while Byron was denoted as belonging to the "Demonic or Satanic School" (for what was seen as a Satanic pride and impiety in his work). Roy Porter and Mikuláš Teich, *Romanticism in National Context* (Cambridge: Cambridge University Press, 1988), 3, 240; Michael Ferber, *A Companion to European Romanticism* (Malden, MA: Blackwell Publishing, Ltd., 2005), 7, 11, 86–87; Aidan Day, *Romanticism* (London: Routledge, 1996), 2; Duncan Wu, *A Companion to Romanticism* (Malden, MA: Blackwell Publishing Ltd., 1988), 4; and Stephen Bygrave, *Romantic Writings* (London: Routledge, 1996), 47.

28. Michael Neve, "Medicine and Literature" in the *Companion Encyclopedia of the History of Medicine*, edited by W. F. Bynum and Roy Porter, Volume 2 (London: Routledge, 2001), pages 1520–1535.

29. Herzlich and Pierret, *Illness and Self in Society*, 123–124.

30. Roy Porter, *Bodies Politic: Disease, Death and Doctors in Britain, 1650–1900* (Ithaca, NY: Cornell University Press, 2001), 61.

31. Porter, *Bodies Politic*, 61.

32. Laura Jean Rosenthal and Mita Choudhury, eds, *Monstrous Dreams of Reason: Body, Self, and Other in the Enlightenment* (Cranbury, New Jersey: Associated University Presses, 2002), 117.

33. Porter, *Bodies Politic*, 61.

34. "The Infirmities of Genius Illustrated," *Tait's Edinburgh Magazine*, Vol. IV (Edinburgh: William Tait, 1834), 49.

35. David Wendell Moller, *Confronting Death: Values, Institutions, and Human Mortality* (Oxford: Oxford University Press, 1996), 12. By the latter part of the eighteenth century, death from suicide was treated as another manifestation of illness (melancholy) and was correspondingly immersed in the elevation of feeling and sensitivity as the principal aesthetic value of Romanticism. This focus on the melancholy passions and grief led to a Romantic fascination with the tragic youthful death, be it the consequence of suicide or the inevitable result of certain illnesses. The death of the young poet Thomas Chatterton at the age of seventeen in 1770 from suicide was deeply influential in linking genius with an early death and in visualizing suicide and other early exits from the mortal plane as a display of increased feeling and sensitivity. Jupp and Gittings, *Death in England*, 212–213. Lawlor has argued of Chatterton that "suicide and madness were other, less godly, fates for over-sensitive poets, their minds overwhelmed by the harshness of an unwelcoming world, especially if they were emanating from the lower ranks of society. At least consumption was involuntary and, in theory, more dignified than unchristian options." Lawlor, *Consumption and Literature*, 124. Madness, suicide, and lingering terminal illnesses, such as tuberculosis, were all poetic options in the Romantic conception, as they were all distinguished by acute and excessive sensibility, which provided the apparatus through which the unavoidable and expected disappointments of life culminated in an early grave. Lawlor, *Consumption and Literature*, 133. See Michael MacDonald and Terrence R. Murphy, eds, *Sleepless Souls: Suicide in Early Modern England* (Oxford: Oxford University Press, 2002). For more on Melancholy see, Clark Lawlor, *From Melancholia to Prozac: The History of Depression* (Oxford: Oxford University Press, 2012)

36. Lawlor, *Consumption and Literature*, 54.

37. Lawlor, *Consumption and Literature*, 54–55, 131–132.

38. Lawlor and Suzuki, "The Disease of the Self," 488.

39. *Hibernian Magazine*, Vol. III (Dublin: Printed by James Potts, 1774), 680.

40. White, *Observations on the Nature and method of cure of the Phthisis Pulmonalis*, 22.

41. Lawlor, *Consumption and Literature*, 121.

42. Thomas Young, *A Practical and Historical Treatise on Consumptive Diseases* (London: B. R. Howeltt, 1815), 43–44.

43. *A Physician's Advice For the Prevention and Cure of Consumption with the Necessary Prescriptions* (London: James Smith, 1824), 123.

44. Herzlich and Pierret, *Illness and Self in Society*, 25.

45. "On the Early Fate of Genius," *The European Magazine and London Review*, Vol. 87 (London: Sherwood, Gilbert, and Piper, 1825), 535–536.

46. Lawlor, *Consumption and Literature*, 53.

47. *The Englishwoman's Magazine and Christian Mother's Miscellany*, Vol. VI (London: Fisher, Son & Co., 1851), 606.

48. Herzlich and Pierret, *Illness and Self in Society*, 46.

49. Lawlor, *Consumption and Literature*, 7.

50. Ron M. Brown, *The Art of Suicide* (London: Reaktion Books Ltd., 2001), 134.

51. James Najarian, *Victorian Keats: Manliness, Sexuality, and Desire* (New York: Palgrave Macmillan, 2002), 27.

52. Percy Bysshe Shelley, *The Complete Works of Percy Bysshe Shelley: Letters of Percy Bysshe Shelley*, ed., Nathan Haskell Dole, Vol. 8 (London: Virtue & Company, 1906), 150.

53. "On the Early Fate of Genius," 536.

54. Timothy Ziegenhagen, "Keats, Professional Medicine, and the Two Hyperions," *Literature and Medicine* 21, No.2 (Fall 2002), 287, 290; Bynum, *Spitting Blood*, 79.

55. Raymond D. Havens, "Of Beauty and Reality in Keats," *ELH*, Vol. 17, No 3 (Sept. 1950), 209.

56. Bynum, *Spitting Blood*, 79.

57. Bynum, *Spitting Blood*, 79–81; Dubos and Dubos, *The White Plague*, 12–13.

58. John Keats, *The Complete Poetical Works and Letters of John Keats*, ed., Horace E. Scudder, Cambridge Edition (Boston: Houghton Mifflin Company, 1899), 338.

59. John Keats, *The Complete Poetical Works of John Keats edited by Harry Buxton Forman* (London: H. Frowde, 1907), 231.

60. Dubos and Dubos, *The White Plague*, 10.

61. Lawlor, *Consumption and Literature*, 136–137.

62. Keats, *The Complete Poetical Works and Letters of John Keats*, 440.

63. John Keats, *Selected Letters of John Keats: Based on the Texts of Hyder Edward Rollins*, ed., Grant F. Scott (Harvard: Harvard University Press, 2005), 484.

64. Joseph Severn, *Joseph Severn Letters and Memoirs*, Grant F. Scott, ed. (England: Ashgate Publishing Ltd., 2005), 113–114.

65. Keats, *Selected Letters of John Keats*, 497.

66. Najarian, *Victorian Keats*, 27.

67. Dubos and Dubos, *The White Plague*, 11.

68. George Noël Gordon Byron, *Life, Letters and Journals of Lord Byron* (London: John Murray, 1844), 520.

69. One of the earliest examples of the consumptive Romantic poet was Henry Kirke White (1785–1806), whose claim to fame derived more from his illness than his poetry. White wrote an ode *To Consumption*, and the disease also figured heavily in some of his fragments. For White, consumption was more than just a subject, it was also a goal, and the young author appeared infatuated with the condition before he ever experienced it. White was heavily steeped in evangelical Christianity and was also conscious of animating the Romantic myth of the consumptive poet. White thus combined his notions of evangelicalism with Romantic ideology to visualize consumption as his ideal "good death." He constructed an illness narrative that not only glamorized the experience of tuberculosis but also explicitly linked the illness and poetic genius. Lawlor, *Consumption and Literature*, 127–128.

70. John Keats, *The Poetical Works and Other Writings of John Keats in Four Volumes,* edited by Harry Buxton Foreman, Vol. III (London: Reeves & Turner, 1883), 374.

71. Percy Bysshe Shelley, *Adonais: An Elegy on the Death of John Keats* (Pisa, 1821), 4.

72. Shelley, *Adonais: An Elegy on the Death of John Keats*, 20.

73. Percy Bysshe Shelley, *Adonais, edited by William Michael Rossetti, a new edition revised with the assistance of Arthur Octavius Prickard* (Oxford: Clarendon Press, 1903), 68.

74. Shelley, *Adonais: An Elegy on the Death of John Keats*, 3–4.

75. Florence Nightingale, *Notes on Nursing: What it is, and What it is Not* (London: Harrison, 1860), 204.

Chapter 5

1. Karen Halttunen, *Confidence Men and Painted Women: A Study of Middle-Class Culture in America, 1830–1870* (New Haven: Yale University Press, 1982), 60. While Halttunen's book is about the United States, a lot that is in it applies equally well to middle-class culture in Britain.

2. Lawlor, *Consumption and Literature*, 153.

3. Halttunen, *Confidence Men and Painted Women*, xiv.

4. Halttunen, *Confidence Men and Painted Women*, xiv.

5. Lawlor and Suzuki, "The Disease of the Self," 492.

6. Fred Kaplan, *Sacred Tears: Sentimentality in Victorian Literature* (Princeton, New Jersey: Princeton University Press, 1987), 58.

7. Religious conviction was a fundamental part of the middle-class imagining of the model family. There was a feminization of religion and an elevation of the status of benevolence and moral purity, qualities explicitly identified as feminine traits. Although the prescriptive ideology of "separate spheres" was not necessarily a reflection of the reality of life for most, the rhetoric was nonetheless pervasive in the life of the nineteenth-century middle-class woman. Upper- and middle-class women were never entirely free of these popular idealizations, which managed to exert influence over the entire social spectrum and helped define individual as well as social respectability. Middle-class women struggled to accommodate their personal circumstances with the idealized model, which apportioned duties for both men and women according to religious guidelines designed to maintain order.

8. The female role developed as part of a larger discourse on sexuality, and sexual ideologies were a vital component of the cultural battles waged in Britain beginning in the 1790s, when two opposing movements arose. The Regency, identified as it was with the character of the Prince Regent and the militarization of society produced by the extended war with France, created an era of debauchery, typified by the obvious libertinism common among the military and noblemen. A reaction to these excesses grew among the respectable, propertied classes, many of whom sought to craft a new imperative for bourgeois morality and so started to foster a new sexual and moral sincerity under the aegis of evangelicalism. This evangelicalism necessitated an alteration in the sexual debate, forcing attention, as Roy Porter has argued, "away from the Georgian 'pleasures of procreation'" and instead in a direction that emphasized public character, civic probity, and "a re-idealization of love over sensuality, or moral law." Roy Porter and Lesley Hall, eds, *The Facts of Life: The Creation of Sexual Knowledge in Britain, 1650–1950* (New Haven: Yale University Press, 1995), 125–126.

9. These changes have been rationalized alternatively as the product of industrialization, with its associated growth in the separation between the work and home spaces; the growth of evangelicalism, which not only re-imagined female spirituality but also elevated female morality; and the emergence of the middle class in England as a group that sought to differentiate itself. All of these circumstances played a role in shaping the new principles of gender that rested upon a dependent female located within the home and a male breadwinner functioning in the wider world. The "cult of domesticity" was an idealized notion of both home and family that embraced its members and provided a buffer to the outside world. It located Christian values within the home while capitalism and competition were kept in the public sphere achieving a relatively comfortable moral balance. Marjorie Levine-Clark, *Beyond the Reproductive Body: the Politics of Women's Health and Work in Early Victorian England* (Ohio State University Press, 2004), 7; Deborah Gorham, *The Victorian Girl and the Feminine Ideal* (Indiana University Press, 1982)

10. Levine-Clark, *Beyond the Reproductive Body*, 2.

11. George Gordon, Lord Byron, was reported to have said to Lord Sligo, upon looking in a mirror after recovering from an illness in 1828 that had left him weak and thin: "How pale I look! I should like, I think, to die of a consumption." When asked for a reason, Byron replied, "Because then the women would all say, 'See that poor Byron—how interesting he looks in dying!'" The article went on to assert that despite the minor nature of the related anecdote "the relater remembered as a proof of the poet's consciousness of his own beauty." *The Literary Gazette and Journal of the Belles Lettres, Arts, Sciences, &c.* (London: James Moyes, 1830), 54.

12. Lady Morgan to her niece, February 6, 1843, In *Lady Morgan's Memoirs: Autobiography Diaries and Correspondence*, Vol. II, 2nd edn. (London: Wm. H. Allen & Co, 1863), 474.

13. Lawlor, *Consumption and Literature*, 107, 154–155.

14. "Life, Letters, and Literary Remains of John Keats," *The British Quarterly Review*, Vol. VIII (London: Jackson & Walford, 1848), 328.

15. Lawlor and Suzuki, "The Disease of the Self," 493.

16. Lawlor, *Consumption and Literature*, 72.

17. Thomas Hayes, *A Serious Address on the Dangerous Consequences of Neglecting Common Coughs and Colds* (London: John Murray and Messrs. Shepperson and Reynolds, 1785), 61.

18. *The World of Fashion*, Vol. XXVII (London, April 1, 1850), 43.

19. Waller, "The Illusion of an Explanation," 411.

20. *The New Monthly Magazine and Literary Journal*, Vol. V, (London: Henry Colburn and Co., 1822), 255–256.

21. November 6, 1836, *Diary of Thomas Foster Barham* (1818–1866), Wellcome Library, London, UK, 17–18.

22. G. M. C. "A Sketch of Two Homes," *The Dublin University Magazine: A Literary and Political Journal*, Vol. XLIX, January to June 1857 (Dublin: Hodges, Smith & Co., 1857), 542.

23. G. M. C. "A Sketch of Two Homes," 545.

24. *Physiology for Young Ladies, In Short and Easy Conversations* (London: S. Highley, 1843), 78–79.

25. Smith-Rosenberg and Rosenberg, "The Female Animal," 112.

26. Davidoff and Hall, argue middle-class ideology developed as a counterpoint to perceived aristocratic degeneration and corruption, rather than as a form of middle-class emulation of aristocratic lifestyles. The nineteenth-century middle class embodied certain expectations, most importantly the desire for improvement, both personal and social. Davidoff and Hall, *Family Fortunes, 1780–1850*, 149.

27. Barnes, *The Making of a Social Disease*, 49.

28. Parker, *The Subversive Stitch*, 20.

29. Lawlor, *Consumption and Literature*, 65–66.

30. Both scientific and medical theories helped shape an ideological structure that was traditional in its direction but also remained accommodating to a variety of particulars utilized to both justify and validate the place assigned to women. Smith-Rosenberg and Rosenberg, "The Female Animal," 112.

31. Ornella Moscucci, *The Science of Woman: Gynecology and Gender in England, 1800–1929* (Cambridge: Cambridge University Press, 1993), 105.

32. Robert Bentley Todd, *The Descriptive and Physiological Anatomy of the Brain, Spinal Cord, and Ganglions, and of their Coverings* (London: Sherwood, Gilbert, and Piper, 1845), 121.

33. Hastings, *Pulmonary Consumption*, 11.

34. Deshon, *Cold and Consumption*, 71–72.

35. Alexander Walker, *Intermarriage; of the Mode in Which and the Causes Why, Beauty, Health and Intellect, Result from Certain Unions, and Deformity, Disease and Insanity, From Others* (London: John Churchill, 1838), 24.

36. Walker, *Intermarriage*, 47, 49.

37. Reid, *A Treatise on the Origin, Progress, Prevention, and Treatment of Consumption*, 172.

38. Walker, *Intermarriage*, 44.

39. Walker, *Intermarriage*, 21.

40. Walker, *Intermarriage*, 21.

41. "Dr. Pring's Principles of Pathology," *The Medico-Chirurgical Review, and Journal of Medical Science*, ed., James Johnson, Vol. IV (London: G. Hayden, 1824), 271.

42. Lawlor, *Consumption and Literature*, 17–18. Although not a new assertion, these ideas were re-popularized in the eighteenth century as part of the debate over the uniqueness of humans in relation to the natural world and the characteristics that defined sex. Phobias over the menstrual blood were of long standing, and contact with it, or even close proximity to it, were thought to have a multitude of negative effects ranging from the souring of wine and other foodstuffs, to the destruction of crops and bees. Closeness to a menstruating female was also believed at one point to

impel madness in dogs, and cause flowers to lose their scent. Menstrual blood itself had also been assigned the ability to function as a poison; for instance, in the thirteenth century the medical scholar Albertus Mangnus was asked by a priest to write about the subject in a work entitled the "Secrets of Woman." The request was most likely made because it was believed that menstruating females produced a poison thought to be able to kill a child still in the cradle. Edward Shorter, *Women's Bodies: A Social History of Women's Encounter with Health, Ill-Health, and Medicine* (New Brunswick: Transaction Publishers, 1997), 287–288; Londa Schiebinger, *Nature's Body: Sexual Politics and the Making of Modern Science* (London: Pandora, An Imprint of HarperCollins Publishers, 1993), 89–91.

43. Robert Thomas, *The Modern Practice of Physic*. Ninth Edition. (London: Longman, Rees, Orme, Brown, and Green, 1828), 540.

44. "Phthisis," *The Penny Cyclopaedia of the Society for the Diffusion of Useful Knowledge*, Vol. XVIII (London: Charles Knight and Co., 1840), 123.

45. C. J. B. Aldis, *An Introduction to Hospital Practice* (London: Longman, Rees, Orme, Brown, Green, and Longman, 1835), 116.

46. Katherine Ott, *Fevered Lives: Tuberculosis in American Culture since 1870* (Harvard: Harvard University Press, 1996), 6.

47. Francis Hopkins Ramadge, *Consumption Curables* (London: Longman, Rees, Orme, Browne, Green, and Longman, 1834), 81.

48. Samuel Dickson, *Fallacies of The Faculty, Being the Spirit of the Chrono-Thermal System*. (London: H. Bailliere, 1839), 180.

49. Dickson, *Fallacies of The Faculty*, 181.

50. Thomas, *The Modern Practice of Physic*, 545.

51. John T. Ingleby, *A Practical Treatise on Uterine Hemorrhage in Connexion with Pregnancy and Parturition* (London: Longman, Rees, Orme, Brown, Green, and Longman, 1832), 89.

52. Marshall Hall, *Commentaries Principally on Those Diseases of Females Which are Constitutional*, 2nd edn. (London: Sherwood, Gilbert, and Piper, 1830), 140.

53. Walker, *Intermarriage*, 7.

54. Jalland and Hooper, *Women From Birth to Death*, 281.

55. Walker, *Intermarriage*, 41.

56. John C. Ferguson, *Consumption: What it is, and What it is not* (Belfast: Henry Greer, 1856), 5.

57. Halttunen, *Confidence Men and Painted Women*, 57.

58. Todd, *The Descriptive and Physiological Anatomy of the Brain, Spinal Cord, and Ganglions*, 121.

59. Caldwell, *The Last Crusade*, 17.

60. Halttunen, *Confidence Men and Painted Women*, 57.

61. Lawlor, *Consumption and Literature*, 24. Although there were certainly instances in which individuals sought to exhibit an increased quantity of sensibility, the affectation of emotional sensibility was looked upon with contempt, or at least derision. This condemnation of affectation had been occurring since the latter part of the eighteenth century when sensibility had begun to grow in importance, and is evident in the description of one such individual, a Miss Williams who "is, I think, without any exception, the <u>most</u> affected of any young lady I ever met with! a sentimental affectation— she sits <u>like a lily drooping</u> in Company, & proposes to dislike any thing that is comic" Charlotte Burney to Susan Burney, 1784, Barrett Collection, Vol. XII, Egerton MS 3700A, folio 127, The British Library Department of Manuscripts, London, UK.

62. Emotions had a long tradition of being significant in the course of tuberculosis as such, keeping the patient calm and in good spirits was believed to be of a vital importance in cases of the disease.

63. Clark, *A Treatise on Pulmonary Consumption*, 236–237.

64. H. D. Chalke, "The Impact of Tuberculosis on History, Literature and Art," *Medical History* VI (1962), 307. For instance, Charlotte Brontë makes consumption a defining feature of Helen Burns' character in *Jane Eyre*.

65. Lawlor, *Consumption and Literature*, 76.

66. For more on this transition see Carolyn A. Day and Amelia Rauser, "Thomas Lawrence's Consumptive Chic: Reinterpreting Lady Manners' Hectic Flush in 1794," *Eighteenth-Century Studies* 49.4 (Summer 2016).

67. Cotton, *The Nature, Symptoms, and Treatment of Consumption*, 80.

68. Rosenthal and Choudhury, *Monstrous Dreams of Reason*, 117.

Chapter 6

1. Sontag, *Illness as Metaphor*, 29.

2. For more on Siddons celebrity see Laura Engel, *Fashioning Celebrity: 18th-Century British Actresses and Strategies for Image Making* (Columbus: The Ohio State University Press, 2011).

3. Philip H. Highfill, *A Biographical Dictionary of Actors, Actresses, Musicians, Dancers, managers & Other Stage Personnel in London, 1660–1800*, Vol. 14 (Southern Illinois University Press, 1991), 23. Although her salary from 1788–1799 was £20 per night, increasing to £31.10s per night in the period from 1799–1800, the Siddons family was faced with financial shortfalls because Sheridan was consistently behind in paying her salary and as late as November 1799 still owed Mrs. Siddons over £2,100.

4. Robert Shaughnessy, "Siddons, Sarah (1755–1831)," in *Oxford Dictionary of National Biography*, ed. H. C. G. Matthew and Brian Harrison (Oxford: OUP, 2004); online ed., ed. Lawrence Goldman, May 2008, http://www.oxforddnb.com/view/article/25516 [accessed January 12, 2009].

5. The punctuation of the letters in this chapter appears as in the original manuscripts. Mrs. Siddons to Mrs. Barrington, London, June 3, 1792, Barrington Collection Add MS 73736, The British Library Department of Manuscripts, London, UK.

6. Highfill, *A Biographical Dictionary of Actors,* 26.

7. Entry dated January 26, 1834, in Charles C. F. Greville, *The Greville Memoirs: A Journal of the Reigns of King George IV and King William IV*, Vol. II (New York: D. Appleton and Company, 1875), 213.

8. Mrs. Siddons to Mrs. Barrington, London, April 7, 1792, Barrington Collection Add 73736, The British Library Department of Manuscripts, London, UK.

9. Thomas Campbell was, unfortunately, for posterity's sake, Mrs. Siddons choice as her biographer, and to whom she turned over the bulk of her writings, journals, and personal correspondence. He used disappointingly few of these items in his *Life of Mrs. Siddons*, a circumstance bemoaned by his contemporaries and historians alike. To make matters worse, he failed to return her papers to the family and they were mysteriously lost.

10. Thomas Campbell, *Life of Mrs. Siddons* (New York: Harper & Brothers, 1834), 224.

11. Mrs. Piozzi to Mrs. Pennington, from Guy's Cliffe, Sunday, October 14, 1792, in *The Intimate Letters of Hester Piozzi and Penelope Pennington 1788–1821,* ed. Oswald G. Knapp (London: John Lane, 1914), 69.

12. The therapy was successful as Sally, according to Mrs. Piozzi, was growing "fat and merry." Mrs. Piozzi, September 9, 1792, in *An Artist's Love Story: Told in the Letters of Sir Thomas Lawrence, Mrs. Siddons, and Her Daughters*, Oswald G. Knapp (London: George Allen, 1904), 9–10.

13. Mrs. Piozzi to Mrs. Pennington, from Guy's Cliffe, Sunday, October 14, 1792, in Knapp, ed., *The Intimate Letters of Hester Piozzi and Penelope Pennington*, 69.

14. William Cullen asserted of asthma, that "in some young persons it has ended soon, by occasioning a phthisis pulmonalis." William Cullen, *First Lines of the Practice of Physic*, Vol. II (Edinburgh: Bell & Bradfute, 1808), 215–216. John Roberton seconded these assertions: "Asthma, also, may occasion this disease [consumption], by producing tubercles." John Roberton, *A Treatise on Medical Police, and on Diet, Regimen, &c.*, Vol. I (Edinburgh: John Moir, 1809), 234.

15. John Fyvie, *Tragedy Queens of the Georgian Era* (New York: E. P. Dutton and Company, 1909), 253.

16. Lawrence was reintroduced to the Siddons' daughters sometime after their return from a finishing school in Calais. The girls had been taken there in 1789 or 1790 and had returned approximately two or three years later. They were still there

in 1792, when Mr. Siddons took his son Harry to Amiens and wrote to his wife of his daughters' appearance. In Parsons, *The Incomparable Siddons* (New York: G. P. Putnam's Sons, 1909), 188.

17. During this period, Sally's health remained precarious as evidenced in December of 1797 when Mr. Siddons related that Sally "has had the worst fit I ever knew, and is still very ill." Her condition was confirmed by Maria in a letter to Miss Bird. "Sally is getting better, I hope; she has been very ill, and is still very weak." Mr. Siddons to Dr. Whalley, December 15 and 17, 1797, in *Journals and Correspondence*, Vol. II (London: Richard Bentley, 1863), 109, and Maria Siddons to Miss Bird, 1797, in Knapp, *An Artist's Love Story*, 14.

18. Sir Walter Armstrong, *Lawrence* (New York: Charles Scribner's Sons, 1913), 42.

19. Mrs. Siddons to Dr. Whalley, January 15, 1798, in Whalley, *Journals and Correspondence* (London: Richard Bentley, 1863), Vol. II, 109–110. Dr. George Pearson was well acquainted with Mrs. Siddons' brother Kemble. The two had met when the doctor was first starting out in Doncaster and continued their acquaintance once Pearson had settled in London. William Munk stated "As a practitioner he was judicious and safe rather than strikingly acute or original." This may help explain his cautious approach to Maria's illness. William Munk, *The Roll of the Royal College of Physicians of London*, 2nd edn, Vol. II (London: Published by the College, 1878), 343.

20. Mrs. Siddons to Mrs. Barrington, May 17, 1798, Barrington Collection Add MS 73736, The British Library Department of Manuscripts, London, UK.

21. Sally Siddons to Miss Bird, January 5, 1798, in Knapp, *An Artist's Love Story*, 16–17.

22. Knapp, *An Artist's Love Story*, 15.

23. Sally Siddons to Miss Bird, January 5, 1798, in Knapp, *An Artist's Love Story*, 17.

24. Sally Siddons to Miss Bird, January 28, 1798, in Knapp, *An Artist's Love Story*, 19.

25. Parsons provides an even shorter window, stating that this change in affections occurred within six weeks of the official engagement. Parsons, *The Incomparable Siddons*, 193. For more on Sally and Lawrence's relationship see Laura Engel (2014) "The Secret Life of Archives: Sally Siddons, Sir Thomas Lawrence, and The Material of Memory," *ABO: Interactive Journal for Women in the Arts, 1640–1830*: Vol. 4: Issue 1, Article 2. DOI: http://dx.doi.org/10.5038/2157–7129.4.1.1 available at: http://scholarcommons.usf.edu/abo/vol4/iss1/2 and Douglas Goldring, *Regency Portrait Painter: The Life of Sir Thomas Lawrence* (London: Macdonald, 1921).

26. Sally to Mr. Lawrence, 1798, in Eliza Priestly, "An Artist's Love Story," *Nineteenth Century and After: A Monthly Review*, 57:338 (April 1905), 645–646.

27. Eliza Priestly, "An Artist's Love Story," 646.

28. Eliza Priestly, "An Artist's Love Story," 646.

29. Fyvie, *Tragedy Queens of the Georgian Era*, 254.

30. Sally Siddons to Miss Bird, March 5, 1798, in Knapp, *An Artist's Love Story*, 26–27.

31. Maria Siddons to Miss Bird, March 14, 1798, in Knapp, *An Artist's Love Story*, 29.

32. This pain was an acknowledged symptom of consumption. Henry Herbert Southey stated, in tuberculosis, there was a "sharp transient pain in the chest which is called a stitch" or "some fixed pain either in the side or below the sternum, or a sense of general soreness in the chest." Southey, *Observations on Pulmonary Consumption*, 7–8.

33. Maria Siddons to Miss Bird, March 14, 1798, in Knapp, *An Artist's Love Story*, 29.

34. Knapp, *An Artist's Love Story*, 29–30.

35. Knapp, *An Artist's Love Story*, 30–31.

36. Mrs. Piozzi to Mrs. Pennington, March 27, 1798, In Knapp, ed., *The Intimate Letters of Hester Piozzi and Penelope Pennington*, 152.

37. Knapp, ed., *The Intimate Letters of Hester Piozzi and Penelope Pennington*, 152.

38. Maria Siddons to Miss Bird, April 8, 1798, in Knapp, *An Artist's Love Story*, 32.

39. Knapp, *An Artist's Love Story*, 33–34.

40. Maria Siddons to Miss Bird, May 6, 1798, in Knapp, *An Artist's Love Story*, 42.

41. Mrs. Siddons to Tate Wilkinson, May 29, 1798, in Campbell, *Life of Mrs. Siddons*, 199.

42. Campbell, *Life of Mrs. Siddons*, 199.

43. Phyllis Hembry, *The English Spa: 1560–1815* (London: The Athlone Press, 1990), 245–246.

44. *The New Bath Guide; or Useful Pocket Companion* (Bath: R. Cruttwell, 1799), 55.

45. William Nisbet, *A General Dictionary of Chemistry* (London: S. Highley, 1805), 76.

46. William Saunders, *A Treatise on the Chemical History and Medical Powers of Some of the Most Celebrated Mineral Waters*, 2nd edn. (London: Phillips and Fardon, 1805), 125–126.

47. Dr. Andrew Carrick (1789), quoted in L. M. Griffiths, "The Reputation of the Hotwells (Bristol) as a Health Resort," *The Bristol Medico-Chirurgical Journal* (March 1902), 22.

48. Julius Caesar Ibbetson, *A Picturesque Guide to Bath, Bristol Hot-wells, the River Avon, and the Adjacent Country* (London: Hookham and Carpenter, 1793), 174.

49. Ibbetson, *A Picturesque Guide to Bath*, 170.

50. Saunders, *A Treatise on the Chemical History and Medical Powers of Some of the Most Celebrated Mineral Waters*, 112.

51. Saunders, *A Treatise on the Chemical History and Medical Powers of Some of the Most Celebrated Mineral Waters*, 125.

52. Robert Thomas, *The Modern Practice of Physic*, 4th edn. (London: Longman, Hurst, Rees, Orme, and Brown, 1813), 425.

53. Thomas, *The Modern Practice of Physic,* 425–426.

54. Jeremiah Whitaker Newman, *The Lounger's Common-Place Book*, Vol. IV (London: 1799), 181.

55. Sally Siddons to Miss Bird, Clifton, June 13, 1798, in Knapp, *An Artist's Love Story*, 45.

56. Dowry Square was situated at the bottom of Clifton Hill on the road to the Hot-well house, and as such, provided an unparalleled location for Maria as an invalid visiting the village. Ibbetson, *A Picturesque Guide to Bath*, 166–166, 167; Parsons, *The Incomparable Siddons*, 197.

57. Sally Siddons to Miss Bird, Clifton, June 13, 1798, in Knapp, *An Artist's Love Story*, 46.

58. Mrs. Siddons to Mrs. Pennington, Worcester, July 26 [1798], Lawrence Siddons Letters Add 6445, Folio 1, Cambridge University Library Department of Manuscripts, Cambridge, UK.

59. Edward Owen, in *Observations on the Earths, Rocks, Stones and Minerals, for some miles about Bristol, and on the nature of the Hot-Well, and . . . its water* (1754), addressed the practice of "riding-double" upon Durdham Down writing: "the best lady attending the Hot well will not refuse riding behind a man, for such is the custom of the country. Numbers of what they call double horses are kept for that purpose." Quoted in John Latimer, *The Annals of Bristol In the Eighteenth Century* (Printed for the Author, 1893), 245.

60. Maria's access to the activities of Clifton would have been total, as her mother's boon companion, Mrs. Pennington's husband William, had attained the position of Master of Ceremonies at the Hot-wells in 1785. Knapp, *An Artist's Love Story*, 36, 38.

61. Sally Siddons to Miss Bird, July 27, 1798, in Knapp, *An Artist's Love Story*, 53.

62. Mrs. Siddons to Mrs. Pennington, c.July 31, 1798, Lawrence Siddons Letters Add 6445, Folio 2, Cambridge University Library Department of Manuscripts, Cambridge, UK.

63. Mrs. Siddons to Mrs. Pennington, c.July 31, 1798, Lawrence Siddons Letters Add 6445, Folio 2, Cambridge University Library Department of Manuscripts, Cambridge, UK.

64. Mrs. Siddons to Mrs. Pennington, Cheltenham, August 9, 1798, Lawrence Siddons Letters Add 6445, Folio 3, Cambridge University Library Department of Manuscripts, Cambridge, UK.

65. Mrs. Siddons to Mrs. Pennington, Cheltenham, August 9, 1798, Lawrence Siddons Letters Add 6445, Folio 3, Cambridge University Library Department of Manuscripts, Cambridge, UK.

66. Sally Siddons to Miss Bird, 1798, in Knapp, *An Artist's Love Story*, 72.

67. "I pray God his phrenzy may not impel him to some desperate action! What he can propose by going thither I know not, but it is fit they should both be on their guard. Mr. S. knows nothing of all this, the situation of dear Sally, when one recurs to her original partiality for this wretched madman, placing her in so delicate a situation, we thought it best to keep the matter entirely conceal'd, as it was impossible that anything cou'd come of it, if ever, NEVER, she was

RESOLV'D, till her sister shou'd be perfectly restor'd. I hope it will always be a secret to Mr. S., as it could answer no end but to enrage him and make us all still more unhappy." Mrs. Siddons to Mrs. Pennington, 1798, Lawrence Siddons Letters Add 6445, Folio 7, Cambridge University Library Department of Manuscripts, Cambridge, UK.

68. Mrs. Siddons to Mrs. Pennington, 1798, Lawrence Siddons Letters Add 6445, Folio 7, Cambridge University Library Department of Manuscripts, Cambridge, UK.

69. Thomas Lawrence to Mrs. Pennington, 1798, Lawrence Siddons Letters Add 6445, Folio 8, Cambridge University Library Department of Manuscripts, Cambridge, UK.

70. Thomas Lawrence to Mrs. Pennington, 1798, Lawrence Siddons Letters Add 6445, Folio 8, Cambridge University Library Department of Manuscripts, Cambridge, UK. Lawrence's attempt to shift blame was not a disavowal of the role of feelings in Maria's illness, but rather of Maria's feelings for him.

71. "The affairs of this unhappy man are very much derang'd. He told me some time ago, when he was as mad about Maria as he is now about Sally, that, if she rejected him, he would fly, to compose his Spirit, to the mountains of Switzerland. Maria reign'd sole arbitress of his fate for two years, or more. The other day he told me, if he lost Sally, SWITZERLAND was still his resource. Oh! that caprice and passion shou'd thus obscure the many excellencies and lofty genius of this man! Tell my sweet girl how infinitely more she deserves than I cou'd ever endure, in tenderness to her repose." Mrs. Siddons to Mrs. Pennington, Fryday 1798, Lawrence Siddons Letters Add 6445, Folio 12, Cambridge University Library Department of Manuscripts, Cambridge, UK.

72. Lawrence was not only motivated by forestalling Maria's interference in he and Sally's relationship but, according to Oswald Knapp, Sally was not fully convinced of his constancy and in protecting her feelings increased Lawrence's insecurity to the point where his jealousy overwhelmed any good sense he might have possessed and he was concerned he might have a rival for her affection in Clifton. In Knapp, *An Artist's Love Story*, 94–95.

73. Mrs. Pennington to Lawrence, September 4, 1798, Lawrence Siddons Letters Add 6445, Folio 19, Cambridge University Library Department of Manuscripts, Cambridge, UK.

74. Knapp, *An Artist's Love Story*, 108.

75. Mr. Lawrence to Mrs. Pennington, Postmark, Sept. 7, 1798, Lawrence Siddons Letters Add 6445, Folio 21, Cambridge University Library Department of Manuscripts, Cambridge, UK.

76. Mrs. Pennington to Mr. Lawrence, Hotwells, Sept. 11, 1798, Lawrence Siddons Letters Add 6445, Folio 23, Cambridge University Library Department of Manuscripts, Cambridge, UK.

77. Parsons, *The Incomparable Siddons*, 199.

78. Mr. Lawrence to Mrs. Pennington, Postmark, Oct. 2, 1798, Lawrence Siddons Letters Add 6445, Folio 26, Cambridge University Library Department of Manuscripts, Cambridge, UK.

79. Letter Mrs. Pennington to Mr. Lawrence, Oct. 8, 1798, Lawrence Siddons Letters Add 6445, Folio 31, Cambridge University Library Department of Manuscripts, Cambridge, UK. The newspapers had to print a correction after prematurely reporting Maria's death: "Miss Maria Siddons, whose death was prematurely stated in the public prints, on Saturday se'nnight expired at Bristol Hot Wells." *Bell's Weekly Messenger* (London, England), October 14, 1798; Issue 129.

80. Letter Mrs. Pennington to Mr. Lawrence, Oct. 8, 1798, Lawrence Siddons Letters Add 6445, Folio 31, Cambridge University Library Department of Manuscripts, Cambridge, UK.

81. Letter Mrs. Pennington to Mr. Lawrence, Oct. 8, 1798, Lawrence Siddons Letters Add 6445, Folio 31, Cambridge University Library Department of Manuscripts, Cambridge, UK.

82. Letter Mrs. Pennington to Mr. Lawrence, Oct. 8, 1798, Lawrence Siddons Letters Add 6445, Folio 31, Cambridge University Library Department of Manuscripts, Cambridge, UK.

83. Letter Mrs. Pennington to Mr. Lawrence, Oct. 8, 1798, Lawrence Siddons Letters Add 6445, Folio 31, Cambridge University Library Department of Manuscripts, Cambridge, UK.

84. Knapp, An Artist's Love Story, 127.

85. Mrs. Pennington to Mr. Lawrence, September 4, 1798, Lawrence Siddons Letters Add 6445, Folio 19, Cambridge University Library Department of Manuscripts, Cambridge, UK.

86. Letter Mrs. Pennington to Mr. Lawrence, Oct. 8, 1798, Lawrence Siddons Letters Add 6445, Folio 31, Cambridge University Library Department of Manuscripts, Cambridge, UK.

87. Letter Mrs. Pennington to Mr. Lawrence, Oct. 8, 1798, Lawrence Siddons Letters Add 6445, Folio 31, Cambridge University Library Department of Manuscripts, Cambridge, UK.

88. Mrs. Pennington to Mr. Lawrence, Oct. 2, 1798, Lawrence Siddons Letters Add 6445, Folio 27, Cambridge University Library Department of Manuscripts, Cambridge, UK.

89. Letter Mrs. Pennington to Mr. Lawrence, Oct. 8, 1798, Lawrence Siddons Letters Add 6445, Folio 31, Cambridge University Library Department of Manuscripts, Cambridge, UK.

90. Letter Mrs. Pennington to Mr. Lawrence, Oct. 8, 1798, Lawrence Siddons Letters Add 6445, Folio 31, Cambridge University Library Department of Manuscripts, Cambridge, UK.

91. Lawrence even participates in assigning Maria a refined, intellectual, delicate, beauty, in a poem entitled simply "For Maria," likely written the eve of her death. "If all of thy Beauty that gives me delight were gone to the Joys that are fled/ And all that enchants in that Intellect bright no more sweetest Influence shed/ Were Genius rare gifts with right Judgment combin'd with Talents, their powers to impart/ By saddest Infirmity, torn from thy mind, And tenderness self From thy Heart/In that delicate Form, while a pulse should remain/ Of that mind, but one ray be preserv'd/ That throb, would thy power undiminish'd retain/ That glance be with reverence observ'd/ Unotice'd- unknown-my devotion, I'd prove/ Till the last emanations expire/ As faithful, when cold e'en the embers of love/ As when cherish'd and blest by its Fire/ Then hope from that Power that permitted thy worth/ Thy last dying prescription forgiven / If the soul, by thy virtues, refin'd on this earth, Such its Angel again in their Heaven." Thomas Lawrence, *For Maria*, LAW/5/537, Royal Academy of Arts, London, UK.

92. Letter Mrs. Pennington to Mr. Lawrence, Oct. 8, 1798, Lawrence Siddons Letters Add 6445, Folio 31, Cambridge University Library Department of Manuscripts, Cambridge, UK.

93. Letter Mrs. Pennington to Mr. Lawrence, Oct. 8, 1798, Lawrence Siddons Letters Add 6445, Folio 31, Cambridge University Library Department of Manuscripts, Cambridge, UK.

94. Letter Mrs. Pennington to Mr. Lawrence, Oct. 8, 1798, Lawrence Siddons Letters Add 6445, Folio 31, Cambridge University Library Department of Manuscripts, Cambridge, UK.

95. Clark Lawlor argues that in this cultural prototype, women were subordinate to and dependent upon men, and love provided the avenue through which women could connect themselves to and bond with men. As a result, Lawlor argued that when this love went awry the woman had no other option except disease and in due course death and, if at all possible, that death should be the beautiful exit provided by tuberculosis. Lawlor, *Consumption and Literature*, 16, 152, 154.

96. Lawlor, *Consumption and Literature*, 16, 152, 154.

97. Richardson's novel had been translated into French in 1751, and Rousseau was certainly familiar with the work as he complimented it in his *Letter to d'Alembert*. Jean-Jacques Rousseau, *La Nouvelle Héloïse: Julie, or the New Eloise*, Translated and Abridged by Judith H. McDowell, 5th Edition (The Pennsylvania State University Press, 2000), 8. Apparently, Rousseau initially planned to have Julie die by drowning, but changed his plans and had her exit life via the tableaux of consumption, as Richardson had done with Clarissa. David Marshall, *The Frame of Art: Fictions of Aesthetic Experience, 1750–1815* (Baltimore: The Johns Hopkins University Press, 2005), 94.

98. Lawlor, *Consumption and Literature*, 59.

99. "Clarissa's illness [was] probably a galloping consumption." Margaret Ann Doody, *A Natural Passion: A Study of the Novels of Samuel Richardson* (Oxford: Oxford University Press, 1974), 171.

100. Lawlor, *Consumption and Literature*, 9.

101. Lawlor, *Consumption and Literature*, 58–59.

102. Samuel Richardson, *Clarissa*. Contained in *The Novelist's Magazine*. Vol. XV. Containing the Fifth, Sixth, Seventh, and Eighth Volumes of *Clarissa* (London: Harrison and Co., 1784), 1140.

103. Richardson, *Clarissa*, Vol. XV, 1145.

104. Marshall, *The Frame of Art*, 95.

105. Mrs. Sarah Siddons to Mrs. Elizabeth Barrington, October 19, 1798, Barrington Collection Add MS 73736, The British Library, London, UK.

106. Oswald Knapp dated this letter as having been written on October 4, 1798, a full three days before Maria's death. Mrs. Piozzi to Mrs. Pennington, October 4, 1798, in Knapp, ed., *The Intimate Letters of Hester Piozzi and Penelope Pennington*, 164–165.

107. Mrs. Piozzi to Dr. Gray, October 14, 1798, in *Autobiography, Letters and Literary Remains of Mrs. Piozzi (Thrale),* A. Hayward, ed., Vol. II, second edition (London: Longman, Green, Longman, and Roberts, 1861), 249–250.

108. Letter Mrs. Siddons to Mrs. Pennington, October 27, 1798, Lawrence Siddons Letters Add 6445, Folio 45, Cambridge University Library Department of Manuscripts, Cambridge, UK.

109. Verse 600, from *Night Thoughts*. Knapp, *An Artist's Love Story*, 128.

110. Mrs. Sarah Siddons to Mrs. Elizabeth Barrington, Cheltenham, May 16, 1803, Barrington Collection Add MS 73736, The British Library Department of Manuscripts, London, UK.

111. Mrs. Siddons to Mrs. Fitzhugh, Cheltenham, June 1803, in *Mrs. Siddons*, Nina A. Kennard (Boston: Roberts Brothers, 1887), 276.

Chapter 7

1. Beddoes, *Essay on the Causes, Early Signs, and Prevention of Pulmonary Consumption*, 178.

2. Rosenthal and Choudhury, *Monstrous Dreams of Reason*, 117.

3. Lawlor, *Consumption and Literature*, 43. Susan Sontag has argued that it was during this period that consumption came to be inextricably tied to appearance. The disease, she wrote, "was understood as a manner of appearing, and that appearance became a staple of nineteenth century manners. The TB influenced idea of the body was a new model for aristocratic looks. The tubercular look had to be considered attractive once it came to be a mark of distinction, of breeding." Sontag, *Illness as Metaphor and Aids and Its Metaphors*, 28–29. While, Jean and Rene Dubos applied these assertions specifically to women arguing that "the distorted picture of consumption drawn by poets and novelists was in keeping with the peculiar ideal of feminine beauty that was then prevailing." Dubos and Dubos, *The White Plague*, 54. See also, Roy Porter "Consumption: Disease of the Consumer Society?" in John Brewer and Roy Porter ed., *Consumption and the World of Goods* (London: Routledge, 1993); and Lawlor and Suzuki, "The Disease of the Self."

4. Roy Porter, *Flesh in the Age of Reason* (New York: W. W. Norton & Co., 2003), 241.

5. *The London Medical and Surgical Journal*, Vol. III (London: Renshaw and Rush, 1833),

6. Herzlich and Pierret, *Illness and Self in Society*, 25.

7. Steven J. Peitzman, "From Dropsy to Bright's Disease to End-Stage Renal Disease," *The Milbank Quarterly*, Vol. 67, Supplement 1, *Framing Disease: The Creation and Negotiation of Explanatory Schemes* (1989), (Published by: Milbank Memorial Fund), 18–19.

8. Peitzman, "From Dropsy to Bright's Disease to End-Stage Renal Disease," 17.

9. Peter McNeil, "Ideology, Fashion and the Darlys' 'Macaroni' Prints," in *Dress and Ideology: Fashioning Identity from Antiquity to the Present*, Shoshana-Rose Marzel and Guy D. Stiebel, eds. (London: Bloomsbury, 2015), 112. See also Hannah Greig, *The Beau Monde: Fashionable Society in Georgian London* (Oxford: Oxford University Press, 2013).

10. Dror Wahrman, *The Making of the Modern Self: Identity and Culture in Eighteenth-Century England* (New Haven: Yale University Press, 2004), 62. Amelia Rauser, building upon Wahrman, has argued that "caricature signified insiderness and sophistication as well as exaggeration and superficiality," as a result caricature marked individualism, but also served "as a warning of its dangerous extremism." Amelia Rauser, *Caricature Unmasked: Irony, Authenticity, and Individualism in Eighteenth-Century English Prints* (Newark: University of Delaware Press, 2008), 76.

11. *The Times*, Monday, March 25, 1793 (London, 1793), 2.

12. For more on corpulence and obesity see Sander L. Gilman, *Obesity: The Biography* (Oxford: Oxford University Press, 2010) and Sander L. Gilman, *Fat: A Cultural History of Obesity* (Cambridge: Polity Press, 2008).

13. Porter, *Flesh in the Age of Reason*, 240, 243. Clark Lawlor has argued this phenomenon was entrenched by 1799. Lawlor, *Consumption and Literature*, 44.

14. Porter, *Flesh in the Age of Reason*, 240.

15. William Wadd, *Cursory Remarks on Corpulence or Obesity Considered as a Disease*, 3rd edition (London: J. Callow, 1816), 54–55.

16. "On Corpulence," *The New Monthly Magazine and Literary Journal*, Vol. X (London: Henry Colburn, 1824), 184.

17. *The Art of Beauty; or the Best Methods of Improving and Preserving the Shape, Carriage, and Complexion. Together with, the Theory of Beauty* (London: Knight and Lacey, 1825), 77–78.

18. Walker, *Intermarriage*, 339.

19. Lawlor, *Consumption and Literature*, 58.

20. For a further discussion of the role of sensibility and nerves in consumption see Carolyn A. Day and Amelia Rauser, 'Thomas Lawrence's Consumptive Chic: Reinterpreting Lady Manners' Hectic Flush in 1794', *Eighteenth-Century Studies* 49.4 (Summer 2016).

21. James Makittrick Adair, *Essays on Fashionable Diseases* (London: T.P. Bateman, 1790), 4.

22. *A Manual of Essays*, Vol. II (London: F. C. & J. Rivington, 1809), 106.

23. Adair, *Essays on Fashionable Diseases*, 3. For more on the commercialization of fashion see Neil McKendrick, John Brewer, and J. H. Plumb, *The Birth of a Consumer Society: The Commercialization of Eighteenth-Century England* (Bloomington: Indiana University Press, 1982) and John Styles, *The Dress of the People: Everyday Fashion in Eighteenth-Century England* (New Haven: Yale University Press, 2007).

24. *The Lady's Magazine*, Vol. XXI (London: 1790), 117.

25. For discussions of eighteenth and nineteenth century beauty see Greig, *The Beau Monde*; Aileen Ribeiro, *Facing Beauty: Painted Women and Cosmetic Art* (London and New Haven: Yale University Press, 2011); Patricia Phillippy, *Painting Women: Cosmetics, Canvases & Early Modern Culture* (Baltimore: The Johns Hopkins University Press, 2006); Caroline Palmer, "Brazen Cheek: Face-Painters in Late Eighteenth-Century England," *Oxford Art Journal* 31 (2008), 195–213; and Richard Corson, *Fashions in Makeup: From Ancient to Modern Times* (New York: Universe Books, 1972).

26. George Cheyne, *George Cheyne: The English Malady*, xxviii.

27. Lawlor, *Consumption and Literature*, 55–58.

28. *The Lady's Magazine*, (London: 1774), 523. Clark Lawlor rightly calls attention to Dr. John Gregory's contribution to this debate, who wrote "But though good health be one of the greatest blessings of life, never boast of it . . . We so naturally associate the idea of female softness and delicacy, with a correspondent delicacy of constitution, that when a woman speaks of her great strength . . . we recoil at the description." Dr. John Gregory, *A Father's Legacy to His Daughters* (Philadelphia: 1795), 32. Also in Lawlor, *Consumption and Literature*, 57.

29. George Keate, *Sketches from Nature*, Vol. II (London: J. Dodsley, 1790), 38–39.

30. Edmund Burke, *A Philosophical Enquiry into the Origin of our Ideas of the Sublime and Beautiful* (Notre Dame: University of Notre Dame Press, 1968), 11.

31. Burke, *A Philosophical Enquiry*, 11.

32. John Leake, *Medical Instructions Towards the Prevention and Cure of Chronic Diseases Peculiar to Women*, Vol. 1, 6th Edition (London: Baldwin, 1787), 302–303.

33. *La Belle Assemblée*, Vol. III, (London: J. Bell, 1811), 202.

34. Davidoff and Hall, *Family Fortunes*, 28.

35. *The Age We Live In: A Fragment Dedicated to Every Young Lady of Fashion* (London: Lackington, Allen, and Co., 1813), 79–80.

36. For instance, Beddoes compared women "to flowers brought forward by the cherishing heat of the conservatory . . . They cannot with impunity bear to be roughly visited by the winds of heaven. The slightest cause disorders them,

and ... they exist in a perpetual state of dangerous weakness. For in this country, by whatever cause women under thirty are weakened, there is always considerable hazard of consumption." Beddoes, *Essay on the Causes, Early Signs, and Prevention of Pulmonary Consumption*, 124.

37. Akiko Fukai, et al., *Fashion: the Collection of the Kyoto Costume Institute: a History from the 18th to the 20th Century* (Taschen, 2002), 151–152.

38. "Scenes of the Ton, No. 1. *Bringing out Daughters*," *The New Monthly Magazine and Literary Journal*, Vol. 25 (London: Henry Colburn and Richard Bentley, 1829), 566.

39. Betty had just recently died due to a "fatal cold by exposure to the night air, in consequence of a blunder of her coachman at Almack's. It was the first time she had been exposed to the air of Heaven five minutes for twenty years before her decease." "Scenes of the Ton," 566.

40. "Scenes of the Ton," 566.

41. Mrs. William Parkes, *Domestic Duties; or Instructions to Young Married Ladies* (London: Longman, Hurst, Rees, Orme, Brown, and Green, 1825), 253.

42. *The World of Fashion*, Vol. IX (London: 1832), 263.

43. *Tait's Edinburgh Magazine*, Vol. 1 (Edinburgh: William Tait, 1834), 54.

44. The use of the imagery of consumption to characterize female beauty became more frequent and can be found throughout imaginative and medical literature in the late eighteenth and early nineteenth centuries. For instance, Samuel Richardson describes his heroine Clarissa in the following manner: "One faded cheek rested upon the good woman's bosom, the kindly warmth of which had overspread it with a faint, but charming flush; the other paler, and hollow, as if already iced over by death. Her hands white as the lily, with her meandering veins more transparently blue than ever I had seen even hers; (veins so soon, alas! To be choaked [sic] up by the congealment of that purple stream, which already so languidly creeps rather than flows through them!) her hands hanging lifelessly." Samuel Richardson, *Clarissa. Contained in The Novelist's Magazine. Vol. XV* (London: Harrison and Co., 1784), 1133. The classic look of consumptive beauty was also that of Lucy Asheton, "the lamp fell upon her beautiful but delicate face, from which the rose had long since departed; the blue veins were singularly distinct on the clear temples, and in the eye was that uncertain brightness which owes not its luster to health. Her pale golden hair was drawn up in a knot at the top of her small and graceful head, and the rich mass shone as we fancy shine the bright tresses of an angel." "An Evening of Lucy Asheton's," *Heath's Book of Beauty* (London: Longman, Rees, Orme, Brown, Green, and Longman, 1833), 248. Lucy's appearance—the gradual emaciation, sparkling eyes, the pronounced blue veins, and flush brought on by a low-grade fever—all mirror consumption.

45. Neville Williams, *Powder and Paint: A History of the Englishwoman's Toilet, Elizabeth I-Elizabeth II* (London: Longmans, Green and Co., 1957), 81.

46. *The Art of Beauty*, 338, 381–382.

47. *The Medical and Physical Journal*, Vol. II (London: William Thorne, 1799), 115.

48. Dubos and Dubos, *The White Plague*, 123–124.

49. *The Monthly Magazine*, Vol. XII (London: Richard Phillips, 1801), 444. These "accounts of diseases" were part of the attempts by the physicians of the Finsbury dispensary to account for morbidity in the metropolis. For more on this practice see Irvine Loudon, *Medical Care and the General Practitioner, 1750–1850* (Oxford: Clarendon Press, 1986).

50. Phillippy, *Painting Women*, 6. Aileen Ribero has argued that the fashion for white skin and red cheeks and lips dates back to antiquity, stating that "By the fourth century BCE, the application of cosmetics was a well-established part of the life of the fashionable woman ... the face was painted (with white lead powder or wheat flour), the cheeks and lips reddened (either with wine lees, red ochre or vermillion-red mercuric sulphide)." Ribeiro, *Facing Beauty*, 38. While Phillippy has stated that by the sixteenth century, European instructional manuals had established "a consensus on ideals of feminine beauty—blonde hair, black eyes, white skin, red cheeks and lips." Phillippy, *Painting Women*, 6.

51. These references to the symptoms of consumption were those that were most commonly mentioned in more than 90 separate medical treatises dating from 1674 to 1860.

52. Charlotte Brontë made specific mention of Emily's hair when discussing the day before she lost her battle with tuberculosis. "Emily sat on the hearth to comb her hair. She was thinner than ever now—the tall, loose-jointed, 'slinky'

Notes

girl—her hair in its plenteous dark abundance was all of her that was not marked by the branding finger of death." Shorter, *The Brontës*, 13.

53. "Eye miniatures were popular at the end of the 18th century as "an attempt to capture 'the window of the soul', the supposed reflection of a person's most intimate thoughts and feelings." Eye Miniature, England, early 19th century (painted), Museum number: P.57-1977. ©Victoria and Albert Museum, London. For more on eye miniatures see Hanneke Grootenboer, *Treasuring the Gaze: Intimate Vision in Late Eighteenth-Century Eye Miniatures* (Chicago: University of Chicago Press, 2012.)

54. "Criticism on Female Beauty," (From the New Monthly Magazine) *The Times*, Thursday, Aug 18, 1825.

55. A. F. Crell and W. M. Wallace, *The Family Oracle of Health; Economy, Medicine, and Good Living*, Vol. I (London: J. Walker, 1824), 176–177.

56. Aileen Ribeiro argues this was a practice with a long history, stating "The appearance of emotion could be created by dilating pupils of the eyes with atropine (from belladonna, extracted from the berries of deadly nightshade), which made the eyes seem darker and more glistening; although dangerous, it was especially popular in the sixteenth century with Italian women—thus the plants name." Ribeiro, *Facing Beauty*, 76.

57. Crell and Wallace, *The Family Oracle of Health*, 176–177.

58. *The Art of Beauty*, 294.

59. Crell and Wallace, *The Family Oracle of Health*, 437.

60. Lampblack was made when a small plate was held above a candle or lamp flame, allowing the smoke to leave a residue that was collected and applied to the eyelashes using a brush to darken their appearance. Williams, *Powder and Paint*, 102.

61. *La Belle Assemblée*, Vol. III (London: J. Bell, 1807), 205.

62. Even more disturbingly, some beauty prescriptions were also behaviors believed to actively bring about tuberculosis. "It is said that nothing tends to whiten the skin so much as walking abroad in the cool of the evening, especially near water. This may be possible; but is not the humidity of the evening productive of ill consequences, which would make those pay very dear who would purchase a fine skin at that rate, especially since it is an advantage that may be procured in so many other ways?" *La Belle Assemblée*, Vol. III, 207.

63. Edward Goodman Clarke, *The Modern Practice of Physic* (London: Longman, Hurst, Rees and Orme, 1805), 219–220.

64. *La Belle Assemblée*, Vol. III, 206.

65. Armstrong, *Practical Illustrations of the Scarlet Fever, Measles, Pulmonary Consumption and Chronic Diseases*, 255–256.

66. *The Atheneum; or Spirit of the English Magazines*, Vol. V (Boston: John Cotton, 1831), 84.

67. *The Edinburgh Magazine*, Vol. XV (Edinburgh: Archibald Constable & Company, 1824), 169.

68. "Bell on the Anatomy of Painting," *The Edinburgh Review*, No. XVI (Edinburgh: 1806), 376.

69. *The Mirror of the Graces; or the English Lady's Costume* (London: B. Crosby and Co., 1811), 43.

70. Colin Jones, "The King's Two Teeth," *History Workshop Journal*, (2008) 65 (1): 79–95, 90–91. For more on the commodification of dentistry see Roger King, *The Making of the Dentiste c.1650–1760* (Aldershot: Ashgate, 1999); A. S. Hargreaves, *White as Whalebone: Dental Services in Early Modern England* (Leeds: Northern Universities Press, 1998); Christine Hillam, *Brass Plate and Brazen Impudence: Dental Practice in the Provinces*, 1755–1855 (Liverpool: Liverpool University Press, 1991); Mark Blackwell, "Extraneous Bodies": The Contagion of Live-Tooth Transplantation in late-Eighteenth-Century England, Eighteenth-Century Life, Volume 28, Number 1 (Winter 2004) 21–68; and Colin Jones, *The Smile Revolution in 18th Century Paris* (Oxford: Oxford University Press, 2014).

71. Jones, *The Smile Revolution*, 73.

72. Andrew Duncan, *Medical Commentaries*, Part I (London: Charles Dilly, 1780), 64.

73. *A Physician's Advice For the Prevention and Cure of Consumption*, 122–123.

74. Rowland's Odonto Pearl Dentifrice claimed not only to exterminate diseases of the teeth and gums but also to render teeth "perfectly sound, arraying in pure whiteness and fixing firmly in their sockets—producing a BEAUTIFUL SET

OF PEARLY TEETH." Hudson's Tooth powder declared that it cured "gum boils, swelled face, and the tooth-ache" and was capable of removing "the scurvy from the gums." *The Court Journal*, (London: Henry Colburn, 1833), 63.

75. Jones, *The Smile Revolution*, 119.

76. *The Art of Beauty*, 149–150.

77. Max Wykes-Joyce, *Cosmetics and Adornment: Ancient and Contemporary Usage* (London: Peter Owen, 1961), 81.

78. *La Belle Assemblée*, Vol. II (London: J. Bell, 1807), 109.

79. *The Art of Beauty*, 104.

80. Williams, *Powder and Paint*, 79.

81. *The Servant's Guide and Family Manual*, 2nd edn. (London: John Limbird, 1831), 99.

82. *The Art of Beauty*, 187.

83. *The Art of Beauty*, 194.

84. Murray, *A Treatise on Pulmonary Consumption its Prevention and Remedy*, 40.

85. *A New System of Practical Domestic Economy* (London: Henry Colburn, 1827), 82.

86. Corson, *Fashions in Makeup*, 295.

87. This was an intensification of an already "entrenched notion that appearance revealed nature." Porter, *Flesh in the Age of Reason*, 247. Early Victorian culture on the whole was swayed by sentimentalism, which provided one avenue for escaping difficult social realities. Halttunen, *Confidence Men and Painted Women*, xvi. The sentimentalists increasingly sought to conceal reality through a refusal to acknowledge the harsher aspects of a situation; a repudiation of the real world which permitted the further elevation of consumption as an ideal of beauty. Lawlor and Suzuki, "The Disease of the Self," 492.

88. Halttunen, *Confidence Men and Painted Women*, 57, 71.

89. Herzlich and Pierret, *Illness and Self in Society*, 147.

90. Thomas Gisborne, *An Enquiry into the Duties of the Female Sex* (London: Printed by Luke Hansard for T. Cadell and W. Davies, 1806), 28. Gisborne, however, refused to grant that the female fortitude to endure suffering was higher than that of their male counterparts, asserting instead that, due to their slighter stature, women did not experience the same degree of suffering as a larger framed man.

91. G. to J. T., June 1814, in Rev. R. Polwhele, *Traditions and Recollections; Domestic, Clerical, and Literary*, Vol. II (London: John Nichols and Son, 1826), 662.

92. Mrs. Ellis, *The Women of England, their Social Duties, and Domestic Habits* (London: Fisher, Son & Co., 1839), 384. Mrs. Sarah Stickney Ellis, a well-known writer of evangelical conduct books, was the wife of Mr. William Ellis, the chief foreign secretary of the London Missionary Society. Mrs. Ellis was extremely interested in the promotion of temperance and what she deemed the proper education of the young ladies of England, principles she elucidated in her numerous works. She was instrumental in defining the middle-class Victorian woman within the context of marriage and promoted women as the guardians of respectability. George Smith, *The Dictionary of National Biography* (London: Oxford University Press, 1964), 714–715.

93. Mrs. Ellis, *The Women of England*, 384–385.

94. Mrs. Ellis, *The Daughters of England, Their Position in Society, Character & Responsibilities* (London: Fisher, Son, & Co., 1842), 181.

95. Mrs. Ellis, *The Daughters of England*, 233–234.

96. Charlotte Brontë to W. S. Williams, January 18, 1849, in Shorter, *The Brontës*, 21.

97. "On the Beauty of the Female Figure," *Blackwood's Lady's Magazine*, Vol. 24 (London: A. H. Blackwood and Page, 1848), 23.

98. *Leigh Hunt's London Journal*, Vol. 1 (London: Charles Knight, 1834), 137–138. "Criticism on Female Beauty" acknowledged that beauty was "a very poor thing unless beautified by sentiment;" most particularly, "affectation and pretension spoil everything." *The New Monthly Magazine and Literary Journal*, Part II (London: Henry Colburn, 1825), 72, 74.

99. Walker, *Beauty*, 4.

100. George Combe, *Lectures on Phrenology* (London: Simpkin, Marshall, & Co., 1839), 325.

101. The verse came from Wordsworth's Excursion Book I, line 503. Theophilus Thompson, *Clinical Lectures on Pulmonary Consumption* (London: John Churchill, 1854), 176–177.

102. Although the assigning of virtue and beauty to those suffering from tuberculosis was already present at the turn of the nineteenth century, these connections continued to intensify, so by the 1840s Charlotte Brontë repeatedly assigned elevated character to both Anne and Emily while they labored under tuberculosis. She stated of Emily, "I looked on her with an anguish of wonder and love. I have seen nothing like it; but, indeed, I have never seen her parallel in anything. Stronger than a man, simpler than a child, her nature stood alone." Shorter, *The Brontës*, 13. Such associations between character and consumption were also evident in the account of Eliza Herbert (1830): "A more delicate and lovely little creature than was Eliza Herbert, at this period, cannot be conceived. She was the only bud from a parent stem of remarkable beauty:—but, alas, that stem was suddenly withered by consumption! ... Little Eliza Herbert inherited, with her mother's beauty, her constitutional delicacy. Her figure was so slight, that it almost suggested to the beholder the idea of transparency; and there was a softness and languor in her azure eyes, beaming through their long silken lashes, which told of something too refined for humanity ... In short, a more sweet, lovely, and amiable being than Eliza Herbert never adorned the ranks of humanity ... and kept Sir.___in a feverish flutter of apprehension every day of his life, was, that his niece was, in his own words, 'too good- too beautiful, for this world.'" "Passages from the Diary of a Late Physician. Chapter IV. Consumption," *Blackwood's Edinburgh Magazine*, Vol. XXVIII (Edinburgh: William Blackwood; London: T. Cadell, 1830), 771. Despite being touted as "Passages from the Diary of a Late Physician" it is not possible to determine whether Eliza's trails derived from an actual case or were simply the product of the author's imagination. Despite this ambiguity, the tale provides insight into accepted contemporary depictions about the illness and Eliza's tale is just one among a multitude of writings (fictional, ostensibly true, or even factual) centered on consumption during the first half of the nineteenth century.

103. *The Englishwoman's Magazine and Christian Mother's Miscellany*, Vol. I (London: Fisher, Son & Co., 1846), 342.

104. *The Ladies Hand-book of the Toilet, a Manual of Elegance and Fashion* (London: H. G. Clarke and Co., 1843), vii.

105. An English Lady of Rank, *The Ladies Science of Etiquette* (New York: Wilson & Company, 1844), 43.

106. An English Lady of Rank, *The Ladies Science of Etiquette*, 43.

107. Gilbert, *Pulmonary Consumption*, 51.

108. Charlotte Brontë to W. S. Williams, February 1, 1849, in Shorter, *The Brontës*, 23.

109. *The Art of Beauty*, 90.

110. *The Art of Beauty*, 116.

111. *The Art of Beauty*, 124.

112. Crell and Wallace, *The Family Oracle of Health*, Vol. I, 293.

113. Alexander Walker, *Beauty: Illustrated Chiefly by an Analysis and Classification of Beauty in Women* (London: Henry G. Bohn, 1846), 232. For more on the impact of Walker's *Beauty* see Aileen Ribeiro, *Facing Beauty*, 232–233.

114. Mrs. A. Walker, *Female Beauty*, 200. Mrs. Walker is thought to be a pseudonym used by physiologist Alexander Walker. Although reflecting Alexander Walker's attitude, by presenting it in the form of a toilet manual these notions were carried to a wider audience. "Walker, Alexander (1779–1852)," Lucy Hartley in *Oxford Dictionary of National Biography*, online edn, ed. David Cannadine, Oxford: OUP, 2004, http://www.oxforddnb.com/view/article/56049 [accessed June 29, 2016].

115. Clark, *A Treatise on Pulmonary Consumption*, 13–14.

116. An English Lady of Rank, *The Ladies Science of Etiquette*, 47–48.

117. An English Lady of Rank, *The Ladies Science of Etiquette*, 47–48.

118. Esther Copley, *The Young Woman's Own Book and Female Instructor* (London: Fisher, Son, & Co., 1840), 378.

119. Corson, *Fashions in Makeup*, 319. An 1837 article in *The Magazine of the Beau Monde* complained: "Instances are not wanting, of young persons attempting to bleach their skins, and beautify themselves ... Mercury and lead manufactured in various forms, are, unhappily, ingredients too common in many of our modern cosmetics ... [and]

occasions … tubercles in the lungs … until at length consumption, either pulmonary or hectic, closes the dreadful scene." "General Observations on Cosmetics," *The Magazine of the Beau Monde,* Vol. 7 (London: I. T. Payne, 1837), 165.

120. *The Art of Dress; or, Guide to the Toilette: With Directions for Adapting the Various Parts of the Female Costume to the Complexion and Figure; Hints on Cosmetics, &c.* (London: Charles Tilt, 1839), 59. For more on these sorts of manuals, see Alieen Ribeiro, *Facing Beauty*, 219–221.

121. *Ladies' Gazette of Fashion* (London: George Berger, 1848), 45.

122. Williams, *Powder and Paint*, 56.

123. Sally Pointer, *The Artifice of Beauty: A History and Practical Guide to Perfumes and Cosmetics* (United Kingdom, 2005), 138.

124. *The London Medical Gazette,* Vol. XII (London: Longman, Rees, Orme, Brown, Green and Longman, 1833), 225.

125. *The New Monthly Belle Assemblée*, Vol. XXVI (London: 1847), 3.

Chapter 8

1. Clothes have been, and continue to be, significantly more than simply a way of covering and protecting the body; instead they are heavily invested with social, political, and moral undertones. The fashioning of the body occurs through make-up, manners, and clothing, and these can also be used to establish social identity, status, and sexuality, all of which become the tools through which the individual is self- and socially-managed. Kaja Silverman has argued that dress "makes the human body culturally visible," while Jennifer Craik has suggested, "we can regard the ways in which we clothe the body as an active process of technical means for constructing and presenting a bodily self." Amy de la Haye and Elizabeth Wilson, eds, *Defining Dress: Dress as Object, Meaning and Identity* (Manchester: Manchester University Press, 1999), 2; Jennifer Craik, *The Face of Fashion: Cultural Studies in Fashion* (London: Routledge, 1994), 46.

2. Craik, *The Face of Fashion*, 44.

3. *La Belle Assembleé,* Vol. I (London: J. Bell, 1806), 79.

4. Mrs. William Parkes, *Domestic Duties; or Instructions to Young Married Ladies* (London: Longman, Hurst, Rees, Orme, Brown and Green, 1825), 172–173.

5. There was a move toward a fluid silhouette, marked by flowing lines and a high waistline, a development often attributed to the effects of the French Revolution; however, the push for simpler lines had already begun before 1789. Ribeiro has argued, "In some respects, it [the Revolution] acted as a catalyst for styles already in the pipeline, but which were pushed to the forefront by the impact of politics." Aileen Ribeiro, *Fashion in the French Revolution* (London: Batsford, 1988), 140. This simplification received impetus from a number of sources, including the works of Jean-Jacques Rousseau and the discovery of Herculaneum and Pompeii. Already by the 1760s, Rousseau had called for a move toward the "natural," including greater informality, simplicity, and a return to "a state of nature." The fascination with the Classical also meant that women's clothing moved to outright emulation, as dresses were often copied directly from the Greek pottery and statuary. Jane Ashelford, *The Art of Dress: Clothes and Society 1500-1914.* (London: National Trust Enterprises Ltd., 1996), 173; Fukai, et al., *Fashion*, 120. For more on Rousseau and the natural body in fashion see Michael Kwass "Big Hair: A Wig History of Consumption in Eighteenth-Century France," *The American Historical Review*, Vol. 111, No. 3 (June 2006), 631–659.

6. The chemise gown, ostensibly named for its resemblance to the undergarment of the same name, was simple in construction, voluminous, with a dropped shoulder and gathered neckline that could be pulled over the head. In 1783, a portrait of Marie-Antoinette wearing this style by Elizabeth-Louise Vigée Lebrun was exhibited. This portrait, and the fashion, created a great scandal; however, the queen's patronage helped popularize the garment, and it spread rapidly across the English Channel. As Kimberly Chrisman-Campbell, has argued "For British tourists—like the Duchess of Devonshire and Mr. Crewe—who flocked to France after the signing of the Treaty of Versailles in 1783, the chemise gown was the quintessential Paris Souvenir." In August 1784, Georgiana Duchess of Devonshire went to a concert attired "in one of the muslin chemises with fine lace that the Queen of France gave me," and the

fashionable elite quickly followed her lead. [Quoted in Ashelford, *The Art of Dress*, 175.] A few months later, *The New Spectator* paid homage to the Duchess's innovation in taste: "I have sometimes been amazed, that those patronesses of taste and fashion in female dress, the Duchesses of Devonshire and Rutland, never procured his *Majesty's Royal Letters Patent*, for the exclusive privilege of wearing, appearing in, and exposing to admiration certain dresses, by them the said Duchesses first invented, formed, fashioned, and worn; for in such words, or in words similar to those, doubtless said Patent would run." *The New Spectator*, No. III (London: 1784), 4. By the latter part of the decade, the chemise dress was an integral part of feminine fashion, and in 1787 *The Lady's Magazine* acknowledged its dominance: "All the Sex now, from 15 to 50 and upwards . . . appear in their white muslin frocks with broad sashes." Quoted in Judith S. Lewis, *Sacred to Female Patriotism: Gender, Class and Politics in Late Georgian Britain* (New York: Routledge, 2003), 176. Kimberly Chrisman-Campbell has argued that "The chemise gown of the 1780s is erroneously equated with the high-waisted, short-sleeved white gowns that became popular in the 1790s and early 1800s. It may have been a precursor of this neoclassical or 'Grecian' gown . . . but it was a much different garment, both in construction and in appearance." Kimberly Chrisman-Campbell, *Fashion Victims: Dress at the Court of Louis XVI and Marie-Antoinette* (New Haven and London: Yale University Press, 2015), 172–175. Ashelford, *The Art of Dress*, 175; Fukai, et al., *Fashion*, 150.

7. Chrisman-Campbell, *Fashion Victims*, 155.

8. It turns out, however, that these contours were not as natural as advertised, relying as they did, upon the undergarment as their "unnatural" predecessors also had done. For more information on cotton textiles see: Beverly Lemire, *Fashion's Favourite: The Cotton Trade and the Consumer in Britain, 1660–1800* (Oxford: Oxford University Press, 1991); Beverly Lemire, *Cotton* (Oxford: Oxford University Press, 2011); George Riello, *Cotton: The Fabric that Made the Modern World* (Cambridge: Cambridge University Press, 2013); Sven Beckert, *Empire of Cotton: A Global History* (New York: Vintage Books, 2014); Jon Stobart and Bruno Blondé, eds, *Selling Textiles in the Long Eighteenth Century: Comparative Perspectives from Western Europe* (Basingstoke: Palgrave Macmillan, 2014); Robert S. DuPlessis, *The Material Atlantic: Clothing, Commerce, and Colonization in the Atlantic World, 1650–1800* (Cambridge: Cambridge University Press, 2016).

9. *La Belle Assemblée,* Vol. IV (London: J. Bell, 1811), 90.

10. Elaine Canter Cremers-van der Does, *The Agony of Fashion,* English Translation Leo Van Witsen (Dorset: Blandford Press, 1980), 73.

11. *La Belle Assemblée,* Vol. I (London: J. Bell, 1806), 614. Susan Sibbald mentions them in her memoirs, describing them as being woven on a stocking-loom and dubbed them "the most uncomfortable style of dress was when they were made so scanty that it was difficult to walk in them." She ran afoul of these undergarments while trying to spring over a small stream when she received "a sudden check" from her tight garments and fell with "her face in the water." Francis P. Hett, *The Memoirs of Susan Sibbald* (Paget Press, 1980), 138.

12. *La Belle Assemblée,* Vol. III (London: J. Bell, 1807), 17.

13. *The Monthly Magazine,* Vol. XXIV (London: Richard Phillips, 1807), 548.

14. Charlotte Burney to Madame d'Arblay, Saturday 23 Vendiemiaire l'an II, Eg MS 3693, Folio 84, The British Library Department of Manuscripts, London, UK.

15. This is not to suggest that there were not options for women seeking to keep warm or that all women ignored the advice of medical authors.

16. *The European Magazine and London Review* (London: J. Sewell, 1785), 23.

17. Early on, the possibility of scanty clothing leading to disease combined with a growing alarm over what was seen as the trespass of decency, in a "Letter to the Editor" of the *Monthly Magazine*, by a gentleman claiming to have just returned to England after a long absence. He expressed dismay that the clothing of the day made the fashionable fair look like members of the Cyprian class, complaining, while at the opera, of the "ladies, whose bosoms were exposed in a manner that I never saw before, except under the piazzas of Covent-Garden of an evening, or in some of the most nocturnal street-walkers. 'Surely (said I,) they are of no other description, unless they are of a higher order of demireps, and kept by men of fashion.'" *The Monthly Magazine*, Vol. XXIV (London: Richard Phillips, 1807), 548.

18. *The Times*, Wednesday, December 11, 1799 (London, 1799), 2. *The Times* is referencing Edmund Burke's indictment of the Jacobins and the French constitutional theorist Emmanuel Joseph Sieyés in his 1795 letter to the Duke of

Bedford. For more information on the letter, see Isaac Kramnick, ed., *The Portable Edmund Burke* (New York: Penguin Books, 1999), 213.

19. Sarah Harriet Burney to Mary Young, December 4, 1792, Barrett Collection, Vol. XII Eg MS 3700 A, folio 226, The British Library Department of Manuscripts, London, UK.

20. Dror Wahrman has examined "Ladies dress, as it soon will be" by James Gillray, arguing it was one of many that satirized the transparency of these fashions and their proclivity for "accentuating the natural female body form." Wahrman, *The Making of the Modern Self*, 65.

21. Beddoes, *Essay on the Causes, Early Signs, and Prevention of Pulmonary Consumption*, 131.

22. *The Fashionable World Displayed*, 2nd edn. (London: J. Hatchard, 1804), 73–74.

23. "A Naked Truth of Nipping Frost," (1803), by Charles Williams, Published by S.W. Fores. Courtesy of The Lewis Walpole Library, Yale University.

24. George Colman, The Younger, *The Gentleman*, (London: Longman, Hurst, Rees, and Orme, 1806), 47.

25. John Roberton, *A Treatise on Medical Police, and on Diet, Regimen, &c.*, Vol. I (Edinburgh: John Moir, 1809), 180–181.

26. Roberton, *A Treatise on Medical Police, and on Diet, Regimen, &c.*, 183.

27. Armstrong, *Practical Illustrations of the Scarlet Fever, Measles, Pulmonary Consumption and Chronic Diseases*, 211.

28. As one journalist acknowledged, "you cannot form your under dress too scanty to exhibit the drapery which may flow over it to advantage." In some instances, women only wore stockings and one tight petticoat. In *La Belle Assemblée*, Vol. I (London: J. Bell, 1806), 614.

29. *La Belle Assemblée*, Vol. I (London: J. Bell, 1810), 246.

30. Ashelford, *The Art of Dress*, 178–179. Fukai, et al., *Fashion*, 150. For more on cashmere shawls see David Brett, "The Management of Colour: The Kashmir Shawl in a Nineteenth-Century Debate," *Textile History*, Vol. 29 (1998); Michelle Maskiell, "Consuming Kashmir: Shawls and Empires, 1500–2000," *Journal of World History*, Vol.13 (Spring 2002); Isabella Fabretti, "Ugly and Very Expensive: The Cashmere Shawls of Empress Josephine," *Piecework*, Vol. 14, (2006); Chitralekha Zutshi, "'Designed for eternity': Kashmiri Shawls, Empire, and Cultures of Production and Consumption in Mid-Victorian Britain," *Journal of British Studies*, Vol. 48 (April 2009).

31. "Passages from the Diary of a Late Physician. Chapter IV. Consumption," *Blackwood's Edinburgh Magazine*, No. CLXXIII, Vol. XXVIII (Edinburgh: William Blackwood; London: T. Cadell, 1830), 780.

32. Armstrong, *Practical Illustrations of the Scarlet Fever, Measles, Pulmonary Consumption and Chronic Diseases*, 211.

33. Armstrong, *Practical Illustrations of the Scarlet Fever, Measles, Pulmonary Consumption and Chronic Diseases*, 213.

34. Saunders, *Treatise on Pulmonary Consumption*, 7.

35. Reid, *A Treatise on the Origin, Progress, Prevention, and Treatment of Consumption*, 203.

36. *La Belle Assemblée*, Vol. III (London: J. Bell, November 1807), 282.

37. *The Monthly Magazine*, Vol. XXIV (London: Richard Phillips, 1807), 549.

38. William Burdon and George Ensor, *Materials for Thinking*, Vol. I (London: E. Wilson, 1820), 75.

39. *La Belle Assemblée*, Vol. I, Part I (London: J. Bell, June 1806), 227.

40. *La Belle Assemblée*, Vol. I, Part I (London: J. Bell, June 1806), 227.

41. Dubos and Dubos, *The White Plague*, 54.

42. *La Belle Assemblée*, Vol. VI (London: J. Bell, 1809), 163–164.

43. Edward Ball, *The Black Robber*, Vol. I (London: A. K. Newman and Co., 1819), 81–82.

44. *La Belle Assemblée*, Vol. I (London: J. Bell, 1806), 502.

45. Reid, *A Treatise on the Origin, Progress, Prevention, and Treatment of Consumption*, 163.

46. *The Ladies Magazine* (Dec. 1818) as quoted in *Robinson's Magazine, A weekly Repository of Original Papers; and Selections from the English Magazines*, Vol. II (Baltimore. Joseph Robinson, 1819), 204–205.

Notes

47. Dorothea Sophia Mackie, *A Picture of the Changes of Fashion* (D.S. Mackie, 1818), 54.

48. *La Belle Assemblée,* Vol. XXI, (London: J. Bell, 1820), 87.

49. Felix M' Donogh, *The Hermit in London, or Sketches of English Manners* (New York: Evert Duyckinck, 1820), 214.

50. *A Physician's Advice For the Prevention and Cure of Consumption*, 123.

51. M' Donogh, *The Hermit in London*, 215–216.

52. *The Ladies Pocket Magazine of Literature & Fashion*, No. VIII (London: Joseph Robins, 1829), 23.

53. Sir Arthur Clarke, *A Practical Manual for the Preservation of Health and of the Prevention of Diseases Incidental to the Middle and Advanced Stages of Life* (London: Henry Colburn, 1824), 62.

54. Sir Arthur Clarke, *A Practical Manual for the Preservation of Health*, 62

55. *La Belle Assembleé,* Vol. VI (London: Geo. B. Whittaker, 1827), 167.

56. Thomas, *The Modern Practice of Physic*, 9th ed., 540.

57. By a Physician, *The Pocket Medical Guide* (Glasgow: W.R. M'Phun, 1834), 56–57.

58. *The Ladies Monthly Museum,* Vol. XVIII (London: Dean and Munday, 1823), 142.

59. *The Ladies Monthly Museum,* Vol. XVIII, 142–143.

60. As Crell and Wallace stated: "Out of the four or five thousand who annually die of consumption . . . in the metropolis, we may safely say that two-thirds can date their complaints, from their attending some crowded assembly. The danger then is when you are heated to perspiration in the theatre, ball-room, &c., that your feet be exposed to some cold stream of air, or become cold from damp . . . This rashness has often caused instant death, and oftener laid the foundation of a lingering and fatal illness . . . bringing on cough and decline." Crell and Wallace, *The Family Oracle of Health*, Vol. I, 258–259.

61. *The London Medical Gazette*, Vol. XII (London: Longman, Rees, Orme, Brown, Green, and Longman, 1833), 234.

62. *The London Medical Gazette*, Vol. XII, 234.

63. Reid, *A Treatise on the Origin, Progress, Prevention, and Treatment of Consumption*, 197.

64. G. Calvert Holland, *Practical Suggestions for the Prevention of Consumption* (London: W. M. S. Orr, 1750), 114. The eighteenth-century "corset" was a rigid long-waisted concoction of closely stitched together casings (intended for whalebone or cane inserts) to give stiffness and form to the garment. These stays generally laced up the rear, had high backs, shoulder straps, and a busk inserted down the front for extra support.

65. George Cheyne to Hans Sloane, Bath, July 11, 1720, Sloane MS 4034, Folio 323, The British Library Department of Manuscripts, London, UK.

66. Benjamin W. Richardson, *The Hygienic Treatment of Pulmonary Consumption* (London: John Churchill, 1757), 38.

67. Dr. John Gregory, *A Comparative View of the State and Faculties of Man with those of the Animal World* (London: J. Dodsley, 1765), 31–32.

68. For instance, William White asserted: "The binding of the body tight with ligatures, by obstructing the free circulation of the blood through the cutaneous vessels, occasions . . . haemoptoe, inflammation, &c. I would therefore forewarn the fair sex of the dangerous tendency of drawing their stays too tight. My sensibility has been much affected on observing several melancholy consequences of such a practice, where the vessels of the lungs, too tender to bear such an increased impetus of the circulation, were ruptured, and a haemoptoe produced." White, *Observations on the Nature and Method of Cure of the Phthisis Pulmonalis*, 26–27.

69. The exposed bosom and projecting shoulders could not be achieved without aid. What nature had failed to gift, artifice could provide. Presumably, a young woman with a naturally slender figure may have been liberated from her stays for a short time at the beginning of the century, while an older, stouter individual would have continued to rely on a corset as part of her effort to accommodate to neoclassical fashions. Norah Waugh, *Corsets and Crinolines* (New York: Routledge/Theatre Arts Books, 2004), 75; Elizabeth Ewing, *Dress and Undress: A History of Women's Underwear* (London: Batsford Ltd., 1978), 57.

70. Ewing, *Dress and Undress*, 57. For an example of trade cards, see: John Arpthorp. Stay & Corsett Maker (c. 1802) and H. Rudduforth, Long Stay Corset & Vest Manufacturer, *JJ Trade Cards 26 (68),* From the John Johnson Collection, ©Bodleian Library 2001. For Caricatures, see James Gillray, "Progress of the Toilet—The Stays" (1810).

71. Waugh, *Corsets and Crinolines*, 75.

72. The corset was cut to fit the body and could be "properly shifted or padded in those parts required for persons to whom nature has not been favorable." Martha Gibbon, Stays for Women and Children, patent number 2457, December 17, 1800. The National Archives, London, UK.

73. Reid, *A Treatise on the Origin, Progress, Prevention, and Treatment of Consumption*, 198–199.

74. Roberton, *A Treatise on Medical Police, and on Diet, Regimen, &c.*, 182–183.

75. Despite the vehemence of the protests, the return of the corset was not as dramatic an occurrence in England as in France, in part because it had never completely disappeared in Britain. David Kunzle, *Fashion and Fetishism: Corsets, Tight-lacing, & Other Forms of Body Sculpture* (United Kingdom: Sutton Publishing, 2004), 80, 82; Waugh, *Corsets and Crinolines*, 75.

76. *La Belle Assemblée,* Vol. II (London: J. Bell, 1811), 213.

77. A Lady of Distinction, *The Mirror of the Graces*, 36.

78. *La Belle Assemblée,* Vol. II (London: J. Bell, 1811), 90–91.

79. Natural waistlines returned in the mid-1820s and Fukai states that "corsets once again became necessary for women's fashions since smaller waists were recognized as an important feature of the new style." Fukai, et al., *Fashion*, 151–152.

80. Phyllis G. Tortora and Keith Eubank, *Survey of Historic Costume: A History of Western Dress*, 3rd edn. (New York: Fairchild Publications, 2004), 278.

81. Ashelford, *The Art of Dress*, 189.

82. Douglas A. Russell, *Costume History and Style* (New Jersey: Prentice-Hall, Inc., 1983), 340.

83. Aileen Ribeiro, *Facing Beauty*, 230.

84. T. Bell, *Kalogynomia, or the Laws of Female Beauty* (London: J. J. Stockdale, 1821), 315–316.

85. Fukai, et al., *Fashion*, 151.

86. The neckline grew during the 1820s and became a broad oval shape. Over the next ten years the shoulder seam dropped, further amplifying the bosom by exposing more of the décolletage and highlighting the long, swanlike neck, a feature increasingly admired in a woman. Even more attention was drawn to the neckline by the tight-fitting bodice below. Francois Boucher, *A History of Costume in the West* (London: Thames and Hudson Ltd., 1987), 366.

87. By 1827, the gigot sleeve had achieved such grand proportions it often required the addition of some form of support provided by whalebone, buckram, horsehair, or even down stuffing to maintain shape. The dimensions of these sleeves reached their pinnacle around 1835.

88. Fukai, et al., *Fashion*, 151.

89. "Bishop Sleeves," *The New Monthly Magazine and Literary Journal*, Part II (London: Henry Colburn and Richard Bentley, 1829), 214.

90. This busk became a major source of concern as one author remarked, "It is not enough that the stays are laced so tight as scarcely to leave room for the women to breathe, but the mischief which such pressure would occasion is greatly increased, by a stiff piece of whalebone, or steel, introduced in front." *The Ladies Pocket Magazine of Literature & Fashion*, No. VIII (London: Joseph Robins, 1829), 27.

91. Waugh, *Corsets and Crinolines*, 75, 79. As the waist lengthened, the number of inserts also increased, and beginning around 1835, the hips were further enhanced by a "basque"-shaped construction.

92. Sarah Levitt, *Victorians Unbuttoned: Registered Designs for Clothing, Their Makers and Wearers, 1839-1900* (London: George Allen and Unwin, 1986), 26.

93. There was a practical innovation in corsetry that concurred in 1823 when Rogers of London took out a patent on corset lacings; however, the style of eyelet that would eventually come into common use in 1828 was invented by Daude of Paris. The Romantic style of corset typically laced in the rear, and shoulder straps continued as a prominent feature until the 1840s. The eyelet and other technical inventions, including the split busk patented in 1829, aided in the achievement of the feminine silhouette. This improvement allowed for the development of a front-fastening corset, although the item did not come into common usage until the middle part of the century. Ewing, *Dress and Undress*, 58.

94. *The Ball; Or, A Glance at Almack's in 1829* (London: Henry Colburn, 1829), 31.

95. Articles on the subject were published in every conceivable venue, from medical journals to fashion periodicals, and they were even distributed in the standalone form of pamphlets. The subject was also discussed in the various books devoted to beauty, dress, health, and hygiene and was even mentioned in household encyclopedias, dictionaries, and the growing genre of general periodicals devoted to "useful and entertaining knowledge" whose audience was taken to be "the educatable woman." Kunzle, *Fashion and Fetishism*, 90.

96. The number of women reported to have died in the annual reports of 1838. *Fraser's Magazine for Town and Country*, Vol. XXV (London: G. W. Nickisson, 1842), 191.

97. Ewing, *Dress and Undress*, 60–61.

98. A great number of these anatomical illustrations, like the one published in *The Penny Magazine of The Society for the Diffusion of Useful Knowledge* (1833), were either direct copies or based upon the work of the German anatomist and physician Samuel Thomas von Sömmerring whose 1788 work on the *Effects of Stays* remained incredibly influential, despite the alterations in the shape of the corset since that date.

99. *The Art of Beauty*, 26.

100. *La Belle Assembleé*, Vol. VI (London: Geo. B. Whittaker, 1827), 308.

101. *A Physician's Advice For the Prevention and Cure of Consumption*, 127.

102. *The Art of Beauty*, 27.

103. *The Art of Beauty*, 28.

104. There were a number of works dedicated to correcting deformities of the spine and those of the trunk of the body, many of which put forth the corset as the originator of these defects.

105. Charles Pears, *Cases of Phthisis Pulmonalis, Successfully Treated Upon the Tonic Plan* (London: Crowder, 1801), 11–12.

106. John Mills, "Elastic Stays for Women and Children," Patented March 14, 1815, The National Archives, London, UK.

107. *The Art of Beauty*, 29–30.

108. *The World of Fashion*, Vol. VIII (London: Mr. Bell, 1831), 59.

109. *The Kaleidoscope; or Literary and Scientific Mirror*, Vol. 9 (Liverpool: E. Smith & Co., 1829), 425.

110. Ramadge, *Consumption Curables*, 21.

111. Halttunen, *Confidence Men and Painted Women*, 65.

112. The 1830s, then, were transitional, as fashion moved from the ebullient Romantic style to a drooping sentimentalism that denoted the emerging silhouette.

113. James Laver, *Costume and Fashion: A Concise History* (London: Thames & Hudson World of Art, 2002), 168.

114. Fukai, et al., *Fashion*, 209.

115. As *Female Beauty* observed, "the beauty of the waist, whether high, intermediate, or low, depends in great measure on the form of the corsets or stays." Mrs. A. Walker, *Female Beauty*, 310.

116. *The Magazine of the Beau Monde*, No 68, Vol. 6 (London: I. T. Payne, 1836), 109.

117. Ewing, *Fashion in Underwear*, 54.

118. The rear-lacing corset remained the common style, and shoulder straps continued as a central feature until the 1840s. Gussets were another important feature of the corset, introduced in the 1830s to help fit the garment to the bust and hips. In France in the 1840s there was another new development in corset making—the creation of a new style. This new corset design excluded gussets and was assembled from between 7 to 13 different pieces, each of which was cut to shape to the waist. This style was lightweight, and remarkably short and though it was exceedingly popular on the Continent it was less so in England. The busk also continued as a corset feature in the center front until the split busk gradually became fashionable, and provided an easier method of getting into and out of the corset. The first split busk, one fastened by catches, was patented in 1829, however the device would not catch on until the middle part of the nineteenth century. The use of this split style of busk and the development of front-fastening corsets occurred as the garment as a whole became stiffer; all of these innovations aided in the laces being drawn tighter and tighter. Kunzle, *Fashion and Fetishism*, 25.

119. Kunzle, *Fashion and Fetishism*, 90.

120. Esther Copley, *The Young Woman's Own Book and Female Instructor* (London: Fisher, Son, & Co., 1840), 371.

121. Francis Cook, *A Practical Treatise on Pulmonary Consumption* (London: John Churchill, 1842), 45.

122. Cook, *A Practical Treatise on Pulmonary Consumption*, 55.

123. *The Art of Dress*, 39.

124. *Blackwood's Lady's Magazine*, Vol. 24 (London: A. H. Blackwood and Page, 1848), 23.

125. *The World of Fashion and Continental Feuilletons*, Vol. XXV, No. 292 (London, 1848), 79.

126. By a Lady, *The Young Lady's Friend; A Manual of Practical Advice and Instruction to Young Females On their Entering upon the Duties of Life, After Quitting School* (London: John W. Parker, 1837), 77.

127. During the height of the Romantic period, ribbons, lace or ruffles often adorned the sleeves and necklines of women's dresses, in an effort to amplify the shoulder line; skirts suffered similar decoration, with the addition of appliqué, ruffles, pleats, tucks and even loops made either from silk or fur. According to many sentimentalists, the Romantic period was one of excessive detail and ornamentation, and that ornament and artifice were associated with a deficiency of character. Thus, one author remarked, "That the gay votaries of a vain world should love to deck themselves with superfluous ornament is but in keeping with their character—though even here I often wonder at the evidence afforded of weak mindedness in those who delight to revel in the variegations of fashion, and the useless encumberment of decoration." *The Christian Lady's Magazine*, Vol. VI (London: R. B. Seeley and W. Burnside, 1836), 314. The heavy detailing that characterized Romantic clothing hid, rather than revealed, the "true" temperament and disposition of the woman, while sentimentalists believed the new style, in contrast, emphasized a sincere simplicity in dress which translated into the revelation of a woman's essence.

128. Janet Dunbar, *The Early Victorian Woman: Some Aspects of Her Life, 1837–57* (London: George G. Harrap & Co. Ltd., 1953), 20.

129. Alfred Beaumont Maddock, *Practical Observations on the Efficacy of Medicated Inhalations in the Treatment of Pulmonary Consumption, Asthma, Bronchitis, Chronic Cough and Other Diseases of the Respiratory Organs and in Affections of the Heart*, 2nd edn. (London: Simpkin, Marshall, & Co., 1845), 33.

130. "Narrow shoulders and broad hips are esteemed beauties in the female figure, while in the male figure the broad shoulders and narrow hips are most admired." In Mrs. Merrifield, *Dress as a Fine Art* (London: Arthur Hall, Virtue, & Co., 1854), 30.

131. Aileen Ribeiro has argued that the "quietened down" dress of the 1840s restricted movement and as such complimented the feminine social role "that a woman should not appear to be capable of any physical effort." Aileen Ribeiro, *Dress and Morality* (Oxford: Berg, 1986), 126.

132. *Blackwood's Lady's Magazine*, Vol. 24, 25.

133. Christopher Breward, *The Culture of Fashion* (Manchester: Manchester University Press, 1995), 149.

134. Russell, *Costume History and Style*, 343; Laver, *Costume and Fashion*, 173.

135. The tight bodices, over even more-tightly laced stays, provided further indicators that physical activity in women was discouraged, though Fukai, et al. argue this "was viewed less as a restrictive element than an indicator of influence." Fukai, et al., *Fashion*, 152.

136. Russell, *Costume History and Style*, 343; Laver, *Costume and Fashion*, 173.

137. Mrs. John Sandford, *Woman, In her Social and Domestic Character* (London: Longman, Rees, Orme, Brown, and Green, 1831), 5.

138. Russell, *Costume History and Style*, 334.

139. The 1830s, then, were transitional, as fashion moved from the ebullient Romantic style to a drooping sentimentalism that denoted the emerging silhouette.

140. Norah Waugh, *The Cut of Women's Clothes, 1600–1930* (London: Faber and Faber Ltd., 1968), 140.

141. Hall, *Commentaries Principally on Those Diseases of Females Which are Constitutional*, 142.

142. Hall, *Commentaries Principally on Those Diseases of Females Which are Constitutional*, 146.

Notes

143. Hall, *Commentaries Principally on Those Diseases of Females Which are Constitutional*, 147.

144. *A Physician's Advice For the Prevention and Cure of Consumption*, 127.

145. Deshon, *Cold and Consumption*, 72.

146. Deshon, *Cold and Consumption*, 72.

147. John Tricker Conquest, *Letters to a Mother on the Management of Herself & Her Children in Health & Disease* (London: Longman and Co., 1848), 231–232.

Epilogue

1. Steele, *Fashion and Eroticism: Ideals of Feminine Beauty from the Victorian Era to the Jazz Age* (Oxford: Oxford University Press, 1985), 57.

2. This move away from both sentimental clothing and mentality was illustrated, in part, by yet another shift in the shape and appearance of head and face, there was a drift from the elongated oval to an appearance of a rounded sphere. The pensive expression characteristic of the sentimental face and demeanor gradually fell out of favor and the face acquired an increasingly animated appearance.

3. Steele, *Fashion and Eroticism*, 91–92.

4. By the early part of the nineteenth century, different disciplines concerned with societal improvement—ranging from the religious, medical, and philosophical to political economy as well as Utilitarianism—all proffered solutions to the problems of population growth, poverty, and observed threats to health. During the nineteenth century, there was a steady extension of governmental authority into new areas. The unending complications brought about by overcrowding gave rise to a number of reform efforts and increased involvement by the government in the domestic lives of a growing number of people. Social policy mimicked larger political and economic trends, as there was an inexorable drift away from laissez-faire attitudes toward increased governmental intervention. The population of the cities had rapidly expanded beyond the coping abilities of existing institutions and structures in all sorts of ways including poor relief, sewer and drainage systems, and housing for the urban working classes. The corresponding social and economic problems created by industrialization prompted a number of responses, and the public intercession into the lives of individuals on the basis of improving, preserving, or managing health was often contentious, leading to debates over individual rights versus public protection. Roy Porter, *The Greatest Benefit to Mankind*, 408–409, 420–421.

5. Alexandre Dumas, The Younger, *The Lady with the Camelias* (London: George Vickers, 1856) and Wilkie Collins, *The Law and the Lady*, edited by David Skelton (London: Penguin Books, 1998), 386.

6. For example, in 1852 *La Dame aux Camélias* was reviewed in both *The Westminster Review* and *Bentley's Miscellany*. Later in the 1850s the work was invading and influencing other aspects of English literary life, for instance in 1858 it was mentioned in other novels, like the *A Lover's Quarrel: or, The Country Ball* and was used as part of *Punch's* social commentary on *The English Churchman*.

7. *Blackwood's Edinburgh Magazine*, Vol. LXXII (London: 1852), 728.

8. Quoted in H. D. Chalke, "The Impact of Tuberculosis on History, Literature and Art," *Medical History* VI (1962), 308.

9. For more on the life of Duplessis, see: Virginia Rounding, *Grandes Horizontales: The Lives and Legends of Four Nineteenth-Century Courtesans* (London: Bloomsbury, 2003.) and Julie Kavanagh, *The Girl Who Loved Camellias: The Life and Legend of Marie Duplessis* (New York: Vintage Books, 2013).

10. John Forester, *The Life of Charles Dickens, in Two Volumes*. Vol. I, 1812–1847 (London: Chapman & Hall, 1899), 522.

11. P. Toussaint, *Maries Dupléssis: la vrai Dame aux Camélias* (Paris, 1958), Quoted in Dormandy, *The White Death*, 62.

12. Porter, ed. *The Cambridge Illustrated History of Medicine*, 107.

13. Porter, ed. *The Cambridge Illustrated History of Medicine*, 107.

14. There was still a palpable rejection of the contagion theory for tuberculosis in England, although the notion was gaining purchase on the continent. This adherence to heredity and miasmata had much to do with the dominance of the sanitary approach to the illness among social reformers and the strength of the life insurance industry in England.

Acceptance of contagion would have led to large payouts of life annuities, additionally, in England many of the top physicians at hospitals for consumption were also on the payroll of the insurance companies. This institutional integration contributed to the longevity of the notion that consumption ran in families. Even after Koch's discovery of the tubercle bacillus there was a continued place for hereditary predisposition in English life tables.

15. Porter, ed. *The Cambridge Illustrated History of Medicine*, 171.

16. Patricia A. Cunningham, *Reforming Women's Fashion, 1850–1920* (Kent, Ohio: The Kent State University Press, 2003), 5.

17. Cunningham, *Reforming Women's Fashion*, 10–11.

18. Susan Sontag argues that during the second half of the nineteenth century there was a reaction against "the Romantic cult of disease." Sontag, *Illness as Metaphor*, 34.

19. A China-aster is a flower with a daisy-like appearance. Thomas Chandler Haliburton, *Nature and Human Nature* (London: Hurst and Blackett, 1859), 196.

20. Ewing, *Dress and Undress*, 74–75.

21. Cremers-van der Does, *The Agony of Fashion*, 90.

22. *The Family Herald; Domestic Magazine of Useful Information and Amusement*, Vol. IX (London: George Biggs, 1851), 317.

23. Steam-molding involved taking the garment, once stitched and boned, and starching it heavily then shaping it with steam over a mold constructed in the preferred silhouette. In Ewing, *Dress and Undress*, 76.

24. Cunningham, *Reforming Women's Fashion,* 6.

25. Ewing, *Dress and Undress*, 64–65.

26. Madame Roxy A. Caplin, *Health and Beauty; or Corsets and Clothing, Constructed in Accordance with the Physiological Laws of the Human Body* (London: Darton and Co., 1856), xi.

27. Caplin, *Health and Beauty*, ix–x.

28. Georgina D. Feldberg, *Disease and Class*, 7.

SELECT BIBLIOGRAPHY

Primary sources

Adair, James Mattkrick. *Essays on Fashionable Diseases*. London: T. P. Bateman, 1790.

Addison, William. *Healthy and Diseased Structure and the True Principles of Treatment for the Cure of Disease, Especially Consumption and Scrofula*. London: John Churchill, 1849.

A Lady of Distinction. *The Mirror of the Graces; Or the English Lady's Costume*. London: B. Crosby, 1811.

A Lady of Rank. *The Book of Costume or Annals of Fashion From the Earliest Period to the Present Time*. London: Henry Colburn, 1846.

Aldis, C. J. B. *An Introduction to Hospital Practice, In Various Complaints*. London: Longman, Rees, Orme, Brown, Green, and Longman, 1835.

An English Lady of Rank. *The Ladies Science of Etiquette*. New York: Wilson & Company, 1844.

Ancell, Henry. *A Treatise on Tuberculosis, the Constitutional Origin of Consumption and Scrofula*. London: Longman, Brown, Green, and Longmans, 1852.

Andrew, Thomas. *A Cyclopedia of Domestic Medicine and Surgery*. Glasgow: Blackie and Son, 1842.

Armstrong, John. *Practical Illustrations of the Scarlet Fever, Measles, Pulmonary Consumption and Chronic Diseases*. London: Baldwin, Cradock, and Joy, 1818.

The Art of Beautifying the Face & Figure, Comprising Instructions, Hints, & Advice, Together with Numerous New and Infallible Recipes in Connexion with the Skin, Complexion, Hair, Teeth, Eyes, Eyebrows, Eyelashes, Lips, Ears, Hands, Feet, Figure, &c. London: G. Vickers, Angel Court, Strand, 18—.

The Art of Beauty; or the Best Methods of Improving and Preserving the Shape, Carriage, and Complexion. London: Knight and Lacey, 1825.

The Art of Dress; or, Guide to the Toilette: With Directions for Adapting the Various Parts of the Female Costume to the Complexion and Figure; Hints on Cosmetics, &c. London: Charles Tilt, 1839.

Barlow, J. *The Connection Between Physiology and Intellectual Philosophy*. Second Edition. London: William Pickering, 1846.

Baron, John. *An Enquiry Illustrating the Nature of Tuberculated Accretions of Serous Membranes; and of the Origin of Tubercles and Tumors in Different Textures of the Body*. London: Longman, Hurst, Rees, Orme, and Brown, 1819.

Baron, John. *Illustrations of the Enquiry Respecting Tuberculous Diseases*. London: T. and G. Underwood, 1822.

Barrow, William. *Researches on Pulmonary Phthisis, from the French of G.L. Bayle*. Liverpool: Printed by G. F. Harris's Widow and Brothers; for Longman, Hurst, Rees, Orme, and Brown, London, 1815.

Bartlett, Thomas. *Consumption: Its Causes, Prevention, and Cure*. London: Hippolyte Bailliere, 1855.

Beddoes, Thomas. *Essay on the Causes, Early Signs, and Prevention of Pulmonary Consumption for the Use of Parent and Preceptors*. Bristol: Biggs & Cottle, 1799.

Bell, T. *Kalogynomia, or the Laws of Female Beauty: Being the Elementary Principles of That Science*. London: J. J. Stockdale, 1821.

Bennet, Christopher. *Theatrum tabidorum: or the Nature and Cure of Consumptions Whether a Phthisis, and Atrophy or an Hectic with Preliminary Exercitations*. London: W. and J. Innys, 1720.

Bernard, Franz. *The Physical Education of Young Ladies*. London: Simpkin, Marshall and Co., 18—.

Black, William. *A Comparative View of the Mortality of the Human Species, At All Ages*. London: C. Dilly, 1788.

Blackmore, Sir Richard. *A Treatise of Consumptions and other Distempers Belonging to the Breast and Lungs*. Second Edition. London: John Pemberton, 1725.

Blanc, Charles. *The Art of Ornament and Dress*. London: Frederick Warne and Co., 18—.

Bodington, George. *An Essay on the Treatment and Cure of Pulmonary Consumption*. London: Longman, Orme, Brown, Green, and Longmans, 1840.

Buchan, William. *Domestic Medicine: or a Treatise on the Prevention and Cure of Diseases by a Regimen of Simple Medicines*. Sixteenth Edition. London: A. Strahan & T. Cadell, 1798.

Burdon, William and George Ensor, *Materials for Thinking*, Vol. I. London: E. Wilson, 1820.

Burke, Edmund. *A Philosophical Enquiry into the Origin of our Ideas of the Sublime and Beautiful*. Edited by James T. Boulton. Notre Dame: University of Notre Dame Press, 1968.

Buxton, Isaac. *An Essay On the Use of a Regulated Temperature in Winter-Cough & Consumption*. London: Cox, 1810.

By A Lady. *The Young Lady's Friend; A Manual of Practical Advice and Instruction to Young Females On their Entering upon the Duties of Life, After Quitting School*. London: John W. Parker, 1837.

By a Physician. *Sure Methods of Improving Health and Prolonging Life*. Third Edition. London: Simpkin and Marshall, 1828.

By a Physician. *The Manual for Invalids*. Second Edition. London: Edward Bull, 1829.

By a Physician. *The Pocket Medical Guide*. Glasgow: W.R. M'Phun, 1834.

Byfield, Robert. *Sectum: Being the Universal Directory in the Art of Cutting; Containing Unerring Principles Upon Which Every Garment May Be Made to Fit the Human Shape With Ease and Elegance*. London: printed for H.S. Mason, 1825.

Campbell, J. S. *Observations on Tuberculous Consumption*. London: H. Bailliere, 1841.

Caplin, Madame Roxy A. *Health and Beauty; or Corsets and Clothing, Constructed in Accordance with the Physiological Laws of the Human Body*. London: Darton and Co., 1856.

Carr, Daniel. *Observations on Consumption of the Lungs*. London: Longman, and Co., 1844.

Carswell, Robert. *Pathological Anatomy. Illustrations of the Elementary Forms of Disease*. London: Longman, Orme, Brown, Green, and Longman, 1838.

Charles, Richard D. *An Essay on the Treatment of Consumptions*. London: G. Hersfield, 1787.

Cheyne, George & Roy Porter (ed.). *George Cheyne: The English Malady (1733)*. London: Routledge, 1991.

Childs, G. B. *On The Improvement and Preservation of the Female Figure*. London: Harvey and Darton, 1840.

Clarke, Sir Arthur. *A Practical Manual for the Preservation of Health and of the Prevention of Diseases Incidental to the Middle and Advanced Stages of Life*. London: Henry Colburn, 1824.

Clarke, Edward Goodman. *The Modern Practice of Physic*. London: Longman, Hurst, Rees and Orme, 1805.

Clark, James. *A Treatise on Pulmonary Consumption Comprehending an Inquiry into the Causes Nature Prevention and Treatment of Tuberculous and Scrofulous Diseases in General*. London: Sherwood Gilbert and Piper, 1835.

Combe, Andrew. *The Principles of Physiology Applied to the Preservation of Health, and to the Improvement of Physical and Mental Education*. Edinburgh: Adam & Charles Black, 1834.

Combe, George. *The Constitution of Man Considered in Relation to External Objects*. Fourth Edition. Edinburgh: William and Robert Chambers, 1836.

Combe, George. *Lectures on Phrenology*. London: Simpkin, Marshall, & Co., 1839.

Congreve, Henry. *Consumption Curable*. Sixth Edition. London: John Nichols, 1837.

Conquest, John Tricker. *Letters to a Mother, On the Management of Herself and Her Children in Health and Disease*. London: Longman and Co., 1848.

Cook, Francis. *A Practical Treatise on Pulmonary Consumption, its Pathology, Diagnosis, and Treatment*. London: John Churchill, 1842.

Copley, Esther. *The Young Woman's Own Book and Female Instructor*. London: Fisher, Son, & Co., 1840.

Cotton, Richard Payne. *The Nature, Symptoms, and Treatment of Consumption*. London: John Churchill, 1852.

Crell, A. F. and W. M. Wallace. *The Family Oracle of Health; Economy, Medicine, and Good Living*. Vol. I. London: J. Walker, 1824.

Crichton, Sir Alexander. *Practical Observations on the Treatment and Cure of Several Varieties of Pulmonary Consumption*. London: Lloyd and Son, 1823.

Cullen, William. *First Lines of the Practice of Physic*. Vol. II. Edinburgh: Bell & Bradfute, 1808.

Curtis, John Harrison. *Simplicity of Living: Observations on the Preservation of Health, in Infancy, Youth, Manhood and Age*. Third Edition. London: Henry Renshaw, 1839.

Deshon, Henry C. *Cold and Consumption or Consumption, its Prevention and Cure*. London: Henry Renshaw, 1847.

East, Rowland. *The Two Dangerous Diseases of England, Consumption and Apoplexy*. London: John Lee, 1842.

Mrs. Ellis. *The Women of England, their Social Duties, and Domestic Habits*. London: Fisher, Son & Co., 1839.

Mrs. Ellis, *The Daughters of England, Their Position in Society, Character & Responsibilities*. London: Fisher, Son, & Co., 1842.

Mrs. Ellis. *The Mothers of England: Their Influence and Responsibility*. London: Fisher, Son & Co., 1843.

Mrs. Ellis. *The Young Ladies' Reader; or Extracts From Modern Authors, Adapted for Educational or Family Use*. London: Grant and Griffith, 1845.

Mrs. Ellis. *Temper and Temperament; or, Varieties of Character*. Vol. I. London: Fisher, Son & Co., 1846.

Mrs. Ellis. *Prevention Better Than Cure; Or the Moral Wants of the World We Live In.* London: Fisher, Son, & Co., 1847.

Mrs. Ellis. *The Education of Character: With Hints on Moral Training.* London: John Murray, 1856.

The English Gentlewoman; or Hints to Young Ladies on Their Entrance into Society. London: Henry Colburn, 1845.

Epps, John. *Consumption: (Phthisis) its Nature and Treatment.* London: Sanderson, 1859.

Etiquette for Ladies; With Hints on the Preservation, Improvement and Display of Female Beauty. Philadelphia: Lea & Blanchard, 1839.

Evans, John T. *Lectures on Pulmonary Phthisis.* London: Longman, Brown and Co., 1844.

The Fashionable World Displayed. Second Edition. London: J. Hatchard, 1804.

The Female Instructor; or the Young Woman's Companion. Liverpool: Nuttall, Fisher, and Dixon, 1815.

Ferguson, John C. *Consumption: What it is, and What it is not.* Belfast: Henry Greer, 1856.

Furnivall, J. J. *On the Successful Treatment of Consumptive Disorders, and Female Complaints Connected Therewith.* London: Whittaker & Co., 1835.

Gardner, John. *Consumption. An Account of Some Discoveries Relative to Consumption.* London: Simpkin, Marshall & Co., 1850.

Gilbert, Henry. *Pulmonary Consumption: Its Prevention & Cure Established on the New Views of the Pathology of the Disease.* London: Henry Renshaw, 1842.

Gisborne, Thomas. *An Enquiry into the Duties of the Female Sex.* London: T. Cadell and W. Davies, 1806.

Graham, Thomas, J. *On the Diseases Peculiar to Females.* London: Simpkin & Marshall, 1834.

Graham, Thomas J. *Modern Domestic Medicine: A Popular Treatise.* Third Edition. London: Simpkin & Marshall, 1827 & Sixth Edition. London: Simpkin & Marshall, 1835.

Gregory, Dr. John, *A Comparative View of the State and Faculties of Man with those of the Animal World.* London: J. Dodsley, 1765.

The Guide of Service; The Lady's Maid, London: Charles Knight and Co., 1838.

Hall, Marshall. *Commentaries Principally on Those Diseases of Females Which are Constitutional.* Second Edition. London: Sherwood, Gilbert, and Piper, 1830.

Hamilton, Alexander. *A Treatise on the Management of Female Complaints.* Eighth Edition. Edinburgh: Peter Hill & Company, 1821.

Harvey, Gideon. *Morbus Anglicus: Or the Anatomy of Consumptions.* Second Edition. London: Nathanael Brook, 1674.

Hasse, Charles Ewald. *An Anatomical Description of the Diseases of the Organs of Circulation and Respiration.* London: C. and J. Adlard, 1746.

Hastings, John. *Pulmonary Consumption, Successfully Treated with Naphtha.* London: John Churchill, 1843.

Hare, Samuel. *Practical Observations on the Causes and Treatment of Curvatures of the Spine.* London: Simpkin, Marshall, & Co., 1838.

Hayes, Thomas. *A Serious Address on the Dangerous Consequences of Neglecting Common Coughs and Colds.* Second Edition. London: John Murray and Messrs. Shepperson and Reynolds, 1785.

Health Made Easy for Young People; or, Physical Training to Make their Lives, In This World, Long and Happy. London: Darton & Clark, 1845.

Holland, G. Calvert. *The Nature and Cure of Consumption, Indigestion, Scrofula and Nervous Afflictions.* London: W. M. S. Orr & Co., 1750.

Holland, G. Calvert. *Practical Suggestions for the Prevention of Consumption.* London: W. M. S. Orr, 1750.

Holmes, John Pocock. *A Treatise on the Employment of Certain Methods of Friction and Inhalation in Consumption, Asthama, and Other Maladies.* London: Samuel Holdsworth, 1837.

Howell, Mrs. M. J. *The Hand-Book of Dress-Making.* London: Simpkin, Marshall, & Co., 1845.

Hull, Robert. *A Few Suggestions on Consumption.* London: Churchill, 1849.

Johnson, James. *A Practical Treatise on Derangements of the Liver, Digestive Organs, and Nervous System.* Second Edition. London: T. and G. Underwood, 1818.

Kilgour, Alexander. *Lectures on the Ordinary Agents of Life, as Applicable to Therapeutics and Hygiene.* Edinburgh: Adam & Charles Black, 1834.

Mrs. King. *The Toilet; or, A Dress Suitable for Every Station, Age and Season.* London: Whittaker & Co., 1838.

Kittoe, W. Hamilton. *Consumption and Asthama.* Second Edition. London: Sherwood, Gilbert & Piper, 1845.

Knapp, Oswald G. *An Artist's Love Story: Told in the Letters of Sir Thomas Lawrence, Mrs. Siddons, and Her Daughters.* London: George Allen, 1904.

Knapp, Oswald G. ed. *The Intimate Letters of Hester Piozzi and Penelope Pennington 1788–1821.* London: John Lane, 1914.

Layard, George Somes. *Sir Thomas Lawrence's Letter-Bag*. London: George Allen, 1906.

The Ladies Hand-Book of Haberdashery and Hosiery. London: H. G. Clarke and Co., 1844.

The Ladies Hand-book of the Toilet, a Manual of Elegance and Fashion. London: H.G. Clarke and Co., 1843.

Leake, John. *Medical Instructions Towards the Prevention and Cure of Chronic Diseases Peculiar to Women*. 6th Edition. London: Baldwin, 1787.

Mackie, Dorothea Sophia. *A Picture of the Changes of Fashion*. D. S. Mackie, 1818.

Madden, William Herries. *Thoughts on Pulmonary Consumption*. London: John Churchill, 1849.

Maddock, Alfred Beaumont. *Practical Observations on the Efficacy of Medicated Inhalations in the Treatment of Pulmonary Consumption, Asthma, Bronchitis, Chronic Cough and Other Diseases of the Respiratory organs and in Affections of the Heart*. Second Edition. London: Simpkin, Marshall, & Co., 1845.

Mansford, John G. *An Inquiry into the Influence of Situation on Pulmonary Consumption*. London: Longman, Hurst, Rees, Orme and Brown, 1818.

May, William. *Essay on Pulmonary Consumptions*. Plymouth: B. Hayden, 1792.

M'Cormac, Henry. *On the Nature, Treatment and Prevention of Pulmonary Consumption, and Incidentally of Scrofula*. London: Longman, Brown, Green, and Longmans, and J. Churchill, 1855.

M'Donogh, Felix. *The Hermit in London, or Sketches of English Manners*. New York: Evert Duyckinck, 1820.

Mrs. Merrifield. *Dress as a Fine Art*. London: Arthur Hall, Virtue, & Co., 1854.

Morton, Richard. *Phthisiologia: or a Treatise of Consumptions Wherein the Difference, Nature, Causes, Signs and Cure of All Sorts of Consumptions are Explained*. London: Sam. Smith and Benj. Walford, 1694.

Murray, John. *A Treatise on Pulmonary Consumption; Its Prevention and Remedy*. London: Whittaker, Treacher, and Arnot, 1830.

Napier, Elizabeth. *The Nursery Governess*. London: T. and W. Boone, 1834.

A New System of Practical Domestic Economy. London: Henry Colburn, 1827.

Pears, Charles. *Cases of Phthisis Pulmonalis Successfully Treated, Successfully Treated Upon the Tonic Plan*. London: T. Crowder, 1801.

A Physician's Advice For the Prevention and Cure of Consumption with the Necessary Prescriptions. London: James Smith, 1824.

Physiology for Young Ladies, In Short and Easy Conversations. London: S. Highley, 1843.

The Polite Lady; Or a Course of Female Education. Third Edition. London: T. Carnan, and F. Newberry, junior, 1775.

Payne, Edwin. *The Preservation of General Health with Some Remarks Upon Healthy Skin*. London: Houlston and Wright, 1862.

Ramadge, Francis Hopkins. *Consumption Curables*. London: Longman, Rees, Orme, Browne, Green, and Longman, 1834.

Reece, Richard. *The Medical Guide, For the Use of The Clergy, Heads of Families, and Seminaries, and Junior Practitioners in Medicine; Comprising a Complete Modern Dispensatory*. London: Longman, Rees, Orme, Brown, and Green, 1828.

Regnault, J. B. *Observations on Pulmonary Consumption*. London: J. Smeeton, 1802.

Reid, John. *A Treatise on the Origin, Progress, Prevention, and Treatment of Consumption*. London: R. Taylor & Co., 1806

Reid, Thomas. *Directions for Warm and Cold Sea-Bathing*. Second Edition. London: T. Cadel, and W. Davies, 1798.

Reid, T. *An Essay on the Nature and Cure of the Phthisis Pulmonalis*. London: T. Cadell, 1782.

Richardson, Benjamin W. *The Hygienic Treatment of Pulmonary Consumption*. London: John Churchill, 1757.

Roberton, John. *A Treatise on Medical Police, and on Diet, Regimen, &c*. Vol. I. Edinburgh: John Moir, 1809.

Robinson, N. *A New Method of Treating Consumptions Wherein all the Decays Incident to Human Bodies are Mechanically Accounted For*. London: A. Bettesworth and T. Warner, 1727.

Mrs. John Sandford. *Woman, In Her Social and Domestic Character*. London: Longman, Rees, Orme, Brown, and Green, 1831.

Saunders, James. *Treatise on Pulmonary Consumption*. Edinburgh: Walker and Greig, 1808.

Saunders, William. *A Treatise on the Chemical History and Medical Powers of Some of the Most Celebrated Mineral Waters*. Second Edition. London: Phillips and Fardon, 1805.

The Servant's Guide and Family Manual. Second Edition. London: John Limbird, 1831.

Shore, [Margaret] Emily, *Journal of Emily Shore*, Barbara Timm Gates, ed. Charlottesville: University Press of Virginia, 1991.

Shorter, Clement. *The Brontës: Life and Letters*, Vol. II. London: Hodder and Stoughton, 1908.

Mrs. L. H. Sigourney. *Letters to Young Ladies*. London: Jackson and Walford, 1841.

Sinclair, Sir John. *The Code of Health and Longevity*. Fourth Edition. London: 1818.

Smyth, James Carmichael. *An Account of the Effects of Swinging Employed as a Remedy in the Pulmonary Consumption and Hectic Fever*. London: J. Johnson, 1787.

Southey, Henry Herbert. *Observations on Pulmonary Consumption*. London: Longman, Hurst, Rees, Orme, and Brown, 1814.

Sydenham, Thomas. *Dr. Sydenham's Practice of Physick. The Signs, Symptoms, Causes and Cures of Diseases*. London: Sam. Smith and Benj. Walford, 1695.

Thackrah, Charles Turner. *The Effects of Arts, Trades, and Professions, and of Civic States and Habits of Living, on Health and Longevity*. Second Edition. London: Longman, Rees, Orme, Brown, Green, and Longman, 1832.

Thomas, Robert. *The Modern Practice of Physic*. Fourth Edition. London: Longman, Hurst, Rees, Orme, and Brown, 1813. Ninth Edition. London: Longman, Rees, Orme, Brown, and Green, 1828.

Todd, Robert Bentley. *The Descriptive and Physiological Anatomy of the Brain, Spinal Cord, and Ganglions, and of their Coverings*. London: Sherwood, Gilbert, and Piper, 1845.

The Toilette; or, a Guide to the Improvement of Personal Appearance and the Preservation of Health. London: John Dicks, 1854.

Turnbull, James. *An Inquiry, How Far Consumption is Curable*. 2nd edition. London: John Churchill, 1850.

Mrs. A. Walker. *Female Beauty: As Preserved and Improved by Regimen, Cleanliness, and Dress*. London: Thomas Hurst, 1837.

Walker, Alexander. *Intermarriage; of the Mode in Which and the Causes Why, Beauty, Health and Intellect, Result from Certain Unions, and Deformity, Disease and Insanity, From Others*. London: John Churchill, 1838.

Walker, Alexander. *Beauty: Illustrated Chiefly By An Analysis and Classification of Beauty in Woman*. Second Edition. London: Henry G. Bohn, 1846.

Walker, Donald. *Exercises for Ladies; Calculated to Preserve and Improve Beauty, and to Prevent and Correct Personal Defects, Inseparable From Constrained or Careless Habits; Founded on Physiological Principles*. Second Edition. London: Thomas Hurst, 1837.

White, William. *Observations on the Nature and Method of Cure of the Phthisis Pulmonalis; or Consumption of the Lungs*. York: Wilson, Spence, and Mawman, 1792.

Woman's Worth: or, Hints to Raise the Female Character. London: H.G. Clarke & Co., 1844.

The Young Ladies Book: A Manual of Elegant Recreations, Exercises, and Pursuits. Second Edition. London: Vizetelly, Branston, and Co., 1829.

Young, Thomas. *A Practical and Historical Treatise on Consumptive Diseases*. London: Thomas Underwood, 1815.

Select secondary sources

Ashelford, Jane. *The Art of Dress: Clothes and Society 1500–1914*. London: National Trust Enterprises Ltd., 1996.

Bailin, Miriam. *The Sickroom in Victorian Fiction*. Cambridge: Cambridge University Press, 1994.

Barker-Benfield, G. J. *The Culture of Sensibility: Sex and Society in Eighteenth-Century Britain*. Chicago: The University of Chicago Press, 1992.

Barker, Hannah and Elaine Chalus. *Women's History: Britain, 1700–1850*. New York: Routledge, 2005.

Barnes, David S. *The Making of a Social Disease: Tuberculosis in Nineteenth Century France*. Berkeley: University of California Press, 1995.

Bates, Barbara. *Bargaining for Life: A Social History of Tuberculosis, 1876–1938*. Philadelphia: University of Pennsylvania Press, 1992.

Beatty, Heather R. *Nervous Disease in Late Eighteenth-Century Britain*. London: Pickering & Chatto, 2012.

Binneveld, Hans and Rudolf Dekker, eds. *Curing and Insuring, Essays on Illness in Past Times: The Netherlands, Belgium, England, and Italy, 16th–20th Centuries*. Rotterdam: Erasmus University, 1992.

Blackwell, Mark. "Extraneous Bodies": The Contagion of Live-Tooth Transplantation in late-Eighteenth-Century England, *Eighteenth-Century Life*, Vol. 28, No. 1 (Winter 2004) 21–68.

Boucher, Francois. *A History of Costume in the West*. London: Thames and Hudson Ltd., 1987.

Breward, Christopher. *The Culture of Fashion: A New History of Fashionable Dress*. Manchester: Manchester University Press, 1995.

Brewer, John & Roy Porter. *Consumption and the World of Goods*. London: Routledge, 1993.

Select Bibliography

Bronfen, Elizabeth. *Over Her Dead Body: Death, Femininity and the Aesthetic*. New York: Routledge, 1992.

Bruna, Denis, ed. *Fashioning the Body: An Intimate History of the Silhouette*. New Haven: Yale University Press, 2015.

Bryder, Lynda. *Below the Magic Mountain: A Social History of Tuberculosis in Twentieth-Century Britain*. Oxford: Clarendon Press, 1988.

Buckley, Cheryl and Hilary Fawcett. *Fashioning the Feminine: Representations and Women's Fashion from the Fin de Siècle to the Present*. New York: I. B. Tauris & Co., Ltd., 2002.

Bynum, Helen. *Spitting Blood: A History of Tuberculosis*. Oxford: Oxford University Press, 2012.

Bynum, W. F. and Roy Porter, eds. *Companion Encyclopedia of the History of Medicine*. London: Routledge, 2001.

Byrde, Penelope. *Nineteenth Century Fashion*. London: BT Batsford, 1992.

Byrne, Katherine. *Tuberculosis and the Victorian Literary Imagination*. Cambridge: Cambridge University Press, 2011.

Caldwell, Mark. *The Last Crusade: The War on Consumption, 1862–1954*, New York: Athenaeum, 1988.

Canter Cremers-van der Does, Elaine. English Translation Leo Van Witsen. *The Agony of Fashion*. Dorset: Blandford Press, 1980.

Clark, G. Kitson. *The Making of Victorian England*. 10th edition. London: Routledge, 2004.

Corson, Richard. *Fashions in Makeup: From Ancient to Modern Times*. London: Peter Owen, 1972.

Craik, Jennifer. *The Face of Fashion: Cultural Studies in Fashion*. London: Routledge, 1994.

Cunningham, Andrew and Roger French. *The Medical Enlightenment of the Eighteenth Century*. Cambridge: Cambridge University Press, 1990.

Cunningham, Patricia A. *Reforming Women's Fashion, 1850–1920*. Kent, Ohio: The Kent State University Press, 2003.

Curtin, Michael. *Propriety and Position: A Study of Victorian Manners*. London: Garland Publishing, Inc., 1987.

Davidoff, Leonore and Catherine Hall. *Family Fortunes: Men and Women of the English Middle Class, 1780–1850*. Chicago: University of Chicago Press, 1987.

de la Haye, Amy and Elizabeth Wilson, eds. *Defining Dress: Dress as Object, Meaning and Identity*. Manchester: Manchester University Press, 1999.

Dormandy, Thomas. *The White Death: A History of Tuberculosis*. London: Hambledon and London Ltd., 1998.

Dubos, Rene and Jean Dubos. *The White Plague: Tuberculosis, Man, and Society*. New Brunswick: Rutgers University Press, 1987.

Elmer, Peter. *The Healing Arts: Health, Disease and Society in Europe 1500–1800*. Manchester: Manchester University Press, 2004.

Ewing, Elizabeth. *Fashion in Underwear*. London: Batsford Ltd., 1971.

Ewing, Elizabeth. *Dress and Undress: A History of Women's Underwear*. London: Batsford Ltd., 1978.

Feldberg, Georgina D. *Disease and Class: Tuberculosis and the Shaping of Modern North American Society*. New Brunswick: Rutgers University Press, 1995.

Fontanel, Beatrice. *Support and Seduction: A History of Corset and Bras*. Harry N. Abrams, Inc.

Fukai, Akiko, et al. *Fashion: the Collection of the Kyoto Costume Institute: a History from the 18th to the 20th Century*. Taschen, 2002.

Gaines, Jane and Charlotte Herzog. *Fabrications: Costume and the Female Body*. London: Routledge, 1990.

Gilbert, Pamela K. *Mapping the Victorian Social Body*. Albany, NY: State University of New York, 2004.

Gordon, John. *Physiology and the Literary Imagination: Romantic to Modern*. Gainesville: University Press of Florida, 2003.

Gorham, Deborah. *The Victorian Girl and the Feminine Ideal*. Bloomington: Indiana University Press, 1982.

Greig, Hannah. *The Beau Monde: Fashionable Society in Georgian London*. Oxford: Oxford University Press, 2013.

Halttunen, Karen. *Confidence Men and Painted Women: A Study of Middle-Class Culture in America, 1830–1870*. New Haven: Yale University Press, 1982.

Hamlin, Christopher. *Public Health and Social Justice in the Age of Chadwick: Britain 1800–1854*. Cambridge: Cambridge University Press, 1998.

Herndl, Diane Price. *Invalid Women: Figuring Feminine Illness in American Fiction and Culture, 1840–1940*. Chapel Hill: University of North Carolina Press, 1993.

Herzlich, C. & Janine Pierret. *Illness and Self in Society*. Baltimore: The Johns Hopkins University Press, 1982.

Hilton, Boyd. *The Age of Atonement: The Influence of Evangelicism on Social and Economic Thought, 1785–1865*. Oxford: Clarendon Press, 1997.

Hollander, Anne. *Seeing Through Clothes*. Berkeley: University of California Press, 1993.

Jalland, Pat and John Hooper. *Women From Birth to Death*. Sussex: The Harvester Press, 1986.

Jones, Colin. *The Smile Revolution in 18th Century Paris*. Oxford: Oxford University Press, 2014.

Jones, Jennifer M. *Sexing La Mode: Gender, Fashion and Commercial Culture in Old Regime France.* Oxford: Berg, 2004.

Jones, Robert W. *Gender and the Formation of Taste in Eighteenth-Century Britain: The Analysis of Beauty.* Cambridge: Cambridge University Press, 1998.

Jupp, Peter C. and Clare Gittings, eds. *Death in England: An Illustrated History.* New Brunswick: Rutgers University Press, 2000.

Kaplan, Fred. *Sacred Tears: Sentimentality in Victorian Literature.* Princeton, New Jersey: Princeton University Press, 1987.

King, Roger. *The Making of the Dentiste c.1650–1760.* Aldershot: Ashgate, 1999.

Köhler, Carl. *A History of Costume.* New York: Dover Publications, Inc., 1963.

Kunzle, David. *Fashion & Fetishism: Corsets, Tight-lacing & Other Forms of Body-Sculpture.* United Kingdom: Sutton Publishing, 2004.

Langland, Elizabeth. *Nobody's Angels: Middle-class Women and Domestic Ideology in Victorian Culture.* Ithaca: Cornell University Press, 1995.

Laver, James. *Costume and Fashion: A Concise History.* London: Thames & Hudson World of Art, 2002.

Lawlor, Clark. *Consumption and Literature: The Making of the Romantic Disease.* New York: Palgrave Macmillan, 2006.

Lawlor, Clark. "It is a Path I Have Prayed to Follow," in *Romanticism and Pleasure*, Thomas H. Schmid and Michelle Faubert, eds. New York: Palgrave Macmillan, 2010.

Lawlor, Clark and Akihito Suzuki. "The Disease of the Self: Representing Consumption, 1700–1830." *Bulletin of the History of Medicine.*, 2000, 74,: 458–494.

Lawrence, Christopher, ed. *Medicine in the Making of Modern Britain, 1700–1920.* London: Routledge, 1994.

Lerner, Barron H. *Contagion and Confinement Controlling Tuberculosis Along the Skid Row.* Baltimore: The Johns Hopkins University Press, 1998.

Levine-Clark, Marjorie. *Beyond the Reproductive Body: the Politics of Women's Health and Work in Early Victorian England.* Ohio State University Press, 2004.

Levitt, Sarah. *Victorians Unbuttoned: Registered Designs for Clothing, Their Makers and Wearers, 1839–1900.* London: George Allen & Unwin, 1986.

Lewis, Judith S. *Sacred to Female Patriotism: Gender, Class and Politics in Late Georgian Britain.* New York: Routledge, 2003.

Lomax, Elizabeth. "Heredity or Acquired Disease? Early Nineteenth Century Debates on the Cause of Infantile Scrofula and Tuberculosis." *Journal of the History of Medicine and Allied Sciences*, 32:4 (October 1977).

Marshall, David. *The Frame of Art: Fictions of Aesthetic Experience, 1750–1815.* Baltimore: The Johns Hopkins University Press, 2005.

Martin, Morag. *Selling Beauty: Cosmetics, Commerce, and French Society, 1750–1830.* Baltimore: The Johns Hopkins University Press, 2009.

Matus, Jill L. *Unstable Bodies: Victorian Representations of Sexuality and Maternity.* Manchester: Manchester University Press, 1995.

McKendrick, Neil, John Brewer, and J. H. Plumb. *The Birth of a Consumer Society: The Commercialization of Eighteenth-Century England.* Bloomington: Indiana University Press, 1982.

Mellor, Anne K. (ed.). *Romanticism and Feminism.* Bloomington: Indiana University Press, 1988.

Moller, David Wendell. *Confronting Death: Values, Institutions, and Human Mortality.* Oxford: Oxford University Press, 1996.

Morgan, Marjorie. *Manners, Morals and Class in England, 1774–1858.* New York: St. Martin's Press, 1994.

Moscucci, Ornella. *The Science of Woman: Gynecology and Gender in England, 1800–1929.* Cambridge: Cambridge University Press, 1993.

Musselman, Elizabeth Green. *Nervous Conditions: Science and the Body Politic in Early Industrial Britain.* Albany: SUNY Press, 2006.

Ott, Katherine. *Fevered Lives: Tuberculosis in American Culture since 1870.* Harvard: Harvard University Press, 1996.

Palmer, Caroline. "Brazen Cheek: Face-Painters in Late Eighteenth-Century England," *Oxford Art Journal* 31 (2008), 195–213.

Parker, Rozsika. *The Subversive Stitch: Embroidery and the Making of the Feminine.* London: The Women's Press, 1984.

Perkin, Joan. *Victorian Women.* New York: New York University Press, 1993.

Phillippy, Patricia. *Painting Women: Cosmetics, Canvases & Early Modern Culture.* Baltimore: The Johns Hopkins University Press, 2006.

Pointer, Sally. *The Artifice of Beauty: A History and Practical Guide to Perfumes and Cosmetics.* United Kingdom, 2005.

Porter, Dorothy. *Health, Civilization and the State. A History of Public Health from Ancient to Modern Times*. London: Routledge, 1999.

Porter, Dorothy and Roy Porter. *Patient's Progress: Doctors and Doctoring in Eighteenth-century England*. Stanford: Stanford University Press, 1989.

Porter, Roy, ed. *Patients and Practitioners: Lay Perceptions of Medicine in Pre-Industrial Society*. Cambridge: Cambridge University Press, 1985.

Porter, Roy. *Doctor of Society: Thomas Beddoes and the Sick Trace in Late-Enlightenment England*. London: Routledge, 1992.

Porter, Roy. *Disease, Medicine and Society in England, 1550–1860*. Second Edition. Cambridge: The Press Syndicate of the University of Cambridge, 1993.

Porter, Roy, ed. *The Cambridge Illustrated History of Medicine*. Cambridge: Cambridge University Press, 1996.

Porter, Roy. *The Greatest Benefit to Mankind: A Medical History of Humanity from Antiquity to the Present*. London: Fontana Press, 1999.

Porter, Roy. *Bodies Politic: Disease, Death and Doctors in Britain, 1650–1900*. Ithaca, NY: Cornell University Press, 2001.

Porter, Roy. *Flesh in the Age of Reason*. New York: W. W. Norton & Co., 2003.

Porter, Roy and Lesley Hall, eds. *The Facts of Life: The Creation of Sexual Knowledge in Britain, 1650–1950*. New Haven: Yale University Press, 1995.

Ribeiro, Aileen, *Dress and Morality*. Oxford: Berg, 1986.

Ribeiro, Aileen, *Fashion in the French Revolution*. London: Batsford, 1988.

Ribeiro, Aileen. *Facing Beauty: Painted Women and Cosmetic Art*. London and New Haven: Yale University Press, 2011.

Rosenberg, Charles E. and Janet Golden, eds. *Framing Disease: Studies in Cultural History*. New Jersey: Rutgers, 1992.

Rosenthal, Laura Jean and Mita Choudhury eds. *Monstrous Dreams of Reason: Body, Self, and Other in the Enlightenment*. Cranbury, New Jersey: Associated University Presses, 2002.

Rousseau, G. S. *Nervous Acts: Essays on Literature, Culture and Sensibility*. London: Palgrave, 2004.

Rousseau, George S. "Nerves, Spirits, and Fibres: Towards Defining the Origins of Sensibility," *Studies in the Eighteenth Century*, R. F. Brissenden and J. C. Eade, eds. Toronto: University of Toronto Press, 1976.

Rousseau, George. "Political gout: dissolute patients, deceitful physicians, and other blue devils." *Notes and Records of the Royal Society of London* 63.3 (2009): 277–296.

Rotberg, Robert I., ed. *Health and Disease in Human History*. Cambridge, Mass: The MIT Press, 2000.

Rothman, Sheila M. *Living in the Shadow of Death: Tuberculosis and the Social Experience of Illness in American History*. Baltimore: The Johns Hopkins University Press, 1994.

Russell, Douglas A. *Costume History and Style*. New Jersey: Prentice-Hall, Inc., 1983.

Schiebinger, Londa. *Nature's Body: Sexual Politics and the Making of Modern Science*. London: Pandora, An Imprint of HarperCollins Publishers, 1993.

Schor, Esther. *Bearing the Dead: The British Culture of Mourning from the Enlightenment to Victoria*. Princeton: Princeton University Press, 1994.

Shorter, Edward. *Women's Bodies: A Social History of Women's Encounter with Health, Ill-Health, and Medicine*. New Brunswick: Transaction Publishers, 1997.

Silver, Anna Krugovoy. *Victorian Literature and the Anorexic Body*. Cambridge: Cambridge University Press, 2002.

Smith, F. B. *The Retreat of Tuberculosis 1850–1950*. London: Croom Helm, 1988.

Smith-Rosenberg, Carroll and Charles Rosenberg. "The Female Animal: Medical and Biological Views of Woman and Her Role In Nineteenth-Century America." *Women and Health in America*. 2nd edition. Ed. Judith Walzer Leavitt. Madison: University of Wisconsin Press, 1999.

Sontag, Susan. *Illness as Metaphor and Aids and Its Metaphors*. New York: Doubleday, 1990.

Stansfield, Dorothy A. *Thomas Beddoes M.D. 1760–1808: Chemist, Physician, Democrat*. Dordrecht, Holland: D. Reidel Publishing Company, 1984.

Steele, Valerie. *Fashion & Eroticism: Ideals of Feminine Beauty from the Victorian Era to the Jazz Age*. Oxford: Oxford University Press, 1985.

Steinke, Hubert. *Irritating Experiments: Haller's Concept and the European Controversy on Irritability and Sensibility, 1750–90*. Amsterdam: Editions Rodopi B.V., 2005.

Strachan, John. *Advertising and Satirical Culture in the Romantic Period*. Cambridge: Cambridge University Press, 2007.

Sturdy, Steve, ed. *Medicine, Health and the Public Sphere in Britain, 1600–2000*. London: Routledge, 2002.

Styles, John. *The Dress of the People: Everyday Fashion in Eighteenth-Century England*. New Haven: Yale University Press, 2007.

Summers, Leigh. *Bound to Please: A History of the Victorian Corset*. Oxford: Berg, 2001.

Taylor, Lou. *The Study of Dress History*. Manchester: Manchester University Press, 2002.

Tortora, Phyllis G. and Keith Eubank. *Survey of Historic Costume: A History of Western Dress*. 3rd ed. New York: Fairchild Publications, 2004.

Wahrman, Dror. *The Making of the Modern Self: Identity and Culture in Eighteenth-Century England*. New Haven: Yale University Press, 2004.

Waksman, Selman A. *The Conquest of Tuberculosis*. Berkeley: University of California Press, 1964.

Waller, John C. "The Illusion of an Explanation: The Concept of Hereditary Disease, 1770–1870." *Journal of the History of Medicine*, 57 (October 2002): 410–448.

Waugh, Norah. *The Cut of Women's Clothes, 1600–1930*. London: Faber and Faber Ltd., 1968.

Waugh, Norah. *Corsets and Crinolines*. New York: Routledge/Theatre Arts Books, 2004.

Williams, Neville. *Powder and Paint: A History of the Englishwoman's Toilet, Elizabeth I-Elizabeth II*. London: Longmans, Green and Co., 1957.

Wykes-Joyce, Max. *Cosmetics and Adornment: Ancient and Contemporary Usage*. London: Peter Owen, 1961.

INDEX

Page numbers in **bold** refer to figures

Index